COMMON PROBLEMS IN

INFECTIONS AND STONES

COMMON PROBLEMS IN

INFECTIONS AND STONES

GEORGE W. DRACH, M.D.
Professor and Chief of Urology
College of Medicine
Department of Surgery
University of Arizona Health Sciences Center
Tucson, Arizona

Mosby
Year Book

St. Louis Baltimore Boston Chicago London Philadelphia Sydney Toronto

Mosby Year Book

Dedicated to Publishing Excellence

Sponsoring Editor: David K. Marshall
Assistant Editor: Julie Tryboski
Assistant Managing Editor, Text and Reference: George Mary Gardner
Senior Production Assistant: Maria Nevinger
Proofroom Manager: Barbara Kelly

Mosby–Year Book, Inc.
11830 Westline Industrial Drive
St. Louis, MO 63146

1 2 3 4 5 6 7 8 9 0 CL MV 96 95 94 93 92

Library of Congress Cataloging-in-Publication Data
Common problems in infections are stones / [edited by] George W. Drach.
p. cm.
Includes bibliographical references and index.
ISBN 0-8151-2909-2
1. Urinary tract infections. 2. Urinary organs—Calculi.
I. Drach, George W.
[DNLM: 1. Kidney Calculi—diagnosis. 2. Kidney Calculi—therapy.
3. Urinary Calculi—diagnosis. 4. Urinary Calculi—therapy.
5. Urinary Tract Infections—diagnosis. 6. Urinary Tract Infections—therapy. WJ 100 C734]
RC901.8.C66 1991 91-28017
616.6—dc20 CIP
DNLM/DLC
for Library of Congress

COMMON PROBLEMS IN

UROLOGY

SERIES EDITOR

Alan J. Wein, M.D.
Professor and Chairman
Division of Urology
University of Pennsylvania School of Medicine
Chief of Urology
Hospital of the University of Pennsylvania
Philadelphia, Pennsylvania

Series Titles:

Rajfer/**Common Problems in Infertility and Impotence**
Gonzales/**Common Problems in Pediatric Urology**
Drach/**Common Problems in Infections and Stones**

CONTRIBUTORS

DEAN G. ASSIMOS, M.D.
Associate Professor of Surgery and Urology, Section of Urology, Bowman Gray School of Medicine, Winston-Salem, North Carolina

RICHARD E. BERGER, M.D.
Associate Professor of Urology, Department of Urology, University of Washington Medical Center, Seattle, Washington

WILLIAM W. BOHNERT, M.D.
Chief of Surgery and Urology, St. Joseph's Hospital and Medical Center, Phoenix, Arizona

WILLIAM BOWIE, M.D.
Professor, Department of Medicine, Division of Infectious Diseases, University of British Columbia, Vancouver, Canada

WILLIAM H. BOYCE, M.D.
Professor Emeritus of Surgery and Urology, Bowman Gray School of Medicine, Winston-Salem, North Carolina

MICHAEL K. BRAWER, M.D.
Associate Professor, Department of Urology, University of Washington, Chief, Section of Urology, Veterans Affairs Medical Center (Seattle), Seattle, Washington

KENNETH BREGG, M.D.
Instructor in Surgery (Urology), The New York Hospital, New York, New York

ANDREW W. BRUCE, M.D.
Professor Emeritus in Urology, University of Toronto, Toronto General Hospital, Toronto, Canada

JOHN R. BURNS, M.D.
Professor, Department of Surgery, Department of Surgery, Division of Urology, University of Alabama at Birmingham, Birmingham, Alabama

CHRISTIAN CHAUSSY, M.D.
Chief, Department of Urology, Staedt, Krankenhaus Harlaching, Germany

GERALD W. CHODAK, M.D.
Professor of Surgery, Department of Surgery, Section of Urology, University of Chicago, Chicago, Illinois

JOSEPH N. CORRIERE, JR., M.D.
Professor and Director, Division of Urology, University of Texas Health Science Center at Houston, Houston, Texas

JOHN M. DONOVAN, M.D.
Assistant Professor of Surgery, Department of Surgery, Section of Urologic Surgery, University of Nebraska Medical Center, Omaha, Nebraska

GEORGE W. DRACH, M.D.
Professor and Chief of Urology, College of Medicine, Department of Surgery, University of Arizona Health Science Center, Tucson, Arizona

STEPHEN P. DRETLER, M.D.
Associate Professor of Surgery, Harvard Medical School, Director of Lithotriptor Unit, Massachusetts General Hospital, Boston, Massachusetts

BRUCE ETTINGER, M.D.
Senior Investigator, Division of Research, Kaiser Permanente Medical Care Program, Oakland, California

JACKSON E. FOWLER, JR., M.D.
Professor and Chief of Urology, University of Mississippi Medical Center, Jackson, Mississippi

FLOYD A. FRIED, M.D.
Chief of the Division of Urology, Rhodes Professor of Surgery, University of North Carolina School of Medicine, Chapel Hill, North Carolina

HUBERT G.W. FROHMULLER, M.D.
Professor and Chairman, Department of Urology, University of Wurzburg Medical School, Luitpoldkrankenhaus, Wurzburg, Germany

GERHARD J. FUCHS, M.D.
Associate Professor of Surgery/Urology, Head, Stone Treatment Center, UCLA Medical Center, Los Angeles, California

JOHN G. GREGORY, M.D.
Private Practice, St. Louis, Missouri

DONALD P. GRIFFITH, M.D.
Professor of Urology, Scott Department of Urology, Baylor College of Medicine, Houston, Texas

WILLIAM O. HARRISON, M.D.
Associate Clinical Professor of Medicine, University of California at San Diego School of Medicine, Consultant Epidemiologist, Department of Health Services, State of California, San Diego, California

ALAN D. JENKINS, M.D.
Associate Professor of Urology, Department of Urology, University of Virginia School of Medicine, Charlottesville, Virginia

THOMAS M. KINKEAD, M.D.
Division of Urology, University of Massachusetts Medical Center, Worcester, Massachusetts

JAMES E. LINGEMAN, M.D.
Director of Research, Methodist Hospital Institute for Kidney Stone Disease, Indianapolis, Indiana

BERNARD LYTTON, M.D.
Professor, Department of Surgery, Section of Urology, Yale University School of Medicine, New Haven, Connecticut

EDWIN M. MEARES, JR., M.D.
Charles M. Whitney Professor and Chairman, Division of Urology, Tufts University School of Medicine, Chairman, Department of Urology, New England Medical Center Hospitals, Boston, Massachusetts

MANI MENON, M.D.
Chairman, Professor of Surgery and Physiology, Division of Urology, University of Massachusetts Medical Center, Worcester, Massachusetts

RICHARD G. MIDDLETON, M.D.
Chairman, Division of Urology, University of Utah Medical Center, Salt Lake City, Utah

ROBERT M. MOLDWIN, M.D.
Assistant Professor, Department of Urology, Long Island Jewish Medical Center, The Long Island Campus for the Albert Einstein College of Medicine, New Hyde Park, New York

S. GRANT MULHOLLAND, M.D.
Professor and Chairman, Department of Urology, Thomas Jefferson University, Philadelphia, Pennsylvania

DANIEL M. NEWMAN, M.D.
Director, Methodist Hospital Institute for Kidney Stone Disease, Indianapolis, Indiana

ROBERT C. NEWMAN, M.D.
Associate Professor, Division of Urology, Department of Surgery, University of Florida College of Medicine, Gainesville, Florida

CHARLES C.Y. PAK, M.D.
Department of Internal Medicine, University of Texas Health Science Center, Dallas, Texas

C. LOWELL PARSONS, M.D.
Professor of Surgery, Division of Urology, University of California at San Diego, San Diego, California

GLENN M. PREMINGER, M.D.
Professor of Urology, Division of Urology, University of Texas Southwestern Medical Center, Dallas, Texas

GREGOR REID, M.D.
Director of Research Services, Associate Professor of Microbiology, University of Western Ontario, Ontario, Canada

MARTIN I. RESNICK, M.D.
Lester Persky, Professor of Urology, Chief, Division of Urology, Case Western Reserve University, Cleveland, Ohio

JAMES A. ROBERTS, M.D.
Professor and Associate Chairman (Research), Department of Urology, Tulane University School of Medicine, New Orleans, Louisiana

ANTHONY J. SCHAEFFER, M.D.
Professor and Chairman, Department of Urology, Northwestern University Medical School, Chicago, Illinois

MARTIN SCHIFF, JR., M.D.
Clinical Professor of Surgery/Urology, Department of Surgery, Section of Urology, University of Arizona Health Sciences Center, Tucson, Arizona

ALLAN D. SEFTEL, M.D.
Division of Urology, Case Western Reserve University School of Medicine, Cleveland, Ohio

JOSEPH W. SEGURA, M.D.
Carl Rosen, Professor of Urology, Department of Urology, Mayo Medical School, Rochester, Minnesota

LINDA DAIRIKI SHORTLIFFE, M.D.
Associate Professor of Urology, Division of Urology, Stanford University Medical School, Stanford, California

ARTHUR D. SMITH, M.D.
Chairman and Professor, Department of Urology, Long Island Jewish Medical Center, The Long Island Campus for the Albert Einstein College of Medicine, New Hyde Park, New York

DAVID T. UEHLING, M.D.
Professor of Surgery, Chairman of the Division of Urology, Department of Surgery, University of Wisconsin Medical Center, Madison, Wisconsin

E. DARRACOTT VAUGHAN, JR., M.D.
James J. Colt, Professor of Urology, The New York Hospital, New York, New York

PREFACE

This text is written for family practitioners, emergency physicians, internists, nephrologists, urologists, and any other physicians who diagnose and treat urinary and genital infections and urinary stones.

This text on urogenital infections and stones was compiled because these diseases are so common in all types of medical practice and because they require special diligence in diagnosis and treatment. In most texts the methods are generalized and not directed toward the problem of a specific patient. In this text we first present the patient's problem, then a consultant discusses the approach to this and related problems.

I would like to suggest a method of chapter review for readers. The chapters in Part I are organized so that urinary tract infections are presented first (Chapters 1 through 12), followed by chapters that deal with infections of the genital systems (Chapters 13 through 20). Part II presents a comprehensive review of diagnosis and treatment of urinary stone disease (Chapters 21 through 50).

If you have a patient with a specific problem, such as an acute stone episode, turn directly to Chapter 21. If after simple metabolic testing you think citrate therapy may be correct for this patient, review Chapter 31. If you wish to review the entire area of infections and stones, then read the text from cover to cover. We have attempted to include all the modern theories of causation and approaches to therapy.

Authors have been selected from experts who have investigated and published in the specific area titled in their chapter(s). I thank them for their chapters, their attention to detail, and for their prompt submission of manuscripts. In addition, I thank the series editor, Alan Wein, M.D., for introducing me to the concepts used in *Common Problems*. The text was organized by Carol Frost, and edited under the direction of David Marshall. They, too, deserve thanks.

Finally, my ongoing thanks to my wife, Paula, who always says, "Not another book!," then spends many hours assisting in its production.

George W. Drach, M.D.

CONTENTS

PART ONE

Urinary Tract Infections

1

Office Bacteriology

Jackson E. Fowler, Jr., M.D.

You open your new office in Surprise, Kentucky, but you find that no laboratory facilities exist in the community. The nearest hospital is 25 miles away. As a service to your patients, you consider establishing office microbiology facilities that will allow you to diagnose the majority of genitourinary tract infections.

This practitioner needs facilities to diagnose the two most common infectious disorders encountered by the urologist—urinary tract infection and infections of the male urethra. Although it is unlikely that he received meaningful exposure to basic bacteriology during residency training, the techniques and interpretations of the tests he will perform are well standardized and not difficult to master. In addition, a variety of available kits permit economically feasible office bacteriology even when the volume of work is limited.

All urologists should have a microscope, a countertop centrifuge, and glass slides and coverslips to perform routine urinalysis. Additional equipment and supplies that will be required to establish the laboratory are listed in Table 1–1.

OFFICE BACTERIOLOGY FOR URINARY TRACT INFECTIONS

Urine Culture

The urine culture documents the presence or absence of bacteria in the urine, provides an estimate of bacterial density, and permits presumptive identification of the bacterial isolates.

A supportive and selective agar media are routinely used for the culture. The plates can be purchased from most medical supply houses and may be stored for several weeks in a refrigerator. The most commonly used supportive medium is sheep blood agar. Gram-negative bacilli and gram-positive cocci that infect or contaminate the urine grow on this medium. MacConkey agar, which contains crystal violet and bile salts to inhibit the growth of gram-posi-

TABLE 1–1.
Equipment and Supplies for the Office Microbiology Laboratory

Equipment
Small incubator
Small refrigerator
Flame or electrical sterilizer for inoculation loops
Supplies
Agar plates or dip slides for urine culture
Platinum or sterile plastic inoculating loops
Agar plates for susceptibility testing
Antibiotic disks and disk dispenser
Nutrient broth and control bacteria for susceptibility testing
API 20E biotyping strips
Reagents for Gram stain
Slides or transport media for *Chlamydia trachomatis* assay
Sterile saline solution, plastic test tubes, and swabs

tive cocci, is a commonly used selective medium. Neutral red, which turns red in an acid pH, is also incorporated to differentiate lactose- and nonlactose-fermenting isolates.

The urine is vigorously mixed to ensure a uniform suspension of bacteria, and 0.05 to 0.001 mL is deposited on the middle of the plate using a calibrated platinum loop that can be sterilized or a disposable sterile plastic loop. The drop is spread in a line from one side to the other and then streaked over the entire surface. This promotes isolated bacterial growth, which facilitates both the counting of colonies and assessment of their morphologic characteristics.

The plate is covered and left undisturbed for 15 to 20 minutes while urine diffuses into the medium and is then incubated in an inverted position at 37°C for 18 to 24 hours. In the inverted position moisture collects on the dependent top rather than on the agar surface. If bacterial growth is not identifiable after 24 hours or if only tiny colonies are seen, the plate is incubated for an additional 24 hours. The plate is discarded if growth is not observed after 48 hours.

The density of bacteria in the urine specimen is estimated by counting the number of colonies on the agar surface and dividing by the volume of the inoculum. Precision in this determination is not necessary. From a diagnostic standpoint, meaningful differences in the estimated density of an isolate are measured by a factor of 10. As such, enormous error in the volume of urine plated or in the counting of colonies is necessary for clinically important miscalculations. There is no need to quantitate growth in densities of greater than 10^4 bacteria/mL, which usually appears as confluent bacterial colonies.

Gram-negative bacilli grow on both the supportive and selective agars (Fig 1–1,A). The appearance of the colonies on MacConkey agar (Table 1–2) is a relatively reliable means for speciation. Note that the reddish colonial discoloration of the lactose fermenters is an important identifying feature. The colonies of gram-negative bacilli on blood agar are gray, convex, and somewhat nondescript.

Gram-positive cocci grow on the supportive sheep blood agar only (Fig 1–1,B). These isolates, which usually reflect contamination of voided urine by commensal vaginal or urethral bacteria, are generally found in densities of less than 10^3/mL. Contamination by more than one gram-positive organism is not unusual, and the morphology of the bacterial colonies is often heterogeneous.

Enterococcus and *Staphylococcus saprophyticus* are the principal urinary pathogens that do not grow on MacConkey agar. However, the density of these organisms in infected urine is usually greater than the density of contaminating gram-positive cocci, and the colonial morphology is homogeneous. This simplifies differentiation between infection and contamination.

Dip-slide culture kits are an alternative method for urine culture that may be more appealing to the urologist. Dip-slide kits consist of a sealed chamber and a slide. One surface of the slide is covered with a supportive agar and the

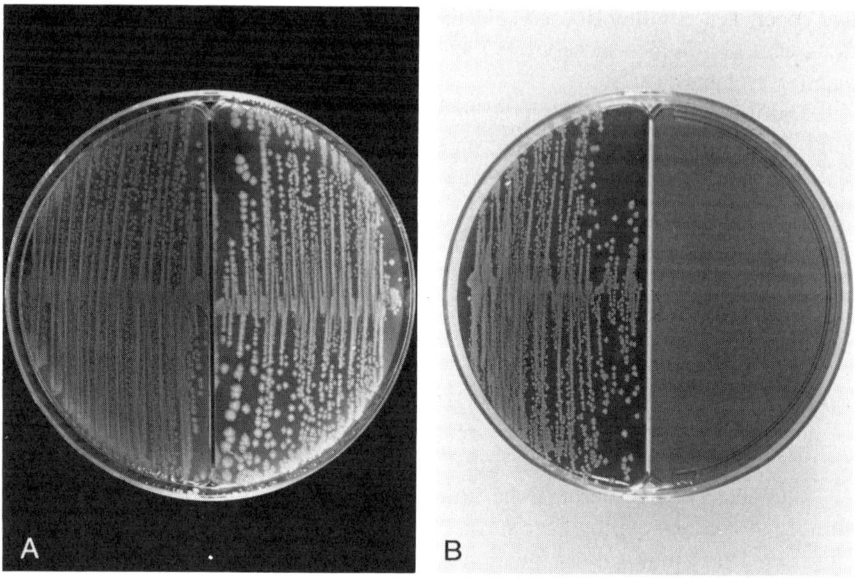

FIG 1–1.
Bacterial growth on agar "biplates." The left sides of the plates contain sheep blood agar, and the right sides contain MacConkey agar. **A,** biplate shows growth of gram-negative bacilli on both sheep blood agar and MacConkey agar. **B,** biplate shows growth of gram-positive cocci on sheep blood agar only. (From Fowler JE Jr: *Urinary Tract Infection and Inflammation.* Chicago, Year Book Medical Publishers, 1989. Used by permission.)

other with a selective agar. The dip slide is inoculated by immersing the slide into a urine specimen or by inserting the slide into the urinary stream. A constant volume of urine is retained on the agar surfaces, and the density of an isolate is estimated from the number of visible colonies that appear after 24 hours of incubation. Figures accompanying dip-slide kits facilitate the correla-

TABLE 1–2.
Colonial Morphology of Gram-Negative Bacilli on MacConkey Agar

Bacterial Species	Colonial Morphology
*Escherichia coli**	Dark pink with central depression
Klebsiella species*	Mucoid, pink
Proteus species	Uncolored, transparent (will swarm on blood agar)
Enterobacter species*	Pink (may be mucoid)
Providencia species	Uncolored, transparent
Serratia marcescens	Uncolored, transparent
Morganella morganii	Uncolored, transparent
Citrobacter species*	Uncolored or pink, transparent
Pseudomonas aeruginosa	Uncolored or metallic green pigmentation

*Lactose fermenter.

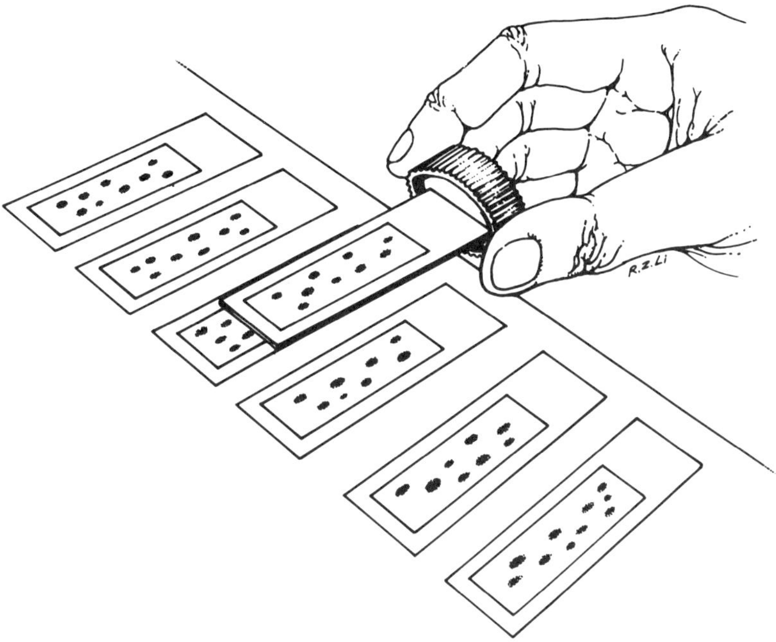

FIG 1–2.
After incubation of a dip slide, the density of bacteria in the urine and the identity of the organism are determined by reference to figures provided by the manufacturer. (From Fowler JE Jr: *Urinary Tract Infection and Inflammation.* Chicago, Year Book Medical Publishers, 1989. Used by permission.)

tion of colony density and bacterial concentration in the urine specimen, and the speciation of gram-negative bacilli based on colony morphology (Fig 1–2). A dip slide costs several dollars and can be stored in a refrigerator for prolonged periods.

Bacterial Speciation With Biochemical Tests

Biochemical testing identifies specific enzymes that are synthesized by bacteria. It is a precise means for the speciation of gram-negative bacilli and an excellent tool for self-assessment of the urologist's abilities to identify organisms on the basis of colonial morphology. The API 20E (Analab Products, Plainview, N.Y.) is ideal for biochemical testing in the office laboratory. Each API 20E strip consists of 20 cupules that contain different dried enzymatic substrates. A suspension of the bacterial isolate (one colony dispersed in 5 mL of sterile saline) is placed in each cupule, the plate is incubated at 37°C overnight, and the results of each reaction are determined by color changes. Some reactions can be identified only after the addition of other reagents. The results are expressed as a seven-digit composite: the biotype of an organism. The genus and species most likely to be associated with a given biotype are determined from a computer-developed profile (analytical profile index) supplied by the manufacturer.

Antimicrobial Susceptibility Testing

Antimicrobial susceptibility testing is a desirable but nonessential procedure in the office laboratory. In most cases an appropriate antibiotic for the treatment of bacteriuria in ambulatory patients can be selected on the basis of the species of the infecting organism. For example, *E. coli* are usually sensitive to all drugs used for the treatment of urinary tract infection, enterococci are almost always susceptible to nitrofurantoin, and *P. aeruginosa* and *Klebsiella* and *Proteus* species are generally susceptible to norfloxacin or ciprofloxacin. However, information obtained from susceptibility testing helps to clarify the reasons for treatment failures.

Susceptibility testing of urinary isolates is most commonly done with the disk diffusion (Kirby-Bauer) assay. The test is based on the observation that the degree of inhibition of bacterial growth on agar medium surrounding an antimicrobial-containing disk correlates with susceptibility to the agent. Conceptually, the assay is a continuum of antimicrobial dilutions in agar because the concentration of drug is inversely related to the distance from the disk. However, no attempt is made to correlate the zone of inhibition with the minimum inhibitory concentration. Rather, the diameter of the zone is used only to estimate susceptibilities to a drug at concentrations achievable in the serum. For nitrofurantoin, which has no antibacterial activity at serum concentrations, the zone of inhibition reflects susceptibility to drug levels in the urine.

Mueller-Hinton agar plates and paper disks impregnated with standardized amounts of an antibiotic and specifically certified for susceptibility testing can be purchased from medical supply houses. In commercial laboratories the infecting organism is isolated from the original culture, subcultured for 4 to 8 hours in a broth medium, adjusted to a density of approximately 10^8 bacteria/mL, and streaked on the agar using a sterile swab on a wooden stick. After standing for 5 minutes, the paper disks are applied with a dispenser and gently pressed onto the agar surface. The plate is then inverted and incubated overnight at 37°C. The diameter of the zone of bacterial growth inhibition around each disk (Fig 1–3) is measured with calipers or templates, and susceptibility or resistance is determined from a standardized table. For most urinary isolates the zone diameters lie well within established ranges of sensitivity or resistance.

A modification of the Kirby-Bauer assay devised by Perez and Gillenwater[1] is recommended for the office laboratory. Urine is streaked directly onto the Mueller-Hinton agar without prior subculture or standardization of the inoc-

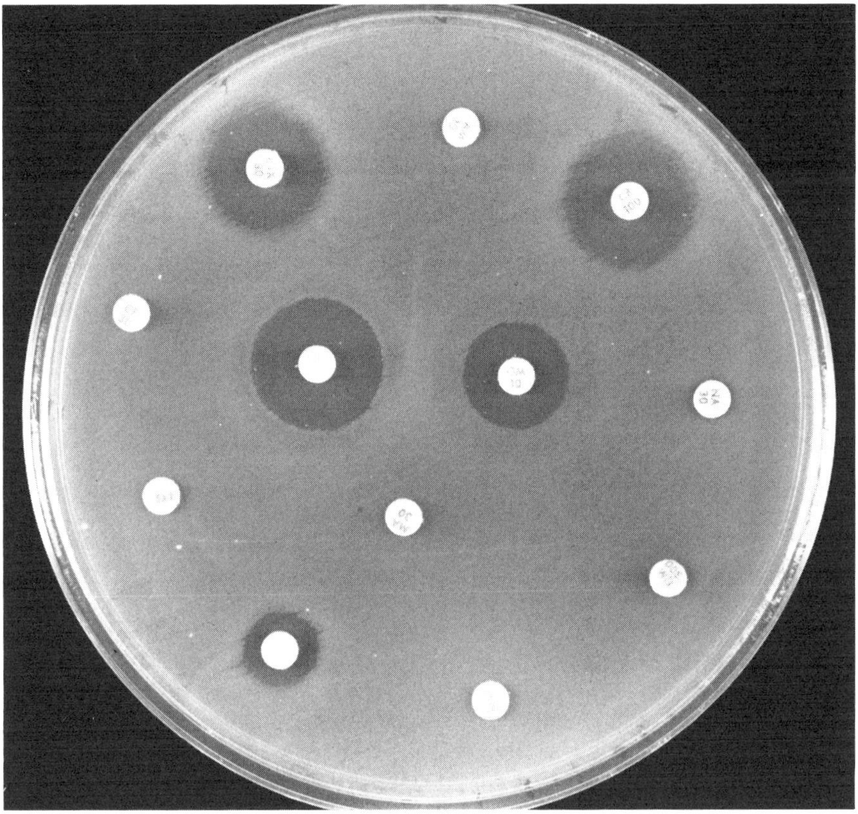

FIG 1–3.
Appearance of zones of inhibition around antimicrobial disks in Kirby-Bauer susceptibility test. (From Fowler JE Jr: *Urinary Tract Infection and Inflammation.* Chicago, Year Book Medical Publishers, 1989. Used by permission.)

ulum density. Antimicrobial disks are then applied, and the methodology previously described is followed. The results obtained with this technique correspond to those of the conventional Kirby-Bauer assay in 97% of specimens with more than 10^5 bacteria/mL. The test is difficult to interpret if there are less than 10^5 bacteria/mL or a polymicrobial infection, and sterile urine is frequently tested. On the other hand, antibiotic sensitivities can be determined within 24 hours, and bacterial subculture is not necessary.

Standard control strains of *E. coli, S. aureus,* and *P. aeruginosa* are used to monitor the accuracy of disk diffusion tests. These organisms are commercially available and can be maintained in a freezer or in a lyophilized state. Before the bacteria are tested, they are incubated for 4 to 18 hours in a nutrient broth and then streaked onto the Mueller-Hinton agar plate. Control tests should be done once each week and on every new batch of Mueller-Hinton agar.

OFFICE BACTERIOLOGY FOR URETHRITIS IN MEN

The etiology, relative incidence, and recommended treatment of primary urethral infections are shown in Table 1–3. Postinfectious urethral inflammation, which may be clinically indistinguishable from primary infections, are of unknown etiology and follow 25% to 50% of gonococcal, chlamydial, and *Ureaplasma* infections. These considerations are relevant because immunoassays are used to detect chlamydial infections, anaerobic culture facilities are required for the diagnosis of *Ureaplasma* infections, and the expenses of these capabilities are prohibitive for most office laboratories. Despite incomplete diagnostic capabilities, however, practical initial management is still feasible because the recommended treatments for chlamydial, *Ureaplasma,* "nonmicrobial," and postinfectious urethritis are identical, and the recommended treatments for diagnosed gonococcal and trichomonal infections are different.

Gonococcal urethritis is documented by the finding of gram-negative intracellular diplococci in the Gram stain smear of the urethral discharge or endourethral swab. The sensitivity of the test is about 95% in symptomatic men, and confirmatory cultures are rarely indicated. Trichomonal urethritis is diagnosed by microscopic visualization of the parasite in a drop of the discharge mixed with saline or in the first 5 mL of voided urine. Trichomonads are pear-shaped organisms that are somewhat larger than squamous epithelial cells. They have a twitching movement and undulating flagella that makes identification straightforward.

It is prudent to document the cure of gonococcal and chlamydial urethritis by culture and immunoassay, respectively. These tests may be advisable also for the evaluation of frequently recurring urethral symptoms. Immunoassays for

TABLE 1–3.
Urethritis in Men

Etiology	Relative Incidence (%)	Recommended Treatment
Neissera gonorrhoeae	40	Cephtriaxone
Trichomonas vaginalis	2	Metronidazole
C. trachomatis	30	Tetracycline or erythromycin
Ureaplasma urealyticum	12	Tetracycline or erythromycin
Nonmicrobial	12	Tetracycline or erythromycin
Postinfectious	—	Tetracycline or erythromycin

C. trachomatis are not dependent on the viability of the organism, and an endourethral specimen that is streaked on a glass slide for immunofluorescent study or deposited in transport media for immunoassay can be sent to a referral laboratory. In contrast, endourethral swabs for *N. gonorrhoeae* cultures must necessarily be obtained at the referral laboratory because isolation of the organism requires inoculation of an agar plate with a fresh specimen.

REGULATION AND QUALITY ASSURANCE

Office laboratories that are used solely for the investigation of a physician's own patients are generally exempt from state and federal regulations imposed on reference laboratories. Nonetheless, this urologist should refer to the *Laboratory Regulation Manual* by Halper and Foster[2] for information that may be applicable in Kentucky.

The urine culture and antimicrobial susceptibility testing are the only procedures described earlier that are subject to guidelines and regulations concerning quality assurance and quality control. A manual that details the methods of tests conducted in the laboratory and a log of clinical and appropriate control results must be kept in the laboratory. The incubator is the only equipment that must be monitored. This requires daily recording of the temperature using a thermometer that is kept within the incubator.

REFERENCES

1. Perez JR, Gillenwater JY: Clinical evaluation of testing immediate antibiotic disk sensitivities in bacteriuria. J Urol 1973; 110:452.
2. Halper HR, Foster HS: *Laboratory Regulation Manual,* Rockville, Md, Aspen Publishers, 1976, vol. 1.

BIBLIOGRAPHY

1. Belsey RE, Baer DM, Statland BE, et al: *The Physician's Office Laboratory.* Oradell NJ, Medical Economics Company, 1986.
2. Fowler JE Jr: *Urinary Tract Infection and Inflammation.* Chicago, Year Book Medical Publishers, 1989.
3. Lennette EH: *Manual of Clinical Microbiology.* Washington, DC, American Society for Microbiology, 1985.
4. Turck M, Lindemeyer RI, Petersdorf RG: Comparison of single disc and tube dilution techniques in determining antibiotic sensitivity of gram negative pathogens. *Ann Intern Med* 1963; 58:56.

2

Recurrent Urinary Tract Infections in Female Children

David T. Uehling, M.D.

A 7-year-old girl presented with a history of day and night urinary incontinence for the past 3 years. Earlier in childhood she seemed to be gaining urinary control. However, in the past 3 years she has had three urinary tract infections and worsening incontinence. Each infection was treated with short-term TMP-SMX, and cleared promptly. The child was bothered by urinating more frequently than her playmates, and also by wetting at school and at night. An intravenous pyelogram was normal. A voiding cystourethrogram showed grade III/V reflux bilaterally. The first recommendation was for low-dose nitrofurantoin prophylaxis to be given for 6 to 12 months. Nine months later the patient again was seen because of persistent frequency, urgency, and enuresis. Repeat voiding cystourethrogram revealed no reflux on the right and grade II/V reflux on the left. The upper urethra appeared dilated on the repeat voiding cystourethrogram (Fig 2–1). At cystoscopy meatal stenosis was not documented. Ureteral catheterization of the left refluxing ureteral orifice showed a 1 cm submucosal tunnel. Both ureteral orifices were somewhat laterally displaced and patulous. Low-dose nitrofurantoin prophylaxis was continued, along with oxybutynin.

DISCUSSION

In this case cystoscopy was done to further evaluate the placement and configuration of the ureteral orifices and to make sure that the abnormal configuration of the urethra seen on the voiding cystourethrogram did not result from an introital or urethral abnormality. No meatal stenosis was found. Both ureteral orifices appeared somewhat abnormal, although reflux had spontaneously subsided on the right and not on the left. The cystoscopy thus was not helpful. The cystoscopy (done with the patient under general anesthesia as an outpatient) involved some risk and expense. What was the gain? In this situation I went against my usual practice, which is not to recommend cystoscopy in girls with recurrent cystitis. I frequently see children who are sent to me after other urologists have done a cystoscopy (and sometimes urethral dilatation or urethrotomy) with no subsequent clinical improvement in the child. Inspection of the perineum can be easily accomplished in most children in this age group as an outpatient with their mothers in the room and the labia spread. The presence of labial adhesions, the position of the urethral meatus, perineal hygiene, and so forth, thus can be ascertained. My own ability to predict which ureteral orifices will spontaneously stop refluxing is limited. If I had made a prediction based

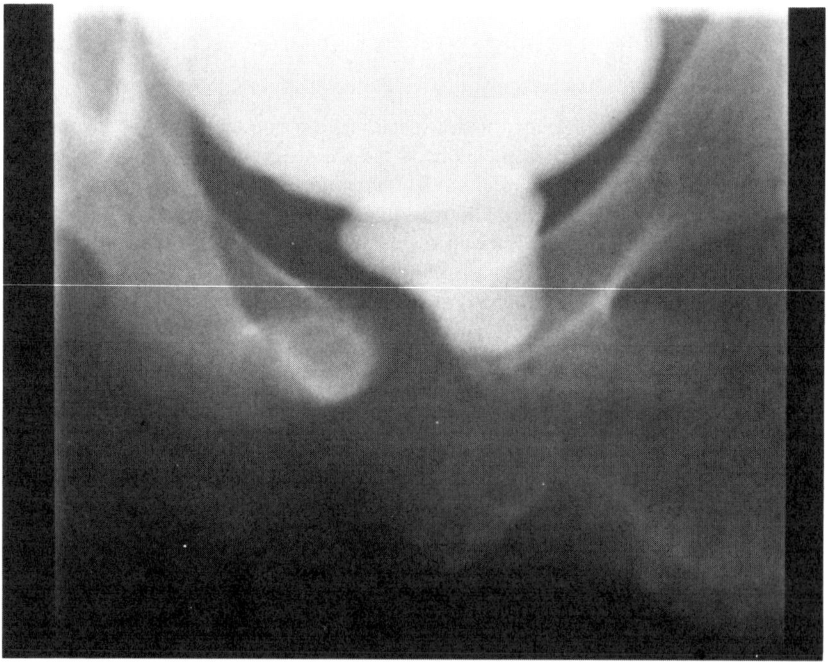

FIG 2–1.
Voiding cystourethrogram in a 7-year-old girl. Note dilated upper urethra.

on cystoscopy findings in this child I would have predicted that both orifices were still refluxing. In fact, only the left continued to do so. The radiographic appearance of the urethra does not diagnose meatal stenosis in girls.[1] Neither urethral dilatation nor urethrotomy is helpful for girls with recurrent UTIs.[2] Urethral caliber is not usually narrower in girls with recurrent infections.[3] My usual indications for antireflux surgery are persistent grade III or greater reflux that persists after 12 to 18 months of prophylaxis. Although there may be variations in opinions on the optimal duration of prophylaxis and degree of reflux for which surgery is indicated, the cystoscopic appearance of the ureteral orifices and the length of submucosal tunnels are only fair predictors of the course of the reflux.

Although characterization of this child's *E. coli* was not carried out further as to its virulence factors or "adhesions," such as O antigens and P type, it was easily treated on three occasions with the usual antimicrobials and did not need to be a virulent or "avidly adhering" organism to cause fever and pyelonephritis in the presence of reflux. Although urinary immunoglobulin levels were not measured in this child, it has been shown that girls with recurrent UTIs have a rise in urinary immunogloblin levels after an infection but low baseline values.[4, 5] Low urinary immunoglobulin levels may be one among many predisposing factors in children with recurrent UTIs. Though local immunity may be sporadically or chronically deficient in these children, it is not easy to augment it by parenteral or local immunization.[6] Thus the goal of increasing local antibodies to have them coat bacteria and thereby prevent bacterial attachment to bladder mucosa remains elusive. Host factors such as the configuration of the carbohydrate "receptors" for bacteria on urothelial cells may be another reason for susceptibility to UTIs. Sheinfeld et al.[7] has reported an association between Lewis blood-group phenotypes and susceptibility to recurrent UTI in women.

The reason for presenting this case is to remind urologists that the indications for cystoscopy in children with recurrent UTIs need to be carefully scrutinized. Although a protracted course of antimicrobials and anticholinergics is not without problems, the clinical course does not get any easier if an unhelpful cystoscopy is interposed. Would it not be better to be honest with parents and referring physicians that much forbearance and long-term medication are the best regimen at such times?

REFERENCES

1. Uehling DT, King LR: Limitations in the diagnostic value of the voiding cystourethrogram. *J Pediatr* 1966; 69:744.
2. Kaplan GW, Sammons TA, King LR: A blind comparison of dilatation, urethrotomy and medication alone in the treatment of urinary tract infection in girls. *J Urol* 1973; 109:917.

3. Graham JB, King LR, Kropp KA, et al: The significance of distal urethral narrowing in young girls. *J Urol* 1967; 97:1045.
4. Uehling DT, Stiehm ER: Elevated urinary secretory IgA in children with urinary tract infections. *Pediatrics* 1971; 47:40.
5. Fliedner M, Mehls O, Rauterberg EW, et al: Urinary IgA in children with urinary tract infections. *J Pediatr* 1986; 109:416.
6. Uehling DT, Hopkins WJ, Jensen J, et al: Vaginal immunization against induced cystitis in monkeys. *J Urol* 1987; 137:327.
7. Sheinfeld J, Schaeffer AJ, Cordon-Cardo C, et al: Association of the lewis blood-group phenotype with recurrent urinary tract infections in women. *N Engl J Med* 1989; 320:773.

3

Recurrent Acute Urinary Tract Infections

S. Grant Mulholland, M.D.

A 24-year-old married woman complains of urinary tract infections (UTIs), which have been recurring three or four times yearly for 2 years. She has had no previous urologic evaluation. Each episode has been diagnosed by urinalysis and treated with antibiotics by her internist. One urinary culture done 3 months ago grew *Escherichia coli* in significant numbers. This organism was pan-sensitive. She has two children (ages 3 and 5 years), products of normal pregnancy and delivery. She had no UTIs during pregnancy, but she states that her mother told her that she had "a couple" of UTIs when she was a child. She is sexually active but expects no pregnancies because she has had tubal ligation. With the exception of this problem, her health has been excellent.

This patient is a 24-year-old woman who is now having three to four UTIs per year. Presumably she is having bacterial infections, but this has been documented only one time. This patient is not at all unusual, because in the 20- to 40-year-old age group or during the childbearing years, about 4% to 6% of women are bacteriuric at any given time, and these women account for about 30% of the cases of symptomatic UTI. Also, women who are found through screening, to have bacteriuria are seven times more likely to develop a symptomatic infection than those who have sterile urine.[1] About 20% of adult women will develop a UTI during their life, and between 3% to 5% of these will go on to experience recurrent UTIs.[2] According to another interesting study, 28% of patients with a first infection will develop a recurrence within 18 months. With a second recurrence, 80% will develop another UTI.[3] There appears to be a population of women who are prone to developing UTIs. We are dealing with literally millions of women in this age group; therefore, it is very important for us not to over evaluate or over treat these patients.

The development of a UTI in the female is preceded by colonization of the vagina. It has been shown quite clearly that rectal bacteria progressively colonize the perineum, then the vagina, urethra, and bladder in a retrograde fashion.[4] The epithelial cells from the mucosal surfaces in women who are prone to have UTI can be shown to have more attachment sites for *E. coli* than epithelial cells from females resistant to UTI.[5] The rate of vaginal carriage of coliform organisms in women prone to UTIs is higher than that in normal women. When one is planning management of these patients, these considerations are important. In younger women, the other reasons for the development of bacteriuria and recurrent UTI may be related to sexual activity, method of contraception, menstruation, and vaginal infections. The vagina appears to be the first area of defense in the development of UTI in women. If the bacteria overcome this defense, the urethra and bladder may be colonized if bacteria are able to adhere to the mucosal surfaces and remain behind after the washing activity of voiding.

DIAGNOSIS

Bacterial cystitis is the leading cause of UTIs, but one must keep in mind that approximately one third of these women may have acute symptoms with sterile urine.[6] Therefore, one must be aware of other causes that can cause acute dysuria and bladder irritation symptoms. It is essential that the patient have her infections documented as bacterial. The method of urine collection is extremely important. A well-instructed patient can usually give a reliable midstream urine specimen via a clean-catch technique. There is a minimum of contamination with this approach. Urethral catheterization is rarely necessary. In about 80%

of the patients with bacterial infections, an office microscope is sufficient to make an accurate diagnosis. Dip sticks that measure the transformation of nitrites to nitrates or measure levels of leukocyte esterase are about 80% accurate. A combination of these dip-stick tests and microscopic analysis probably achieves an accuracy of better than 80%. If the patient has pyuria accompanied by bacteriuria, this makes the diagnosis of bacterial cystitis more suspect. Usually a culture is not necessary with repeated bacterial infections in a known patient who has acute symptoms. Often the microscope can be used to save time and expense. A quantitative bacterial count of greater than 10^5/mL was thought to be necessary to diagnose a UTI. Counts less than 10^5/mL have been demonstrated in 20% to 50% of patients with documented UTIs. Stamm et al.[7] found that 47% of patients with UTIs had counts less than 10^5/mL and, 30% had counts less than 10^4/mL.

EVALUATION OF THE PATIENT

To treat UTI, one definitely should attempt to obtain an accurate history and concentrate on etiologic aspects. This patient had UTIs presumably as a child and now has begun to have them again during her childbearing years. She did not have UTIs with pregnancy, which is a valuable clue. The patient has never had clinical pyelonephritis. Presumably she had no difficulty with bed-wetting or toilet training. Adult women should be evaluated if they meet any of the following criteria:

1. Recurrent UTIs in a patient with a childhood history of UTIs.
2. A rather lengthy history of recurrent UTIs or multiple UTIs in short periods of time
3. A history of pyelonephritis
4. Unusual organisms cultured
5. A poor clinical response to treatment
6. Persistent microhematuria

If one evaluates only these patients, a higher percentage of pathologic conditions will be found at a reduced expenditure in time and money. The way in which these patients are evaluated has changed dramatically during the past decade. Identification of organisms and antimicrobial sensitivity tests are necessary in individuals who have multiple reinfections or in patients who have infections that are difficult to treat. Intravenous pyelograms (IVPs) are virtually obsolete in evaluating most adults.[8] Ultrasound evaluation of the upper urinary tracts and ureters is adequate for most patients. If a patient has hematuria or some other reason to outline the collecting system carefully, there may be a need for an IVP. Cystoscopy adds very little in the diagnostic evaluation of these patients.[9, 10] If the ultrasound evaluation of the adult's upper urinary tracts and ureters is normal, a cystogram usually adds very little information.

TREATMENT

This patient has had multiple acute community UTIs confined to the lower urinary tract. She is autoinfected from fecal flora. The infections occur sporadically enough that probably her fecal flora is not altered with resistant *E. coli* or other gram-negative organisms. Patients who have truly recurrent UTIs (UTIs that occur within 2 to 3 weeks of each other) will have a high exposure to antimicrobials and therefore develop resistant *E. coli* and other gram-negative organisms in their fecal flora. This patient therefore is probably infected with a fairly sensitive *E. coli* organism every 3 to 4 months. She certainly could be treated with a very well-tolerated inexpensive antimicrobial. Our objective in this type of patient is to sterilize the urine and rid her of symptoms. The medical significance of recurrent UTIs in women with an otherwise normal urinary tract is minimal. It was thought in the past that these UTIs resulted in gradual deterioration of the kidneys because of chronic pyelonephritis, but this has been shown to be an extremely rare event. Only in a woman who has some complicating medical or urologic disorder would the deterioration of the upper urinary tracts become an important factor.

Antimicrobial selection in all patients is extremely important. The ideal antimicrobial is readily available, well tolerated, not associated with allergic or untoward reactions, and low in cost. The drug must be well absorbed in the upper GI tract so that there will be a minimal affect on the bowel flora with the subsequent development of diarrhea or resistant organisms. The drug should be well concentrated in the urine within a short time of administration and have little or no effect on the vaginal flora. These antimicrobial drugs also must have a good gram-negative spectrum with little chance of development of resistance.

Ampicillin is a fairly commonly used antimicrobial, but is a poor selection because only 50% is absorbed in the upper GI tract and therefore does have an effect on bowel flora. It also may be associated with vaginal overgrowth of monilia. Amoxicillin is more acceptable if one wants to use an antimicrobial in this family. The nitrofurantoins are 90% absorbed in the upper GI tract and are rapidly excreted in the urine. There is little difficulty with resistant organisms or large bowel flora problems with this drug. The sulfa drugs are 75% absorbed in the upper GI tract and are well excreted in the urine. They do affect the bowel and vaginal flora, especially with prolonged use. Trimethoprim is well absorbed in the upper GI tract and excreted well in the urine. Its spectrum when used alone is moderately good, but the combination of trimethoprim with sulfamethoxazole improves the spectrum, and there is decreased development of resistance. Other antimicrobials such as cephalosporins, newer penicillins, and fluoroquinalones are rarely necessary in this type of patient. They are expensive and should be used in more complicated cases.

It has been well documented by numerous authors that short-course therapy is ideal for a patient such as this one. Probably the ideal length of time is 2 days. Eighty percent of patients who have an acute infection will respond to a short course of therapy. This eliminates secondary side effects such as diarrhea, flora changes in the bowel, and monilial overgrowth. After the clinician becomes familiar with the patient, it is probably best to have the patient self-medicate, especially one who has three to four infections per year. I have had good success with reliable patients who are carefully instructed on the use of the antimicrobial. They are told to begin therapy when they feel the onset of their symptoms; usually they are very aware of the earliest symptoms. They call the office and notify the nurse of each infection. With development of bleeding, fever, flank pain, and so forth, they are asked to come into the office. The patients take the medication for 2 days and then discontinue treatment. In this way the patients are seen far less often in the office. From an economic standpoint, this saves the patient the expense of an office visit and culturing of the urine. The patients are usually seen in the outpatient office once each year to review their treatment and symptoms over the years.

My preference of antimicrobials for self-medication are nitrofurantoin macrocrystals, trimethoprim, and trimethoprim-sulfamethoxazole. I have placed these in order of preference because of the numerous qualifications mentioned earlier, the most important being cost, tolerance, absorption, excretion, spectrum, and development of resistance. Other antimicrobials such as cephalosporins and fluroquinalones can be used carefully in short courses without any adverse effects on the bowel or secondary overgrowth. I do not believe the latter are necessary in the majority of patients, and they are not worth the expense.

It also is extremely important to look for a weak link in the patient's history. If a patient is becoming infected repeatedly because of sexual activity, one antimicrobial after intercourse will obviate the development of these infections. Occasionally patients will become infected only during certain parts of their menstrual cycle. In these patients, treatment at that particular time or change in the type of tampon or sanitary napkin used will help.

FOLLOW-UP

The follow-up in these patients should not be complicated. As mentioned earlier, patients who have recurrent UTIs and normal upper urinary tracts rarely have any complications from their infections. Patients with recurrent acute UTIs should be seen yearly. A complete physical examination, urinalysis, and culture are essential. Periodic examinations to make sure that the urinary tracts are not deteriorating may be necessary on occasion in a patient with a long history. The goal in the majority of these patients is a rather simplified conservative approach that maintains the patient's urine sterile. The treatment should be low cost, safe, and a minimum of inconvenience to the patient.

REFERENCES

1. Gaymans R, Haverkorn MJ, Valkenberg HA, et al: A prospective study of urinary tract infections in a Dutch general practice. *Lancet* 1976; 2:674.
2. Kass EH, Savage WD, Santamarina BAG: The significance of bacteriuria in preventive medicine, in Kass EH (ed): *Progress in Pyelonephritis*. Philadelphia, FA Davis Co, 1964, vol 1, p 3.
3. Harrison WO, Holmes KK, Belding MD, et al: A prospective evaluation of recurrent urinary tract infection in women. *Clin Res* 1974; 22:125A.
4. Stamey TA, Sexton CC: The role of vaginal colonization with enterobacteriaceae in recurrent urinary infections. *J Urol* 1975; 113:214–217.
5. Fowler JE Jr, Stamey TA: Studies of introidal colonization in women with recurrent urinary infections: VII. The role of bacterial adherence. *J Urol* 1977; 117:472–476.
6. Johnson JR, Stamm WE: Diagnosis and treatment of acute urinary tract infections. *Infect Dis Clin North Am* 1987; 1:773.
7. Stamm WE, Wagner KF, Amsel R, et al: Causes of the acute urethral syndrome in women. *N Engl J Med* 1980; 303:409.
8. Pollack HM, Bonner MD: Current status of excretory urography. A premature epitaph. *Urol Clin North Am* 1985; 12:585.
9. Engel G, Schaeffer AJ, Grayhack JT, et al: The role of excretory urography and cystoscopy in the evaluation and management of women with recurrent urinary tract infection. *J Urol* 1980; 123:190.
10. Corriere JN: Avoiding "overkill" in the diagnosis and treatment of lower urinary tract infections. *Urology* 1988; 32(suppl):17.

4

Interstitial Cystitis

C. Lowell Parsons, M.D.

This 62-year-old woman consults you because of 20 years or more of urinary frequency (20 minutes), urgency, and suprapubic pain. She has no evidence of urinary tract infections, and has been told in the past that she has interstitial cystitis. Urinalysis is unremarkable except for 3 to 5 red blood cells/high-power field. Your cystoscopic examination reveals ureters normal in position with clear efflux. She has an area of redness of about 1.5 cm with a central ulceration, located superiorly and somewhat anteriorly on the bladder mucosa. Throughout the bladder surface blood vessels are attenuated, and after hydrodistention, multiple bleeding points are noted. Her capacity during distention is 350 mL. Urinary cytologies obtained at this time are subsequently reported as normal, and biopsy results of the ulcer indicate acute and chronic inflammation.

This individual represents the patient with what I would call severe interstitial cystitis. In the discussion of this case, it is best to review what is currently understood concerning the pathogenesis of this disorder, how she would be staged in terms of severity, and, finally, what type of management options are currently available to treat someone with such a severe form of this disease.

In terms of severity, the case presented here does represent an advanced form of the disease and probably has an incidence in the United States currently estimated at somewhere between 40 and 70 per 100,000 individuals. There are probably five or six times as many people afflicted with milder forms of the disorder that are intermittent in nature and hence harder to track.

The pathogenesis of nonbacterial cystitis has long been believed to be related to the immune system in some form, including autoimmune phenomenon and mast cell problems, and it has also been suggested to be neurologic or psychologic in origin. What currently appears to be true is that perhaps one third of these individuals do have increased numbers of mast cells, and the question is whether or not they represent etiologic factors or a protective mechanism of the host. One thing that has been discovered most recently is that the majority of these patients have significant epithelial dysfunction and a "leaky epithelium."[1] Normal individuals were found to have an epithelial absorption of urea placed in the bladder of approximately 5%, whereas the patients averaged 30%. Causes for this epithelial dysfunction are not yet known and are being investigated in several centers. It may well be, though, that this leaky epithelium leads to solutes diffusing into the subepithelial spaces and setting up the symptoms of inflammation and eliciting a mast cell response in some people.

In an analysis of a large volume of patients with this disease[2] who were referred to a university center for evaluation (thus, probably representing a more significant form of the disease), clinical observations were made concerning the patients. These observations will help sort out the case that was presented here in terms of severity.

Ninety percent of the patients had continuous symptoms present for greater than 1 year and voided an average of ten times per day and 1 to 2 times per night. Eighty-two percent complained of pain associated with their bladder. The average number of daily voids was 16, with an average voided volume of 106 mL (as determined by a 3-day voiding diary). The cystometrogram findings showed that 90% of the patients had bladder capacities of less than 350 mL, and 95% of patients had increased sensory urgency. The cystoscopic evaluation showed an anesthetic bladder capacity of less than 850 mL in 90% of the patients. The average capacity when patients were under anesthesia was 561 mL. Fewer than 20% of patients had a bladder capacity of less than 400 mL. Eight percent of patients had a Hunner ulcer present.

In terms of the case reported here, the individual had a bladder capacity in the bottom 20% of patients and had a Hunner ulcer, which only 8% of patients have. Patients with Hunner's ulcer tend to have significantly worse pain and longer duration of disease.[2] This patient also had numerous glomerulations present after the distention of her bladder to maximum capacity while she was under anesthesia. From studies performed at our university, as many as 50% of patients with Hunner's ulcers have no glomerulations. If any consequence, perhaps this represents long-standing disease with loss of many of the small vessels that normally would rupture following distention.

The most important question to the clinician is how can one successfully improve this particular patient, and what is her prognosis? In general, one can determine from the histories of several hundred patients that about 60% of these patients will have a significant response of their symptoms in terms of hydrodistention of the bladder while they are under anesthesia. Remissions last on average 6 to 12 months. Individuals with more severe disease tend to have less of a response and shorter remission; hence, this individual is less likely to have a good response but may have some amelioration of her symptoms after dilatation of her bladder. Should she have a significant response, one can anticipate that within a few months she will be back to her full-blown symptom complex.

Other treatment options are available for this individual should she fail to respond to dilation or relapse after successful therapy. Dimethylsulfoxide (DMSO) may give her significant remission; therapy would be to place 50 mL of DMSO into her bladder for 5 to 10 minutes weekly for 6 to 10 weeks. This therapy will induce amelioration of symptoms in approximately 30% of patients, but patients such as this one are likely to relapse within a few months after therapy. Unfortunately, although DMSO tends to be active in the first course of the treatment, it becomes less and less active with subsequent courses. One may also see individuals who have severe pain associated with the instillation of DMSO. This is best managed by giving narcotic analgesics just before instillation and encouraging the patient to continue because in spite of the discomfort they feel initially, they still have a good chance to respond to the therapy.

The application of sulfated polysaccharides has been advocated.[3, 4] It is believed that these substances may help prevent the leaks that occur at the bladder surface[5, 6] and may even "detoxify" certain substances in urine that are capable of biochemically interacting with the bladder surface and causing the sulfated polysaccharides to be inactivated (quaternary amines). They have been reported to aid between 30% and 45% of patients when administered orally. The substance used, pentosanpolysulfate, is not currently available in the United States.

Intravesical instillation of the sulfated polysaccharide heparin has been found to be successful in treating as many as 50% of patients with significant forms of the disorder (unpublished data, 1989). The method by which intravesical heparin is used is to place 10,000 mL in 10 mL of sterile water into the bladder 3 days per week for approximately 1 hour. Because the medication is extracorporeal, it can be used indefinitely. It is recommended, however, that serum prothrombin and partial thromboplastin times be obtained for 3 weeks in a row to rule out any unusual antiheparin antibodies.

Bladder distention, DMSO, or heparin therapy could result in significant ameliorations of symptoms in up to 70% to 75% of patients, amelioration being a significant reduction in their pain and reduction in their urgency. There is a very important point to be made at this stage of therapy. Individuals such as this patient have spent years with chronic low-volume voiding and as a result have a reduced bladder capacity purely from that behavioral pattern. They void because of their markedly increased pain and urgency, but nonetheless they wind up with a reduced bladder capacity that has to be addressed independently. If one gets significant amelioration of the pain and urgency, the individual still has the small bladder capacity. We have discovered that by having the patients undergo behavioral modification individuals gradually increase their bladder capacity over many months. They not only get significantly better, but one can maintain remissions in patients who previously would break through, even in patients with fairly advanced disease such as this patient.[7]

The method by which this is performed is to have a long discussion with the patient to explain the concept that frequent low-volume voiding results in a small bladder capacity. The individual should be informed that to increase the intervals between their voids, they have to gradually hold their urine for progressively longer periods of time between voids. Many patients are disbelieving at this point, and they need constant reassurance that it will indeed improve their symptoms and maintain remission. The initial phase of the therapy involves analyzing their voided profiles to see how often they void. If the average patient is voiding hourly, they are then encouraged to wait 1½ hours between voids. This schedule is to be maintained for 1 month, at which point the patient is to revisit the physician for review of the patient's progress. At the end of that month, the interval between voids should be increased by ½ hour. This scenario is to be repeated for approximately 3 to 4 months until the time between voids has been increased to 3 to 4 hours. It has been noted that once patients reach this level, they do have a marked diminution of their symptoms and tend to have very prolonged remissions. There is a very high dropout rate from the patient's point of view first by initial disbelief and second by attempting to take too large a step too quickly. The bladder muscle will not respond except over many months to this type of therapy. Progress has to be slow but forward. Patients are encouraged that 3 months of significant discomfort associated with attempting to do this can result in years of reduced symptoms and potentially save their bladder.

As suggested earlier, to improve patient compliance, one should recommend that they be brought back monthly for at least 3 months to review their progress. It would also be helpful to have a behavioral psychologist involved who could help them over the initial phases, which can be quite uncomfortable. *It is not recommended that patients with severe pain attempt this protocol.* It is not possible for them to pursue it. One must first obtain significant relief of the symptom of pain by either dilatation, DMSO, or polysaccharide therapy before such an endeavor can be undertaken.

In terms of the case presented herein, it represents less than 20% of patients seen at a university center with the syndrome. Historically she had a very poor prognosis in terms of any significant remission. Today, with distention, DMSO, or polysaccharide therapy, this individual has as high as a 50% to 60% chance of obtaining significant relief from her pain. Then by a behavioral modification program of gradually increasing intervals between voids, she has an even better chance of obtaining and maintaining a remission. Patients with ulcers tend to have much worse disease and pain, and they are encouraged to be on some form of polysaccharide therapy indefinitely to help maintain pain at a low level.

Finally, at what point does one say that this individual is not going to respond to conservative therapy and requires definitive surgical management (urinary diversion or cystectomy). If the patient fails to respond to any of these regimens and continues to have severe urinary frequency and pain, considering the long time that she has had it, the patient should definitely be given the option of surgery. It would greatly improve the quality of her life and should be so presented to her so that she may ultimately make the decision. This is an elective decision of the patient because it is not a disease associated with significant mortality. It is a disorder associated with severe symptoms, and as such, only the patient knows if she is able to tolerate it. It is the sufferer who says, "I can no longer tolerate it," for whom the urologist should not hesitate to perform surgery. The only caution here is that augmentation surgery is definitely not a procedure to be considered because this patient does not have a problem with a low-volume bladder and, hence, all her symptoms. She has all of her symptoms first and develops the low bladder volume secondarily. Augmentation would merely leave her unable to void but with all of the severe discomfort she currently has. A more definitive procedure such as cystectomy is recommended.

REFERENCES

1. Parsons CL, Lilly JD: Epithelial dysfunction in nonbacterial cystitis (interstitial cystitis). *J Urol* 1991; 145:732.
2. Parsons CL: Interstitial cystitis: Clinical manifestations and diagnostic criteria in over 200 cases. *Neurourol Urodynam* 1990; 9:241.

3. Parsons CL, Mulholland SG: Successful therapy of interstitial cystitis with pentosanpolysulfate. *J Urol* 1987; 138:513.
4. Parsons CL, Schmidt JD, Pollen J: Successful treatment of interstitial cystitis with sodium pentosanpolysulfate. *J Urol* 1983; 130:51.
5. Lilly JD, Parsons CL: Bladder surface glycosaminoglycans: A human epithelial permeability barrier. *Surg Gynecol Obstet* 1990; 171(b):493.
6. Parsons CL, Boychuk D, Jones J, et al: Bladder surface glycosaminoglycans: An epithelial permeability barrier. *J Urol* 1990; 143:139.
7. Parsons CL, Koprowski PF: Interstitial cystitis: Successful management by a pattern of increasing urinary voiding intervals. *Urology* 1991; 37:207.

5

Catheter-Related Urinary Tract Infection

Anthony J. Schaeffer, M.D.

This 62-year-old man has just undergone a triple-vessel coronary artery bypass. His respiratory function required 5 days of assisted respiration in the intensive care unit. During that time an indwelling urinary catheter remained in place. It was removed on the sixth postoperative day after a urinary culture was obtained. On the seventh postoperative day, he was febrile and complained of dysuria. Urinary culture grew more than 100,000 colony-forming units (CFUs)/mL of *Enterobacter* resistant to ampicillin, cephalothin, cefoxitin, and cephazolin.

Approximately 80% of nosocomial urinary tract infections (UTIs) are preceded by some form of urologic instrumentation, most often indwelling bladder catheterization. The prevalence of indwelling urinary catheters among hospitalized patients is 7% to 16%; therefore, a large population of patients are susceptible to catheter-associated bacteriuria. Although many of these episodes are caused by asymptomatic bacterial colonization, a significant portion of patients develop cystitis, pyelonephritis, bacteremia, or septicemia, which may cause or contribute to death.

DEFINITION

Catheter-associated bacteriuria refers to the presence of 100 or more CFU/mL of urine aspirated from the catheter. Because patients with indwelling catheters have a short urine transit time and are frequently well hydrated, these low counts of bacteria are just as diagnostic as the traditional count of 10^5 CFU/mL. Once small numbers of microorganisms gain access to the catheterized bladder, unless suppressive antimicrobial therapy is being given or started, progression to concentrations greater than 10^5 CFU/mL may occur rapidly and usually within 72 hours.

Catheter-associated bacteriuria is a microbiologically defined term and indicates bacterial colonization of the urinary tract. A UTI implies bacterial invasion of host tissue associated with an inflammatory response. Fever, chills, and flank pain usually indicate acute pyelonephritis. However, complications such as chronic pyelonephritis, impairment of renal function, or infection stones frequently develop in asymptomatic patients with persistent catheter-associated bacteriuria. Pyuria and hematuria are better discriminators, but either infection or irritation from the catheter can cause a similar response. Because it is frequently difficult clinically to distinguish colonization from infection, persistent bacteriuria is regarded as an indication of a probable UTI and potential clinically significant sequelae.

PATHOGENESIS

Catheter-associated bacteriuria is caused by bacteria acquired by the patient from several sources. *Escherichia coli,* other Enterobacteriaceae, and enterococci present in normal colonic flora or acquired during hospitalization have been associated with subsequent UTI in patients with catheterized bladders.

Other pathogens such as *Serratia marcescens* are probably acquired by cross-contamination from sources extrinsic to the patient.

After insertion of an indwelling catheter, bacteria may ascend to the urinary tract by either extraluminal migration from the urethral meatus or intraluminal migration after disconnection of the distal catheter-proximal drainage tube junction or contamination of the drainage bag.

The incidence of catheter-associated bacteriuria depends on the type and duration of catheterization. After a single short-term catheterization, bacteriuria is seen in 1% to 5% of hospitalized patients. The incidence of bacteriuria after single catheterization is even higher in high-risk populations such as those who are pregnant, elderly, or debilitated patients and those with urologic abnormalities.

A much more significant risk occurs in the 7% to 16% of hospitalized patients with indwelling urethral catheters. The incidences of catheter-associated urinary tract bacteriuria in studies of large numbers of patients and a variety of hospital services range from 10% to 20%.

Risk factors predisposing to catheter-associated bacteriuria are listed in Table 5–1.

An unalterable risk factor should alert the clinician to patients who are highly susceptible to catheter-associated bacteriuria and who therefore should be closely monitored. Alterable risk factors may be modified to reduce the incidence and complications of catheter-associated infection.

The duration of catheterization is probably the most significant alterable risk factor for catheter-associated bacteriuria. The cumulative percentages from four epidemiologic studies of patients with catheterized bladders acquiring bacteriuria are shown in Figure 5–1.[1–5] These data demonstrate that the risk of acquiring catheter-associated bacteriuria clearly relates to the duration of catheterization and ranges from 4% to 7.5% per day during the first 10 days of catheterization.

TABLE 5–1.

Risk Factors Predisposing to Catheter-Associated Bacteriuria

Unalterable Risk Factors	Alterable Risk Factors
Female sex	Indication for catheterization
Advanced age	Duration of catheterization
Severe underlying disease	Quality of catheter care
	Cross-contamination

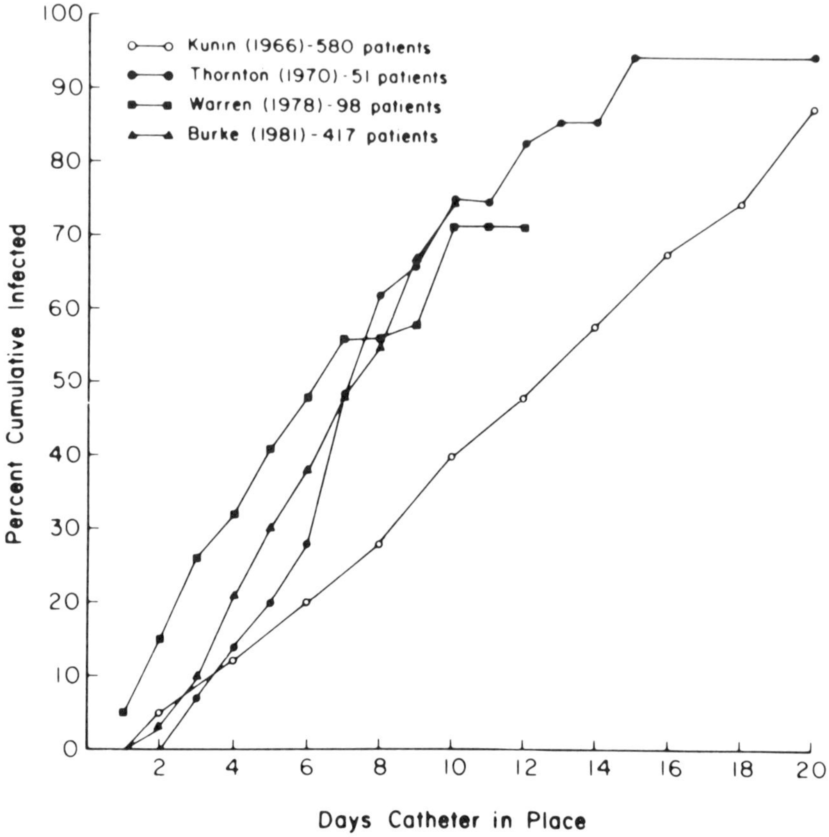

FIG 5–1.
Cumulative percent of catheterized patients acquiring urinary tract infections. (From Fowler JE Jr, Marshall V: *Infect Surg* 1983; 2:43–53. Used by permission.)

SEQUELAE

It is usually assumed that catheter-associated bacteriuria is asymptomatic and benign and will resolve spontaneously after removal of the catheter or after removal of antimicrobial therapy. Although this is frequently true, catheter-associated bacteriuria may be associated with significant morbidity and mortality. Platt et al.[6] observed that the acquisition of UTI during indwelling catheterization was associated with a nearly threefold increase in mortality among hospitalized patients. Approximately 1% of patients with nosocomial UTIs will experience bacteremia that will cause or contribute to death in approximately 10%. The majority of patients who develop bacteremia are more than 50 years of age, and the frequency of this complication is three to four times greater in men than in women. The possibility that catheter-associated bacteriuria may contribute to infections at other sites such as a surgical wound has also been proposed. Finally, catheter-associated UTIs have been shown to increase significantly the duration of hospitalization and hospital cost.

PREVENTIVE MEASURES

Catheter and Drainage System Care

Aseptic insertion of the catheter is obviously important. Once the catheter has been connected to the drainage system, inadvertent disconnection of the catheter-drainage bag junction or contamination of the drainage bag should be avoided. If the junction must be disconnected, sterile technique should be used. Urine specimens should be obtained aseptically by needle aspiration through the catheter drainage bag aspiration port. The drainage port spigot should be kept closed, and the drainage bag should be maintained in a dependent position below the patient and off the floor to prevent contamination of the drainage bag spigot by bacteria from the hospital environment. Separate vessels should be used to collect the urine.

Meatal Care

Daily cleansing of the urethral meatus–catheter junction with water is recommended, but antimicrobial solutions should not be used because they may encourage growth of resistant bacteria.

Urinary Drainage System

Improvements of the urinary drainage system have led to the most striking effect on reduction of catheter-associated bacteriuria. Most sterile drainage systems have been shown to maintain sterile urine in 50% of men and women for 13 and 11 days, respectively. Recently efforts to prevent contamination of the drainage bag by instillation of antimicrobial agents such as chlorhexidine or hydrogen peroxide have been shown to further reduce the rate of contamination of the drainage bag and acquisition of catheter-associated bacteriuria. This approach should be used if bag contamination occurs frequently (e.g., clusters of patients with long-term indwelling urethral catheters). If the drainage bags are unlikely to be contaminated or if the patient is on antimicrobial therapy, instillation of antimicrobials into the drainage bag is not warranted.

Systemic Antimicrobial Agents

The efficacy of prophylactic systemic antimicrobials in catheterized patients remains unclear. In most studies, when patients receive systemic antimicrobials, the incidence of bacteria was reduced during the first 4 days of catheterization and thereafter acquisition of bacteria occurred at the same rate as was observed in patients without systemic antimicrobials. Prophylactic antimicrobial therapy appears prevalent for patients who require short-term catheterization and are at high risk of complications from UTI. However, the potential for adverse drug reactions, selection of resistant organisms, and increased cost argue against the routine use of antimicrobial agents for full prophylaxis against UTI in all patients at low risk of complications from UTIs and in high-risk patients who require long-term catheterization.

All patients with symptomatic catheter-associated UTI should receive systemic antimicrobial therapy. Antimicrobials will eradicate UTI in approximately 80% of patients who are infected at the time of catheterization or who acquire catheter-associated bacteriuria, and 65% of these patients will subsequently maintain sterile urine during catheterization.

Recommendations for Urinary Catheter Care

Indwelling urethral catheters should be used only when absolutely necessary and left indwelling for as short a period as possible. The catheter should be inserted only by adequately trained personnel using aseptic techniques. The drainage bag should be kept in a dependent position and suspended off the floor to prevent bacterial contamination of the drainage tube. The urinary catheter and drainage tube should not be disconnected unless specifically indicated for bladder irrigation or cystometric studies. Urine samples should be obtained through the aspiration port using aseptic technique. The urethral meatus should be cleansed daily with water to reduce encrustations. If possible, bacteriuric and nonbacteriuric patients should be separated. The catheter should not be changed except when obstruction or other malfunction occurs.

Recommendations for Discontinuing Catheterization

The decision concerning whether to culture the urine before removal of the catheter depends on the duration of catheterization and risk status of the patient. Because the incidence of catheter-associated bacteriuria is a fairly predictable 5% to 7% of patients catheterized per day, approximately 15% to 25% of patients will become bacteriuric within 3 to 4 days of catheterization. For patients whose bladders are catheterized less than 3 to 4 days and who are not at high risk of catheter-associated infection, the catheter can be removed without prior culture of the bladder urine. If the patient is at increased risk of complications of UTIs, or if the catheter has been left in place for longer than 3 to 4 days, it is prudent to obtain a urine culture 1 day before the day planned for removal of the catheter. If the culture of the urine demonstrates more than 100 CFU/mL, the catheter should not be removed until antimicrobial sensitivity testing is available and the patient has received specific drug therapy. Empiric therapy is not advisable, because many nosocomial UTIs are caused by resistant bacteria.

Even if the urine shows no growth at the time the catheter is removed, the patient may harbor bacteria in the urethra. For this reason I frequently give antimicrobial prophylaxis for several days and always obtain a urinalysis or urine culture approximately 7 days after removal of the catheter.

If these guidelines are followed, the incidence of sequelae of catheter-associated UTIs can be reduced.

REFERENCES

1. Fowler JE Jr, Marshall V: Nosocomial catheter-associated urinary tract infection. *Infect Surg* 1983; 2:43–53.
2. Kunin CM, McCormack RC: Prevention of catheter-induced urinary tract infections by sterile closed drainage. *N Engl J Med* 1966; 274:1155–1161.
3. Thornton GF, Andriole VT: Bacteriuria during indwelling catheter drainage: II. Effect of a closed sterile drainage system. *JAMA* 1970; 214:339–342.
4. Warren JW, Platt R, Thomas RJ, et al: Antibiotic irrigation and catheter-associated urinary tract infections. *N Engl J Med* 1978; 299:570–573.
5. Burke JP, Garibaldi RA, Britt MR, et al: Prevention of catheter-associated urinary tract infections: Efficacy of daily meatal care regimens. *Am J Med* 1981; 70:655–658.
6. Platt R, Polk BF, Murdock B, et al: Mortality associated with nosocomial urinary tract infection. *N Engl J Med* 1982; 307:637–642.

ADDITIONAL READING

1. Schaeffer AJ: Catheter-associated bacteriuria. *Urol Clin North Am* 1986; 13:735–747.

6

Chronic Pyelonephritis

James A. Roberts, M.D.

Mrs. Jonas, a 54-year-old woman, comes to your office because she has had multiple urinary tract infections (UTIs) in the past 3 years. They began after an anteroposterior bladder repair just before that time. All cultures done thus far have shown the same organism, *Klebsiella pneumoniae*. Cystogram shows no reflux, and intravenous urogram has been interpreted as "focal pyelonephritic change of the right kidney." On further questioning, the patient describes episodes of right flank and abdominal pain that she attributes to "indigestion."

This patient has had multiple UTIs caused by the same species of bacteria. Whether this is a persistent infection that is only temporarily suppressed with the antibiotics or instead recurrent infection with the same species but not the same strain of *K. pneumoniae* would depend on further testing. The first step, therefore, would be to look at the antibiotic sensitivity pattern and biotype of the bacteria found in new and previous infections to determine if they are actually the same strain of *K. pneumoniae*. This information may usually be found in the microbiology laboratory workbooks. A persistent infection would suggest a need for further evaluation, whereas recurrent infection can be more easily handled medically.

EVALUATION OF THE LOWER URINARY TRACT

It is of interest that there is no history of fever associated with the infections. This would therefore suggest lower UTI. *Klebsiella pneumoniae* is an uncommon cause of UTIs until early adulthood, when it becomes more common. It still, however, is much less common than either *Escherichia coli* or *Proteus mirabilis* in women with simple UTIs. However, *Klebsiella* is a common cause of nosocomial UTIs,[1] and it is noted that the infections followed an anterior colporrhapy. Pelvic examination is the first important evaluation, in which one looks for changes suggesting abnormal mucosa secondary to the postmenopausal state. In the postmenopausal woman, changes in vaginal pH and the vaginal cells themselves seem to increase the chances of recurrent infection. Local replacement therapy with estrogen in the form of conjugated estrogen cream will decrease the incidence of infection after menopause.[2] A catheter used at the time of the surgical procedure may well have introduced the organism originally. Urethritis from catheters can lead to abscess formation in periurethral glands and thus the formation of a urethral diverticulum, which can then be a cause of recurrent UTIs. Pelvic examination should evaluate for urethral diverticula, stripping the urethra to look for meatal purulence as a suggestion of the presence of a diverticulum. On occasion, chronic skenitis can also be a cause for such recurrent infections, thus evaluation of Skene's glands should be included in this pelvic examination. Although reabsorbable sutures are usually used for an anterior repair and the bladder is rarely entered, a cystoscopy would be indicated to look for the possibility of suture foreign body in the bladder or urethra, as well as the orifice of a urethral diverticulum.

NONINVASIVE EVALUATION OF THE UPPER URINARY TRACT

If the lower urinary tract is normal, one must consider the fact that some renal infections occur without fever. Antibody coating of bacteria would be highly suggestive of a renal source, though the test has both false positive and false negative results. This is done by adding antisera labeled with fluorescein to human IgG and IgM to bacteria obtained directly from the infected urine and looking for fluorescence of the bacterial cell walls with a fluorescence microscope.

The patient's periodic episodes of flank pain sound colicky and suggest obstruction, especially in the presence of associated nausea ("indigestion"). This raises the possibility that she has passed ureteral stones or even papilla after papillary necrosis. Some species of *K. pneumoniae* produce urease, thus the possibility of infection stones is real. I thus would take plain film tomograms of the kidney, looking for stone. Because of the possibility of papillary necrosis, a glucose tolerance test should be done to determine the presence or absence of diabetes mellitus because papillary necrosis, although occurring from infection, usually does not occur unless the patient is also diabetic. Noninvasive radiologic evaluation of the kidneys as a source of the infection is possible if the patient develops acute pyelonephritis; computer-assisted tomography of the kidneys should be performed to look for inflammatory changes. These are linear areas of low density in a striated pattern after contrast is given. Renal abscess can be seen as multiple or single oval, nonlobar lucencies, whereas the low-density areas are seen in a lobar distribution in acute pyelonephritis. I have also used the scintillation camera because acute pyelonephritis on a quantitative study with hippuran iodine 131 shows decreased blood flow, delayed peak activity, and delayed excretion of radionuclide.[3]

RENAL LOCALIZATION OF INFECTION

The patient shows changes in the right kidney of chronic pyelonephritis similar to those shown in the left kidney of the woman in Figure 6–1. The renal cortical scars with underlining calyectasis are the classical radiologic signs of chronic pyelonephritis. It has been shown that such renal scars with significant renal damage will occur if treatment is significantly delayed during childhood. Our patient does not have vesicoureteral reflux, and reflux is found in only one third of children with renal scars. Eighty percent of these children had a significant delay in treatment, and this delay in treatment is thought to be the cause. Although it was at first thought that these scarred kidneys occurred only by infection during early childhood, it has been more recently shown that recurrent

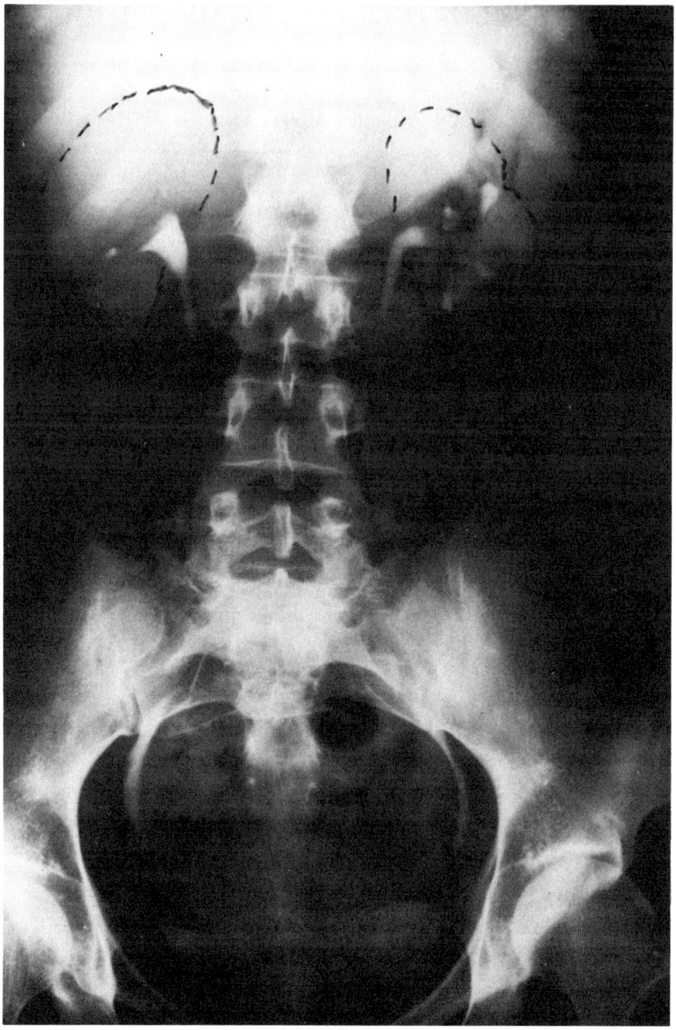

FIG 6–1.
Intravenous pyelogram shows chronic pyelonephritis of the left kidney. Caliectasis with overlying cortical scars *(dashed lines)* makes the radiologic diagnosis.

pyelonephritis leads to further renal scarring and loss of renal function in women as well.[4] This frequently is the result of recurrent infection, but it could well be the result of persistent infection.

Should the evaluation of bacteria from the several episodes of infection show the same strain of *K. pneumoniae* to be persisting and the lower urinary tract be found to be normal, localization studies should be done. In this instance the patient must have active bacteriuria. The bladder washout method uses a Foley catheter to introduce 50 mL of 0.1% neomycin containing two ampules of fibrinolysin-desoxyribonuclease (Elase). This is left in place for 30 minutes, and the bladder is washed with 2 L of sterile water. Urine is then collected for culture every 10 minutes for 30 minutes. Patients with renal infection will have 1,000 to 10,000 bacteria/mL in each of the postwashout specimens. A more direct and accurate method is that of cystoscopic localization, as previously described by Stamey and Pfau.[5] Urine is taken for culture when the cystoscope is introduced, and the bladder is then washed with 2 L of saline solution. The last wash evacuated is cultured, and then ureteral catheters are passed to each renal pelvis and urine collected for culture and urinalysis. As soon as this collection is completed, parenteral antibiotics to which the organism is sensitive are given and continued to eradicate the infection. Should positive ureteral urine cultures localize the infection to the kidney, a nephrectomy will cure a persistent infection caused by organisms residing in the area of chronic pyelonephritis if medical therapy is not successful and the function of the remaining kidney is sufficient to maintain life.

MEDICAL TREATMENT REGIMENS

Medical treatment might involve at-home patient-directed therapy. At the onset of lower urinary tract symptoms, therapy with antibiotics such as trimethoprim-sulfamethoxazole, nitrofurantoin (Macrodantin), or one of the newer fluoroquinolones could be initiated by the patient with either single-dose or 3-day therapy. Follow-up in the office is important to assure eradication of the bacteria. Indeed, failure to cure the infection is one indicator that the infection is probably renal, and some would use this treatment method as a first step in the localization of an infection. An additional method of treatment is low-dose suppressive medication, in this case, trimethoprim alone or nitrofurantoin at bedtime. A breakthrough from this therapy might lead one to more frequently consider nephrectomy, assuming that total renal function is normal.

REFERENCES

1. Roberts JA: Pyelonephritis, cortical abscess, and perinephric abscess. *Urol Clin North Am* 1986; 13:637–645.
2. Roberts JA: Urinary tract infections. *Am J Kidney Dis* 1984; 4:103–117.
3. Fischman NH, Roberts JA: Clinical studies in acute pyelonephritis: Is there a place for renal quantitative camera study? *J Urol* 1982; 128:452–455.

4. Jacobson SH, Lindvall N, Lins L: Renal size, glomerular function and urinary excretion of albumin and 2-microglobulin in patients with renal scarring due to pyelonephritis. *Acta Med Scand* 1987; 222:261–266.
5. Stamey TA, Pfau A: Some function, pathologic, bacteriologic, and chemotherapeutic characteristics of unilateral pyelonephritis in man: II. Bacteriologic and chemotherapeutic characteristics. *Invest Urol* 1963; 1:162–172.

7

Reflux Pyelonephritis

Joseph N. Corriere, Jr., M.D.

You find evidence of complete grade 2 reflux (Fig 7–1) in a voiding cystourethrogram performed on a 3-year-old girl. She has had two proved urinary tract infections (UTIs) in the past year. The last was 6 weeks ago and was treated orally with 7 days of trimethroprim-sulfamethoxazole. No other health problems are known.

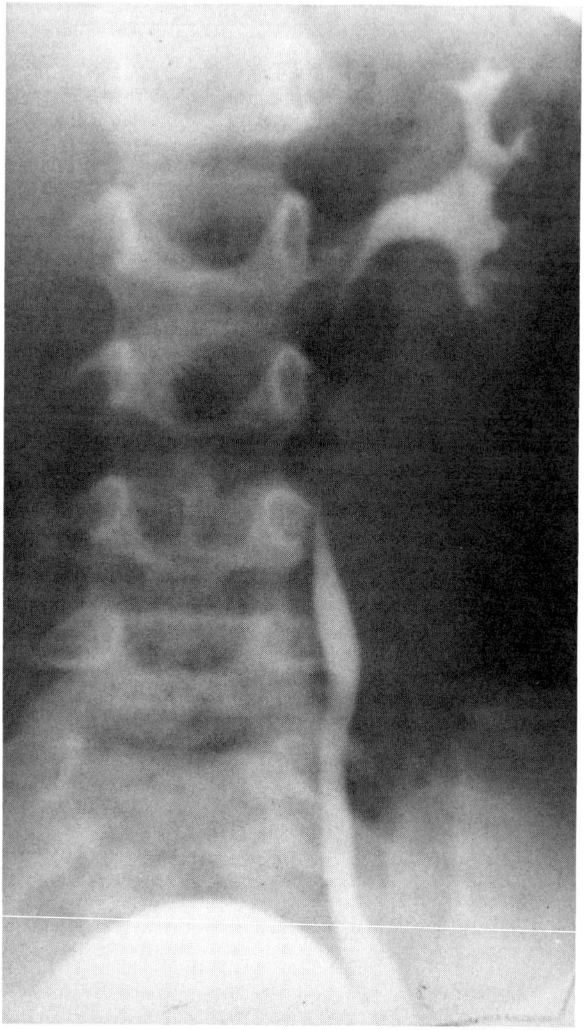

FIG 7–1.
Voiding cystourethrogram of 3-year-old girl with left-sided grade 2 reflux.

REFLUX PYELONEPHRITIS

One of the most difficult decisions regarding therapy of the child with vesicoureteral reflux is deciding between medical and surgical management. If one believes in the water-hammer theory that sterile reflux can cause damage of the upper urinary tract and that children will not outgrow reflux, then surgical therapy is the most likely option. There are also those physicians who believe that long-term antibacterials have significant complications that outweigh the risk of a few hours in the operating room.

However, I believe that if the patient has normal bladder function, only infected reflux will cause damage, and children can with time outgrow reflux. Therefore, I prefer a wait-and-see attitude, particularly regarding this patient who has only grade 2 reflux and has never been treated with suppressive medication. Of the numerous children I am following who are on long-term antibacterial therapy, none has had a significant complication caused by this method of treatment.

Between 60% and 85% of grade 2 reflux will cease spontaneously if infection is controlled. My routine is to use 25 mg of nitrofurantoin at bedtime, which, aside from occasional gastrointestinal distress, is well tolerated long term. And because it reaches a high urine concentration with low blood level, it has no effect on the bowel flora. Reported reactions of interstitial pneumonitis, pulmonary fibrosis, dermatitis, hemolytic anemia, and peripheral neuropathies are rare.

In the patient with reflux and voiding dysfunction, primarily frequency, urgency, and daytime and nighttime wetting, I believe that the addition of 25 mg of imipramine three times daily is helpful in controlling the voiding dysfunction. The subsequent return to a normal voiding pattern probably decreases the chances of recurrent UTI and subsequent reflux. I usually stop the imipramine therapy after 3 months to see if the normal voiding pattern will remain without medication.

All of my patients with grade 2 reflux use antibacterial suppression for at least 6 months, at which time I repeat the voiding cystourethrogram. If the reflux has disappeared, I will stop the medication. If it continues, I resume suppression (25 mg of nitrofurantoin at bedtime) for another 12 months and repeat the cystourethrogram at that time. I do not bother performing renal scans, renal ultrasound, or intravenous pyelograms to look for subsequent scar development because I do not use these as criteria for reimplantation in the asymptomatic child who has kept a sterile urine.

If reflux is still present 18 months after the initiation of this treatment protocol and the grade of reflux has not become worse, I will wait another 18 months before repeating the voiding cystourethrogram. I have been impressed that most of the time within 2 to 2½ years, reflux ceases when the urine is kept sterile and bladder dysfunction is corrected.

I think it is important to discuss with the parent and the referring physician the plan of attack. My rationale for this program is (1) the high rate of resolution of low-grade reflux and (2) my belief that sterile reflux does not damage the upper urinary tracts. Drug therapy should be continued until the age of 6 to 7 years. After this age renal scars do not develop if infection occurs.

Once I make the decision to stop the continuous drug therapy, I recommend urine cultures be done every 3 to 6 months until puberty and at any time a fever of unknown origin develops. Most of the time the patients are being seen by their pediatrician at frequent enough intervals that a urine culture can easily be obtained. I have not set up home culture programs with these patients.

My indications for abandoning conservative therapy and recommending surgery are dependent on (1) multiple breakthrough infections during a regimen of suppressive medication, (2) deterioration of the upper urinary tracts, or both. In this patient with grade 2 reflux, upper urinary tract deterioration is unlikely. Usually grade 3 or higher reflux seems to be the lesion that deteriorates. If breakthrough infection occurs and is not accompanied by fever, I believe a short course of therapy of no more than 5 days is all that is needed to sterilize the urine. If frank pyelonephritis occurs, I then would treat the patient for at least 10 days and begin to lay groundwork with the family for reimplantation surgery.

I have adopted the Cohen procedure for reimplantation in children and have been very pleased with the results. The patients usually come without breakfast the morning of surgery and need only a hemoglobin analysis as a preoperative laboratory test. I use a no. 12 French Foley catheter for 24 hours and no other tubes or drains. If the patient is fully awake and cooperative by the next morning, I will remove the Foley catheter. If voiding is spontaneous and the patient is not too uncomfortable, I will discharge her from the hospital that evening. If there is any question about the postoperative course, I might leave the catheter in the bladder an additional 24 hours and keep the patient in the hospital until I am sure she is voiding properly.

Rarely, after bilateral ureteroneocystostomy, I have seen urinary retention, which is probably secondary to a temporary neuropraxis. I have never seen this become a permanent problem. I think it very important, however, to be sure the patient is voiding to completion before discharge. Bedtime antibacterial suppression is continued for 6 months, at which time an excretory urogram and voiding cystourethrogram are done. Then urine cultures are performed at 6- to 8-week intervals for 6 months and every 3 to 6 months thereafter for a few years.

The hardest decision to make about the desirability of surgery does not occur when the child stops refluxing or when she gets breakthrough infections or upper urinary tract deterioration but when she does not and continues to have sterile, stable vesicoureteral reflux. I do not believe that (1) reflux present at puberty will never resolve (2) reimplantation is technically easier in a child than an adult, or (3) reflux after puberty is more of a concern than before puberty. On the other hand, I think that (1) low-grade reflux in the adult with normal bladder function is of little clinical significance, (2) reflux can remit or improve to a lower grade after puberty, and (3) the technical aspects of ureteroneocystostomy are as easy in the adult as in the child.

SUMMARY

The best prescription for a successful outcome in the child with grade 2 reflux is keeping the urine uninfected, maintaining normal voiding, and carefully monitoring for anatomic changes of the urinary tract. If low-grade reflux is present past puberty, it is best ignored with the caveat that the girl be aware of the possibility of an increased risk of pyelonephritis if cystitis should occur and the need for prompt evaluation and therapy of lower urinary tract voiding symptoms.

BIBLIOGRAPHY

1. Cohen SJ: Ureterozystoneostomie, eine neue antirefluxtechnik., *Aktuell Urol* 1975; 6:1.
2. Duckett JW: Vesicoureteral reflux: A "conservative" analysis. *Am J Kidney Dis* 1983; 3:139.
3. Edwards D, Normand ICS, Prescod N, et al: Disappearance of vesicoureteric reflux during long-term prophylaxis of urinary tract infection in children. *B M J* 1977; 2:285.
4. McLorie GA, Aliabadi H, Churchill BM, et al: Technetium-dimercapto-succinic acid renal scanning and excretory urography in diagnosis of renal scars in children. *J Urol* 1989; 142:790.

8

Perioperative Antibiotic Prophylaxis

Gerald W. Chodak, M.D.

This 73-year-old man developed urinary retention in another city 3 weeks ago. Indwelling catheter was placed, then removed, and replaced twice after he failed to urinate. This catheter has been in place for 2 weeks. His health is good except for urinary retention, and he takes no medications other than 0.25 mg of digoxin/day for mild heart disease. He has no known drug allergies. Your examination of the abdomen and genitalia is normal. On rectal examination, the prostate is 40 g and benign in consistency. Urinalysis of catheter specimen reveals 20 to 30 white blood cells (WBCs)/high-power field (HPF), and no obvious bacteria. You propose a transurethral prostatectomy to him.

This case raises an important issue concerning prophylaxis of patients undergoing surgical procedures. The concept of prophylaxis to prevent infection has been well established for many operations. The principle is quite simple. Provide a satisfactory level of antibiotic in the wound at the time of potential contamination, and infection may be prevented. The studies by Burke[1] clearly showed that the timing of prophylaxis is critical; initiating the drug after contamination will not prevent infection.

Considerable debate has occurred over the years regarding the value of antibiotic prophylaxis for men undergoing transurethral surgery. An extensive critical review revealed that few studies before 1979 were well designed, which made firm conclusions impossible.[2] Those studies that satisfied strict design criteria suggested a potential benefit from prophylaxis, although the exact duration and ideal medication were never well established. More recently, a number of well-designed studies demonstrate that systemic antibiotic prophylaxis will prevent urinary tract infection after this operation.[3–7]

The ideal antibiotic should have broad coverage of gram-negative bacilli, which are the most common pathogens associated with this operation. Usually a first-generation cephalosporin will suffice. The optimum duration of prophylaxis may be much shorter than initially expected. At a recent international symposium on prophylaxis, one perioperative dose was sufficient to prevent infections after this operation. Other studies using antibiotics for less than 24 hours also showed significant improvement compared with controls.[4–6] It is evident from these studies that antibiotics need not be continued until the catheter is removed. All of these results apply to patients who have sterile urine at the time of surgery.

Some patients, however, pose a higher risk for infection. They include men with a recent infection, multiple catheterizations, urinary retention, and most important, an indwelling catheter at the time of surgery. The longer the duration of catheterization preoperatively, the greater the likelihood that significant bacteria may already be present. In the case of this 73-year-old patient, who was in retention several weeks before surgery, he required three catheterizations and then had an indwelling catheter for several weeks before surgery. The fact that his urinalysis showed 20 to 30 WBCs/HPF suggests that significant bacteria was probably already present. The optimal method of managing patients such as these is to obtain a urine culture several days before surgery to initiate proper therapy before the operation is begun. Administering antibiotics before surgery in this case is not true prophylaxis because an infection probably already existed. Furthermore, if a positive culture is obtained, a full course of therapy is needed, and one dose or 24 hours of antibiotics is probably not adequate. In a patient who is allergic to both penicillin and cephalosporins, the drug selected should be based on the sensitivity of the bacteria growing on the urine culture. In the event that no infection is present, a single dose of an aminoglycoside would probably be quite reasonable.

Other principles that will help reduce the infection rate include using good surgical technique, avoiding breaks in the catheter connection, and removing the catheter as early as possible. Although relatively safe, transurethral prostatectomy may cause septicemia, which is still a lethal event in many patients. The use of prophylactic antibiotics is one approach to minimize this problem.

REFERENCES

1. Burke JR: The effective period of preventive antibiotic action in experimental incisions and dermal lesions. *Surgery* 1961; 50:161.
2. Chodak GW, Plaut ME: Systemic antibiotics for prophylaxis in urologic surgery: A critical review. *J Urol* 1979; 121:695–699.
3. Nielsen OS, Maigaard S, Frimodt-Moller N, et al: Prophylactic antibiotics in transurethral prostatectomy. *J Urol* 1981; 126:60–62.
4. Prokocimer P, Quazza M, Gibert C, et al: Short-term prophylactic antibiotics in patients undergoing prostatectomy: Report of a double-blind randomized trial with 2 intravenous doses of cefotaxime. *J Urol* 1986; 135:60–64.
5. Charton M, Vallancien G, Veillon B, et al: Antibiotic prophylaxis of urinary tract infection after transurethral resection of the prostate: A randomized study. *J Urol* 1987; 138:87–89.
6. Shah PJR, Williams G, Chaudary M: Short-term antibiotic prophylaxis and prostatectomy. *Br J Urol* 1981; 53:339–343.
7. Williams M, Hole DJ, Murdoch RWG, et al: 48-Hour cephradine and post-prostatectomy bacteriuria. *Br J Urol* 1980; 52:311–315.

9

Localization of Urinary Tract Infection

Jackson E. Fowler, Jr., M.D.

Mr. Carlton, who has been paraplegic (T10) for 7 years, continues to have chronic urinary tract infections (UTIs) in spite of lengthy antibiotic therapy and spontaneous voiding with complete bladder emptying. The responsible organism is *Pseudomonas aeruginosa*. Cystogram indicates no reflux. Intravenous (IV) urogram reveals normal left upper urinary tracts and bladder and smaller (8-cm) right kidney with pyelonephritic scarring. Nuclear medicine renal function studies assign 9% of total renal function to the right kidney. A right nephrectomy has been advised, but the patient is concerned that the surgery will not cure the infection.

This patient has sequential urinary tract infections caused by the same organism, or persistent bacteriuria. Persistent bacteriuria almost always results from a focus of infection within the urinary system that is resistant to conventional antimicrobial therapy. Potential sites of focal infection in this case include the atrophic, scarred right kidney and the prostate gland. The patient's concerns that nephrectomy may not cure the infection are well-founded, but can be clarified with lower and upper tract bacterial localization studies. The antibody-coated bacteria test is another technique for the diagnosis of invasive infection within the urinary system, but would not differentiate between chronic renal infection and chronic prostatic infection.

I would conduct the lower urinary tract localization study first. Convincing evidence of chronic bacterial prostatitis might obviate the rationale for the proposed surgery and, by inference, the upper urinary tract localization studies. Conversely, it can be argued that if the prostate gland is not infected an upper tract localization study is superfluous, because focal infection of the right kidney is the only other reasonable explanation for the persistent bacteriuria. The legitimate concerns of patients with complex urologic disorders, however, always should be respected, and decisions about performance of upper urinary tract localization studies left to the patient.

LOWER URINARY TRACT LOCALIZATION STUDIES

The lower urinary tract localization study is the only means for definitive diagnosis of chronic bacterial prostatitis. The test involves quantitative culture of systematically collected clinical specimens, and is an exercise in futility unless performed with established clinical and bacteriologic techniques.

Chronic bacterial prostatitis always should be suspected as the cause of persistent bacteriuria when the intravenous pyelogram is normal. However, confirmatory culture documentation is advisable, because recommended treatment involves an 8- to 12-week course of oral antimicrobial therapy at full dosage. The potential side effects and expense of this treatment are not inconsequential, and the physician may be vulnerable if severe toxicity develops in patients without proved prostatic infection.

The possibility of chronic bacterial prostatitis also should be entertained in men with abnormalities of the upper tracts that are potential sites of chronic infection. As in the case that forms the basis for this discussion, information concerning the bacteriologic status of the prostate gland helps to clarify the anticipated outcome of treatment for the upper tract abnormality, and may influence therapeutic decision making.

There is little reason to perform lower tract localization studies in men with no history of urinary tract infection, because the likelihood of chronic bacterial prostatitis is extremely remote. Indeed, the misconception that all symptoms suggesting prostatic inflammation should be investigated with lower tract localization cultures has obscured the value of the test in clinical practice.

Technique

Bacterial infection of the prostate gland is proved by demonstrating that the density of pathogenic bacteria in the prostatic fluid is greater than in the first voided urine specimen. Untreated bacterial infection of the prostate gland, however, inevitably is accompanied by colonization of the urethra and bladder urine with the infecting organism. For this reason nitrofurantoin, penicillin G, or tetracycline is administered for 5 to 7 days before investigation to amplify differences in the density of bacteria in the two specimens. These drugs suppress or eliminate extraprostatic colonization but have no impact on bacteria within the prostate gland. When the infecting organism is resistant to oral antibiotics, the urine usually can be sterilized with several days of therapy with a parenteral aminoglycoside. Trimethoprim, trimethoprim-sulfamethoxazole, norfloxacin, and ciprofloxacin, however, should not be used for this purpose. Each of these agents may reach therapeutic levels in the prostatic fluid and effectively reduce the difference between bacterial densities in the prostatic fluid and first voided urine specimen.

Clinical specimens for lower tract localization studies are obtained with the assistance of the urologist. To reduce the possibility of contamination the foreskin is retracted, the glans penis is cleansed with tap water, and the samples are collected in wide-mouth sterile containers. The first 10 mL of voided urine (voided bladder 1, or VB_1, specimen) and a midstream urine specimen (voided bladder 2, or VB_2, specimen) are obtained first. Prostatic fluid (expressed prostatic secretions, or EPS, specimen) is procured by digital massage of the prostate gland. It is usually possible to express at least 1 drop of EPS if patience is exercised while the fluid traverses the urethra. Ten milliliters of voided urine (voided bladder 3, or VB_3, specimen) is collected immediately after the EPS specimen.

Each of the samples is cultured using conventional quantitative techniques. To identify the infecting organism in densities of 100 to 1,000 organisms per milliliter, the agar media is inoculated with 0.01 to 0.05 mL of the fluids.

Microscopic examination of the EPS is an important complementary diagnostic investigation, because almost all patients with chronic bacterial prostatitis have more than 20 leukocytes per high-power field in the EPS. However, noninflammatory disorders of the prostate gland also may produce increased EPS leukocyte density, and the definitive diagnosis of chronic bacterial prostatitis cannot be made on the basis of microscopic investigations alone.

Interpretation

The VB_1 culture identifies the urethral flora and provides an estimate of the contribution of urethral bacteria to subsequent specimens. If there is no colonization of the urethra by gram-negative bacilli, sterile urine, and an uninfected prostate gland, all of the cultures will be free of gram-negative bacilli (Fig 9–1,A). If gram-negative bacilli colonize the urethra only, the density of the organism in the EPS usually is equal to or less than the density in the VB_1 (Fig 9–1,B). Regardless of the bacteriologic status of the prostate gland, if the bladder urine is infected the density of gram-negative bacilli in all specimens will be equivalent and the study will be uninterpretable (Fig 9–1,C and D). However, if the prostate is infected and bacterial growth in the urine and urethra are suppressed with preinvestigation antimicrobial therapy (Fig 9–1,E), localization of the infection to the prostate gland is relatively straightforward. In most cases the density of bacteria in the EPS is 10 to 1,000 times greater than in the VB_1 or VB_2.

If EPS is not obtainable the VB_3, which should contain varying amounts of prostatic fluid, is compared with the VB_1. However, this approach is less reliable, because dilution of intraurethral prostatic fluid by voided urine is not quantifiable and may lead to false negative test results.

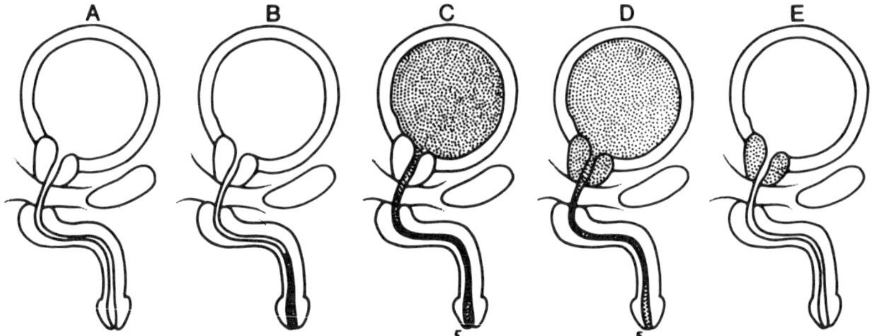

	A	B	C	D	E
VB_1	0	100	10^5	10^5	10
VB_2	0	0	10^5	10^5	0
EPS	0	10	10^5	10^5	10^3
VB_3	0	0	10^5	10^5	10

FIG 9–1.
Characteristic results of lower urinary tract localization cultures (expressed as gram-negative bacilli/mL) in men with no urethral colonization by gram-negative bacilli *(A)*, urethral colonization only by gram-negative bacilli *(B)*, bacteriuria but no prostatic infection *(C)*, prostatic infection and coexisting bacteriuria *(D)*, and prostatic infection with suppression of bacterial growth in the urine by antimicrobial therapy *(E)*. (From Fowler JE Jr: *Urinary Tract Infection and Inflammation.* Chicago, Year Book Medical Publishers, 1989. Used by permission.)

False positive lower tract localization study results are uncommon, because gram-negative bacilli usually do not colonize the male urethra and bacteriuria in the absence of prostatic infection generally leads to uninterpretable, rather than erroneous, culture results. False negative cultures may occur because infection of the prostate gland is a focal process and sampling errors are inevitable. For this reason, more than one culture may be required to document a prostatic infection. Recent or ongoing treatment with trimethoprim, trimethoprim-sulfamethoxazole, norfloxacin, or ciprofloxacin also may cause false negative results, and the clinician must be certain that these drugs have not been used for 2 to 4 weeks before the investigation.

The infecting organism in chronic bacterial prostatitis is as likely to be isolated from the seminal fluid as from the EPS specimen. However, the seminal fluid is more susceptible to contamination than is the EPS, and established criteria for the diagnosis of chronic bacterial prostatitis based on quantitative culture of the seminal fluid and VB_1 are not available.

UPPER URINARY TRACT LOCALIZATION STUDIES

Focal infection of the upper urinary tract always is accompanied by bacterial colonization of the ipsilateral ureteric urine. Such colonization can be documented by the culture of supravesical urine specimens obtained from ureteral catheters or from a urethral catheter after "washout" of the bladder. These upper urinary tract localization studies are analogous to lower urinary tract studies because contamination of the specimen of interest by infected bladder urine is either eliminated or quantitated. However, the urine must necessarily be infected for meaningful test results and antibiotics cannot be used to reduce the density of bacteria in the vesical urine. As with lower tract localization studies, the results of upper tract studies usually are meaningless unless done with established clinical and bacteriologic techniques.

Focal infection within the upper urinary tract is a common cause of persistent bacteriuria, but the clinical indications for localization studies are exceedingly limited. This reflects the relative ease with which bacteriuria and bacterial nephritis can be cured with antimicrobial therapy, the infrequency of persistent bacteriuria from an indeterminate site in the upper tract, and the availability of extracorporeal shock wave lithotripsy for treatment of infected renal stones. The tests may be of value in renal transplantation candidates with persistent bacteriuria, because infection localized to the upper tract is best managed by nephrectomy. In many cases, however, the culture results are difficult to interpret because of severe oliguria.

Ureteral Catheterization Method

Direct sampling of the ureteric urine permits lateralization of supravesical bacteriuria, but requires endoscopic manipulation and in some patients anesthesia. In this case the left kidney is an exceedingly unlikely site of focal infection, and localization of bacteria to the right ureteric urine is not necessary. Nonetheless, information derived from the ureteral catheterization method for upper tract localization will address the patient's concerns with the most precision, and the test probably can be done without anesthesia.

Technique

Colonization of the urine by the infecting organism must be documented by culture the day before the investigation; the procedure is cancelled if the urine is sterile. A cystoscope is inserted into the bladder and a urine sample (catheterized bladder, or CB, specimen) is obtained (Fig 9–2). The bladder then is irrigated with 2 to 3 L saline solution or endoscopic irrigant, and two ureteral catheters are introduced into the bladder through the catheterization ports of the cystoscope. Five milliliters of irrigant draining from each catheter

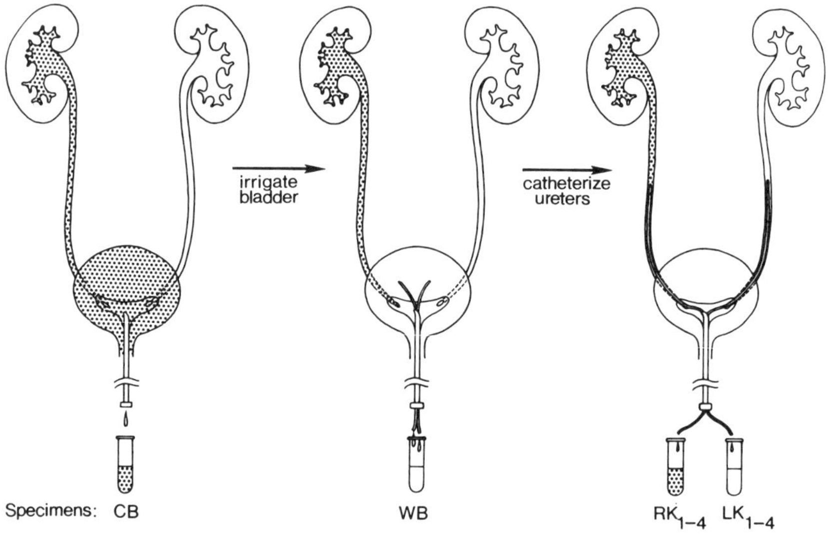

FIG 9–2.
Ureteric catheteterization technique for upper urinary tract bacterial localization. Note that colonization of the supravesical urine can be localized to one or both sides. *CB* = catheterized bladder specimen; *WB* = washed bladder specimen; RK_{1-4} = right kidney specimens 1 to 4; LK_{1-4} = left kidney specimens 1 to 4. (From Fowler JE Jr: *Urinary Tract Infection and Inflammation.* Chicago, Year Book Medical Publishers, 1989. Used by permission.)

is collected as one specimen (washed bladder, or WB, specimen) before intubation of the ureters. Each catheter is advanced to the level of the midureter or renal pelvis, and the initial 10 mL urine that drains from the catheters is discarded. Four sequential 5 to 10 mL specimens then are collected from each catheter: the right kidney (RK_{1-4}) specimens and the left kidney (LK_{1-4}) specimens.

Antibiotic is administered parenterally immediately after procurement of the last RK and LK specimens, to reduce the risks of obstructive bacterial nephritis that may be precipitated by ureteral trauma or edema. Routine techniques are used to culture 0.01 mL of each urine specimen.

Interpretation

The CB specimen documents the presence or absence of infected bladder urine, and the WB specimen provides an estimate of the contribution of residual bladder bacteria to the RK and LK specimens. In most instances the WB specimen either is sterile or contains less than 10 to 100 bacteria per milliliter. If there is colonization of the supravesical urine, the bacterial density in the RK and/or LK specimens usually is 10^4 to 10^5 mL and parallels the density of bacteria in the CB specimen.

False negative culture results are unusual unless the urine has been inappropriately sterilized with antibiotics before investigation. False positive results, however, are problematic. Approximately 25% of men and women with bacteriuria but no clinical evidence of renal infection or potential sites of focal infection in the upper urinary tract will have infected urine in one ureter, and about 25% in both ureters. Nonetheless, it has been my experience that the test results correlate with the anticipated bacteriologic status of the upper tract when there is a unilateral abnormality that is a probable site of focal infection.

Bladder Washout Method

The bladder washout test is more practical and convenient than the ureteric catheterization study, but infection of the supravesical urine cannot be localized to one side or the other. For the reasons elaborated above, however, the rationale for precise localization of infection to this patient's right kidney is not compelling, and the washout technique is a reasonable alternative if catheterization studies are not feasible.

Technique

Urinary tract infection is documented by culture the day before the investigation. The bladder is catheterized, and a portion of the evacuated urine is used as the CB specimen (Fig 9–3). Fifty to 100 mL 1% neomycin solution then is introduced into the bladder, and the catheter is clamped. After 30 min-

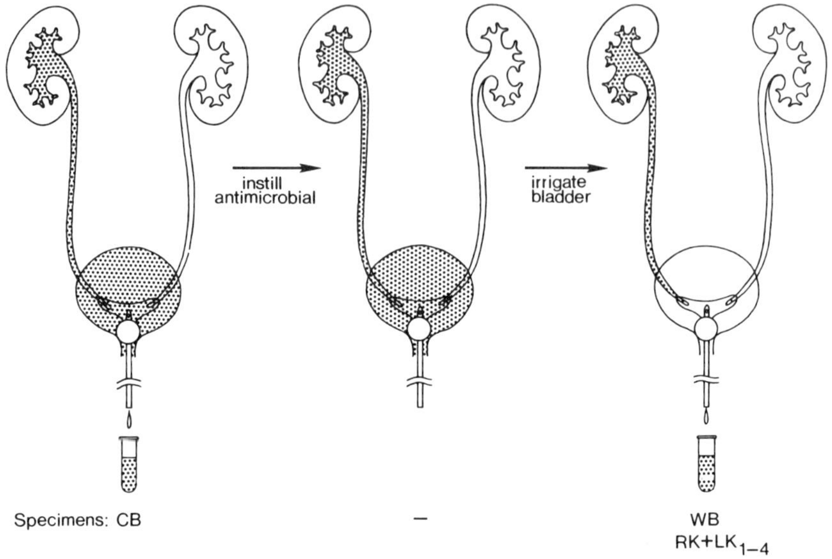

FIG 9–3.
Bladder washout technique for upper urinary tract bacterial localization. Note that colonization cannot be localized to one side or the other. *CB* = catheterized bladder specimen; *WB* = washed bladder specimen; *RK* + *LK* $_{1-4}$ = right and left kidney specimens 1 to 4. (From Fowler JE Jr: *Urinary Tract Infection, and Inflammation.* Chicago, Year Book Medical Publishers, 1989. Used by permission.)

utes the solution is drained and the bladder washed with 2 L sterile saline solution. The last 5 to 10 mL irrigant is used for the WB specimen. Four sequential 5 to 10 mL urine specimens are then collected from the catheter. These samples represent supravesical urine draining into the bladder, and for uniformity are called the RK + LK $_{1-4}$ specimens.

Interpretation

When there is colonization of the supravesical urine the density of bacteria in the RK + LK specimens usually is 10 to 1,000 times greater than in the WB specimen. The potential for false positive and false negative test results parallels that described for the ureteric catheterization technique.

ANTIBODY-COATED BACTERIA TEST

The antibody-coated bacteria test (ACB test) is used primarily for the localization of bacterial infection to the renal parenchyma. The test is based on the observation that infection of the kidney induces an immunologic response that results in the binding of antibody to the infecting organism in vivo. Infection that is confined to the urine elicits a minimal immune response, and in vivo binding of antibody to the infecting organism is unusual. The test does not require urine cultures, and the results are not influenced by colonization of the supravesical urine in the absence of renal infection.

The ACB test would not provide information useful in the management of this case, but the urologist should be familiar with the techniques and interpretation of the assay.

Technique

An infected voided urine specimen is centrifuged, and the bacteria are harvested, washed, and incubated with a solution containing fluorescein-conjugated antibodies directed against human immunoglobulins G, A, and M (Fig 9–4). The fluorescein-conjugated antibodies link with antibody on the surface

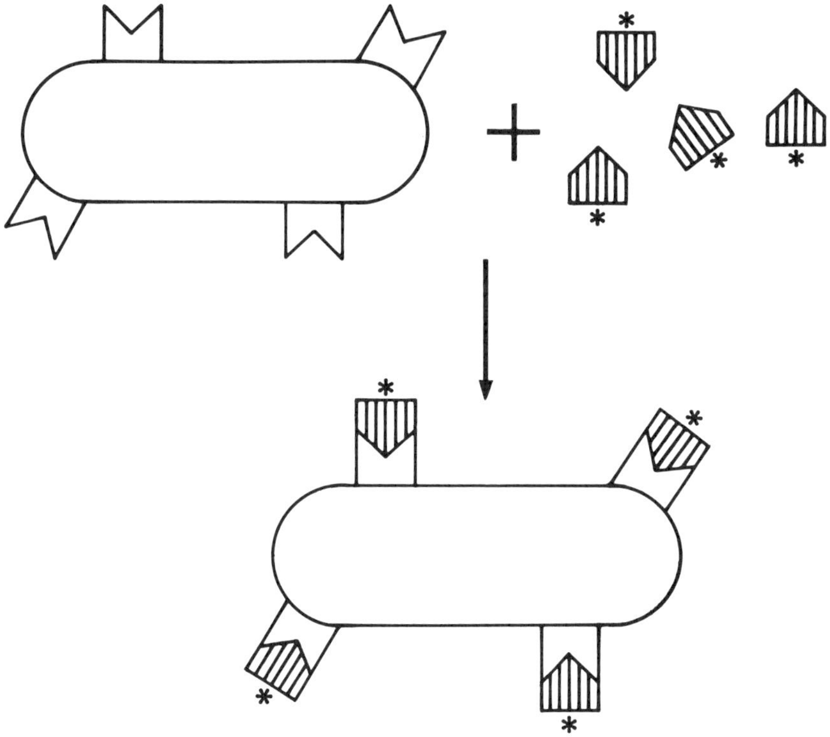

FIG 9–4.
Antibody-coated bacteria test. Bacteria from urine are washed and then incubated with fluorescein-conjugated antibody directed against human IgG, IgA, and IgM. The fluorescein-conjugated antibody binds to antibody on the surface of a bacterium, and the organism fluoresces when viewed with a fluorescent microscope. (From Fowler JE Jr: *Urinary Tract Infection and Inflammation.* Chicago, Year Book Medical Publishers, 1989. Used by permission.)

of the bacteria, and the organisms fluoresce when viewed with a fluorescent microscope.

Interpretation

There are no uniform criteria for designating ACB test results as positive or negative. Some investigators consider only one fluorescing bacterium on a slide as a positive result; others believe that as many as 20% of the visible bacteria must fluoresce for a positive test result.

Regardless of the criterion used for assessing the test results, false positive and false negative test results are not uncommon. Antibody-coated bacteria are seen in children with infected urine but no evidence of bacterial nephritis, and in persons with prolonged bacteriuria, bacterial prostatitis, hemorrhagic cystitis, or intestinal urinary diversions. Cross-reactivity of antibody induced by prior renal infection, autofluorescence, or nonspecific binding of the fluorescein-conjugated antibody to bacteria, and contamination of voided urine specimens by antibody-coated bacteria from the vaginal mucosa are other reasons for false positive results. False negative results have been reported in patients with bacterial nephritis of recent onset or with renal infections caused by bacteria with limited antigenicity.

SUGGESTED READING

1. Fairley KF, Grounds AD, Carson NE, et al: Site of infection in acute urinary tract in general practice. *Lancet* 1971; 2:615.
2. Fowler JE Jr: *Urinary Tract Infection and Inflammation*. Chicago, Year Book Medical Publishers, 1989.
3. Meares EM Jr, Stamey TA: Bacteriologic localization patterns in bacterial prostatitis and urethritis *Invest Urol* 1968; 5:492.
4. Stamey TA, Pfau A: Some functional, pathologic, bacteriologic, and chemotherapeutic characteristics of unilateral pyelonephritis in man: II. Bacteriologic and chemotherapeutic characteristics. *Invest Urol* 1963; 1:162.
5. Thomas VL, Forland M: Antibody-coated bacteria in urinary tract infections. *Kidney Int* 1982; 21:1.

10

Renal and Perirenal Abscess

Martin Schiff, M.D.

You consult with your internist colleague about a 54-year-old woman with left flank pain and intermittent fever. She has adult-onset diabetes treated orally with antidiabetic agents, hypertension, and mild heart disease controlled with medications. She has developed gradual onset of aching left flank pain and afternoon fever with a temperature of 38.8° C. Urinalysis is unremarkable. On examination, you find she is moderately obese and has deep palpation tenderness of the left flank. Computed tomography (CT) scan reveals a 3.5-cm mass on the lateral lower border of the kidney, which on ultrasonic examination has a thick wall and mixed central echoes. Percutaneous needle aspiration biopsy reveals pus, which grows *Staphylococcus aureus*. A small (no. 12 French) silicone catheter is left in the cavity. After 5 days of drainage and antibiotic therapy, the patient continues to have intermittent fever and pain.

Inflammatory lesions of the kidney and surrounding tissues are uncommon but potentially lethal conditions. Modern imaging techniques, including ultrasonography, CT, and occasionally renal arteriography, have enhanced early diagnosis and treatment, thus reducing mortality rates that approached 50% as recently as 20 years ago. These imaging studies have also resulted in a more accurate delineation of precisely which portions of the kidney and perirenal spaces were involved with the inflammatory process, allowing for a better definition of terms.

A *renal carbuncle* is defined as an infection confined to the cortex of the kidney, forming from a coalescence of multiple microbscesses, whose pathogenesis is almost invariably caused by a *Staphylococcus* species. This entity, which appears on imaging studies as a solid or semisolid mass lesion (see later discussion), is akin to a cellulitis or phlegmon and is usually treatable by means of antibiotics without need for surgical drainage.

As the infectious areas forming a renal carbuncle enlarge and become confluent, a *renal abscess* arises, in which there is a well-defined cavity filled with liquefied material. This mass lesion may be confined within the renal cortex, or it may expand into the perinephric space to produce a *perinephric abscess*. Further expansion of the infectious process through Gerota's fascia to involve the ipsilateral psoas/or quadratus lumborum muscles will result in a *retroperitoneal abscess*.

It should be noted that none of the spectrum of inflammatory processes under discussion in this context should be confused with abscesses of the renal medulla, which are usually caused by gram-negative urinary pathogens, frequently produce severe perinephritis and retroperitoneal purulence, and invariably require surgical drainage.

CLINICAL CHARACTERISTICS

The characteristic initial complaints of patients with renal and perirenal inflammatory processes are fever, chills, and flank pain. Usually leukocytosis is present, and the erythrocyte sedimentation rate is elevated. However, neither the urinary sediment nor the urine culture should be necessarily abnormal, because these cortical lesions do not communicate directly with the urinary collecting system. At times, a positive blood culture may be noted. Occasionally changes on a chest x-ray film such as a lower lobe infiltrate, an elevated hemidiaphragm, or a pleural effusion may serve as subtle findings to heighten the clinician's suspicion as to the presence of a renal or perirenal inflammatory process. Similarly, a plain abdominal x-ray film may demonstrate an indistinct renal border or psoas margin.

Renal cortical infection in the absence of any underlying abnormality, such as calculus disease or obstructive uropathy, is likely to be a secondary lesion, disseminated by hematogenous spread. The primary site, which is usually cutaneous but healed, is frequently not elicited in the patient's history. Besides skin lesions, a recent history of dental work and the presence of diabetes mellitus may be other preexisting factors contributing to the initiation of renal cortical infection.

IMAGING STUDIES

A renal carbuncle or abscess appears on an intravenous (IV) urogram as a mass of diminished density, often associated with distortion of the calyces, infundibulum, and renal outline. A carbuncle or an abscess that extends to the periphery of the renal cortex may produce enough edema of the renal capsule to obliterate a segment of the perirenal fat shadow. A perinephric abscess is much more difficult to diagnose by IV urography, since its only manifestations radiographically may be displacement of the kidney or obliteration of the perirenal and psoas fat shadows.

Ultrasonography compliments the IV urogram in that it can demonstrate the boundaries of an intrarenal or perirenal mass, imparting information about the size of the lesion and its location with respect to the kidney. Internal echoes may be present early in the development of a renal carbuncle, giving the appearance of a solid or semisolid mass. After coalescence, however, an abscess can be identified ultrasonographically as a fluid-filled mass with a relatively thick wall. Ultrasonography may be especially valuable in small children not only because it avoids irradiation exposure but also because it obviates the need for special patient preparation or sedation. Once the diagnosis is established, if nonsurgical therapy is attempted (see later discussion), ultrasound provides an excellent means of following any changes in the size, consistency, or wall thickness of the abscess.

If IV urography or ultrasonography indicates the possibility of a renal abscess, or if clinical suspicion persists despite normal screening studies, CT scanning should be performed. With the use of this modality and administration of contrast material, an intrarenal abscess is usually seen as a mass of decreased attenuation surrounded by an enhancing rim (Fig 10–1). Extension of the inflammatory process to the perirenal tissues can be appreciated on CT, with changes noted in Gerota's fascia and the retroperitoneal musculature.

Although largely supplanted by CT, selective renal arteriography can show anatomic details not apparent on any other imaging study. In selected patients this modality may still prove helpful, especially because the mass seen on CT may be indistinguishable from others of similar density, such as cysts or hematomas. A renal carbuncle can be identified angiographically as a mass that pro-

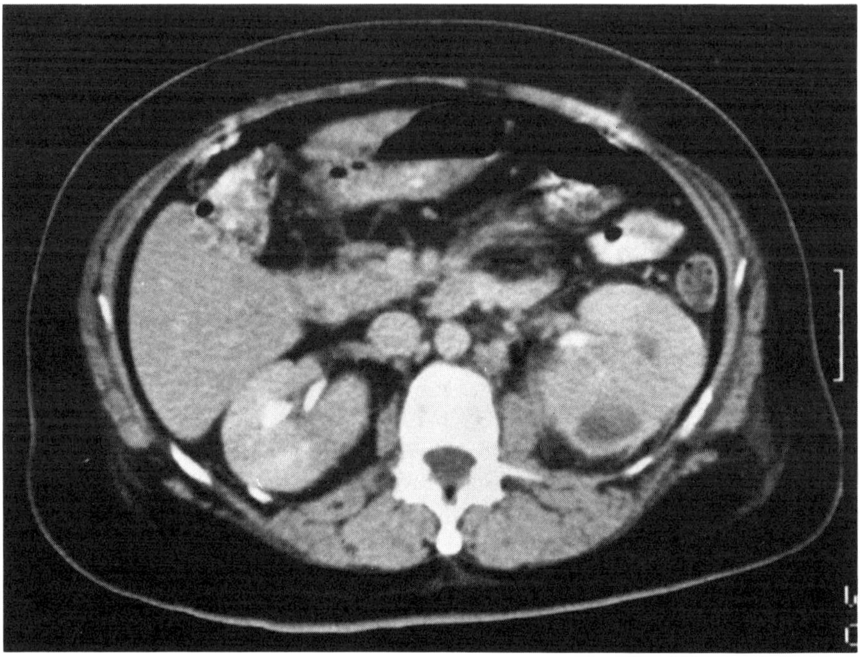

FIG 10–1.
Computed tomography scan with contrast in patient with left intrarenal abscess. Note intrarenal mass in posterior portion of left kidney with blurring of overlying cortical outline.

duces arcing, stretching, and attenuation of adjacent arteries, with the vessels located around the circumference rather than within the mass, which itself is avascular (Fig 10–2,A). Early in the course of development the rim around the carbuncle is poorly visualized, but arterial circulation to the periphery gradually increases with time so that a late study may identify a dense rim in the parenchymal phase (Fig 10–2,B). An untreated abscess may progress to a stage where the rim is thick and poorly vascularized.

Renal and perirenal abscesses can be arteriographically distinguished from tumors because the major portion of an abscess is avascular, whereas the wall of the abscess is hypervascular. Renal carcinoma may be hypervascular or hypovascular but rarely both. In an abscess the arteries may be displaced or angulated by the inflammatory mass or encased by fibrosis, but they retain their normal organization and branching pattern. Tumor neovascularity, on the other hand, consists of intrinsically abnormal vessels. Tumor vessels have no recognizable organization, may enlarge instead of taper as they course peripherally, and have an abnormal branching pattern.

Occasional chronic inflammatory lesions may mimic tumors angiographi-

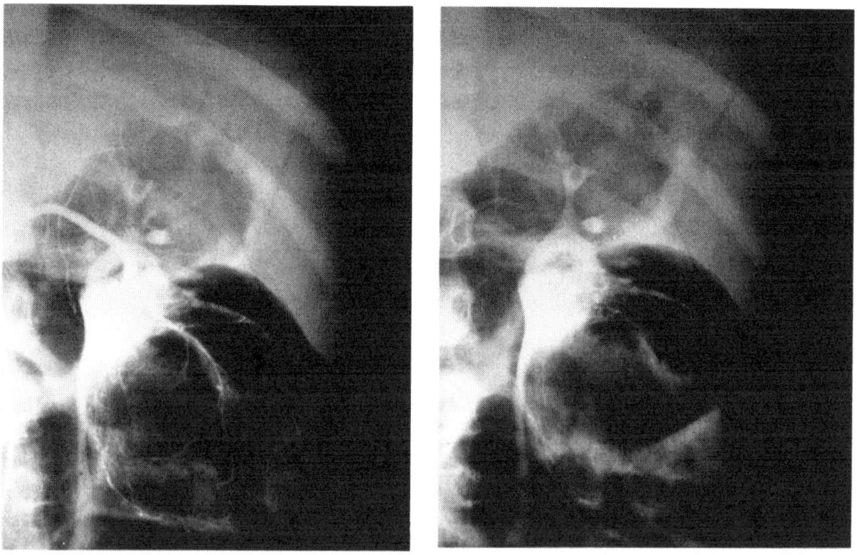

A B

FIG 10–2.
A, selective left renal arteriogram in a patient with an inflammatory mass lesion involving the lower pole of the left kidney. Note the avascularity of the mass itself, with stretching of the vessels around the mass. **B,** nephrographic phase reveals the dense rim surrounding the avascular mass.

cally, especially if the mass is solid and contains central vascularity. However, with the presence of intrinsically normal peripheral arteries and absent central vascularity, a diagnosis of abscess can be accurately established. Oblique projections may be necessary to verify the absence of central vascularity.

Radionuclide imaging using leukocytes with labeled gallium or indium, which accumulate in areas of inflammation, has severe limitations in rapidly and accurately delineating specific intrarenal lesions.

MANAGEMENT

After the diagnosis of renal carbuncle or renal abscess is established based on the clinical findings and uroradiographic studies, it is reasonable to attempt a trial of medial therapy. Although, as noted earlier, a positive blood culture may occasionally be obtained, bacteriologic studies are usually unrevealing. However, because the pathogenic organism in these renal cortical infections is most frequently a penicillin-resistant *Staphylococcus* species, the antibiotic of choice is obviously a penicillinase-resistant penicillin. A reasonable empiric treatment regimen is 4 to 12 g of oxacillin given intravenously each day for the first 10 to 14 days, followed by oral therapy of 1 to 2 g of dicloxacillin each day for 2 to 4 additional weeks. If a history of penicillin hypersensitivity is present, the recommended alternatives are vancomycin or a cephalosporin.[1-3]

Patients treated with antibiotics alone should be significantly improved clinically within 24 hours of initiating therapy. This kind of prompt response justifies continuing antibiotic therapy without surgical intervention using serial ultrasonographic or CT studies to help monitor the clinical response. An unfavorable early clinical course should lead one to suspect misdiagnosis or noncontrol of infection with development of perinephritis, perinephric abscess, or possibly infection with a resistant organism.

Percutaneous drainage of intrarenal or perirenal abscesses has become an attractive approach, with placement of the drainage catheter facilitated by ultrasound or CT monitoring.[4, 5] This technique, which was originally used as a means of obtaining a specimen for bacteriologic examination, is most effective when used in conjunction with antimicrobial therapy, especially when a well-defined, nonloculated lesion is present. A multiloculated intrarenal abscess and most perirenal abscesses are usually managed best by open surgical drainage through a subcostal incision.[6] When multiple intrarenal abscesses are present or the patient is critically ill (especially insulin-dependent diabetic patients), prompt nephrectomy is the procedure of choice, assuming the function of the contralateral kidney has been assessed to be satisfactory.

CASE IN CONTEXT

The case history presented at the outset of this discussion exemplifies many of the characteristic features seen in patients with renal cortical infection.

The somewhat insidious onset, the patient's obesity, and the unrevealing urinalysis all serve to make early diagnosis extremely difficult, allowing renal infection to progress to frank abscess formation. The correct diagnosis was made on renal imaging studies in conjunction with percutaneous aspiration of the abscess cavity. Thus, it was entirely appropriate, especially in a hemodynamically stable patient, to attempt to treat this condition nonsurgically. Although it is always somewhat discouraging to note the continued presence of intermittent fever and pain after 5 days of therapy, in my experience this clinical course is not atypical, especially in diabetic patients. It would seem reasonable to continue the original treatment plan on a day-to-day basis using one's best clinical judgment to determine whether improvement, however slow, is continuing to occur. Monitoring the diminution in size of the abscess cavity with serial ultrasonography or instillation of contrast material via the percutaneous catheter may provide objective evidence of improvement in the situation.

Both the physician and the patient should remain aware that a change from medical to surgical treatment may be required at any time. An episode of bacteremia, a progressive rise in the white blood cell count, or deterioration of the patient's clinical condition should lead promptly to surgical exploration and drainage or possibly nephrectomy.

REFERENCES

1. Schiff M, Glickman M, Weiss RM, et al: Antibiotic treatment of renal carbuncle. *Ann Intern Med* 1977; 87:305.
2. Rives RK, Harty JI, Amin M: Renal abscess: Emerging concepts of diagnosis and treatment. *J Urol* 1980; 124:446.
3. Hantman IE, Berger BW: Nonsurgical treatment of renal cortical abscess. *Urology* 1981; 17:415.
4. Pedersen JF, Hancice S, Kristensen JK: Renal carbuncle: Antibiotic therapy governed by ultrasonically guided aspiration. *J Urol* 1973; 109:777.
5. Gerzof SG: Percutaneous drainage of renal and perinephric abscess. *Urol Radiol* 1981; 2:171.
6. Lytton B: Surgery of the kidney, in Harrison JH, et al (eds): *Urology,* ed 4. Philadelphia, WB Saunders Co, 1979, vol 3.

11

Fungal Urinary Tract Infections

John M. Donovan, M.D.

During your hospital rounds, a colleague asks you to review the intravenous (IV) pyelogram of his 34-year-old female patient who has been admitted with left flank pain, pyuria, and apparent fungi in the urine. The films show no stones, prompt bilateral function, but calyectasis of the middle pole, left kidney, with an irregular lucent filling defect in the renal pelvis. The right kidney is normal. You are informed that the patient has juvenile diabetes and requires insulin twice daily. In view of the filling defect, you are asked to see the patient. On your examination, you find that she is slightly obese and has marked percussion and palpation pain in the left posterior and lateral flank. Urinary cultures performed on two catheter specimens grew *Candida*.

Positive fungal urine cultures in the immunocompromised patient represent a dilemma to urologists. Does this represent colonization or signify serious infection? Because candidal infection may cause obstruction, sepsis, or death, it is important to differentiate colonization from invasive infection. Recently it has been found that patients with candiduria alone from systemic infections had a 63% mortality rate. Patients with candiduria plus other sites of infection had 100% mortality. Thus, persistent candiduria, particularly in the debilitated patient, should mandate a thorough assessment.

INITIAL EVALUATION

When evaluating patients with candiduria, one needs to keep in mind underlying risk factors. Recent antibiotic therapy, the presence of an indwelling catheter, stent, nephrostomy tube or recent tube presence, diabetes mellitus, or a history of a urinary tract infection (UTI) are the most common risk factors found in patients with fungal infection. Other risk factors include an operation within the previous 3 months, recent urologic procedures, cancer, or patients receiving total parenteral nutrition. Renal insufficiency, obstructive uropathy, urolithiasis, previous radiation therapy or chemotherapy, or immunosuppressive medications are additional factors to consider.

FEVER AND SYSTEMIC FINDINGS

Apart from symptoms referable to the urinary tract, such as urgency, frequency, and dysuria, the presence or absence of abdominal or flank pain and fever should be noted. A search should be made for any mucocutaneous lesions and saprophytic foci as reservoirs of potential *Candida* infection. Oral thrush, perlèche, onychia, paronychia, and intertrigo are not uncommon, especially in diabetic patients.

FUNGURIA

The criteria for the evaluation and treatment of funguria is unclear. Fungal colony counts of 10,000 to 15,000/mL or more are considered as the upper limit between infection and colonization. Most authors believe that clean-catch midstream collections in male patients or single catheterized urine samples in female patients are required to accurately evaluate the urine fungal culture results.

Asymptomatic urinary colonization is not unusual. *Candida albicans* is the most common fungal isolate. Asymptomatic candiduria implies colonization without tissue invasion. Pyuria is present in almost 90% of urine of patients with serious infections but is seen in only 47% of patients believed to have asymptomatic colonization. When evaluating a positive urine culture, one should also remember the possibility of contamination of an improperly collected specimen. Therefore, reports of candiduria cannot be evaluated unless the method of collection of the urine specimen and the presence or absence of a Foley catheter are specified. The presence of an indwelling Foley catheter promotes candiduria regardless of the presence or absence of renal candidiasis, and there is a marked overlapping of the incidence of *Candida* in both groups.

DIAGNOSIS

A diagnosis of significant fungal UTI should be based on a clinical presentation of irritative voiding symptoms, defined physical signs, and positive fungal urinary cultures. Like bacterial infections, a likelihood of an invasive fungal infection is increased when the patient has either lower urinary tract irritative voiding symptoms or flank pain. Patients with flank pain, fever, and an elevated white blood cell (WBC) count usually suggest fungal pyelonephritis; however, these symptoms may be indistinguishable from those of bacterial pyelonephritis. Another diagnostic feature should include bacterial and fungal cultures of other sites such as blood, wounds, IV lines, pharynx, stool, and cerebrospinal fluid. Fungal serology or antigen levels may be used to distinguish infection vs. colonization.

Cystoscopy and bladder biopsy may be helpful to differentiate overt cystitis from bladder colonization. Cystoscopy, retrograde pyelography, and divided urine cultures from the renal pelvis may help determine upper vs. lower urinary tract involvement. Renal ultrasound or computed tomography (CT) scan can be used to evaluate the renal parenchyma in those patients suspected of having upper UTIs. If a solitary filling defect is noted within the pelvis, the density of the defect by CT scan can be determined. The radiodensity of a fungal coagulum is similar to soft tissue. Radiographic evaluation is also important to rule out obstruction of the upper urinary tracts.

THERAPY

In the absence of symptoms or the evidence of tissue invasion, candiduria is relatively nonpathogenic; therefore, antifungal therapy is not indicated. Usually the funguria disappears when predisposing factors such as antibiotic therapy or indwelling catheters are eliminated.

Antifungal therapy is indicated for symptomatic patients. Again, an attempt should be made to first eliminate the preexisting factors by removing catheters or stones and relieving obstruction. In patients with fungal cystitis, urinary alkalization alone may be therapeutic.

Amphotericin B has been used as an effective irrigant in fungal cystitis and noninvasive upper urinary tract colonization.[1] Irrigation may be intermittent or continuous. Fifty milligrams of amphotericin B in 1 L of sterile water infused over 24 hours are routinely recommended. The amphotericin B solution needs to be shielded from light. Local irrigation may also be used along with systematic antifungal therapy. It should be mentioned that amphotericin B given intravenously is excreted poorly in urine and is indicated only for invasive soft tissue fungal infections.

Systemic antifungal therapy is required for invasive infections. 5-Flurocytosine or ketoconazole alone may suffice for lower UTIs. Usually 2 to 3 g of 5-flurocytosine taken daily in four divided doses for 4 to 6 weeks is indicated for lower UTIs. However, higher doses of 5-flurocytosine up to 7 g/day may be required for upper tract or systemic infections. The side effects of 5-flurocytosine are more commonly seen with larger doses and can occur in 30% of patients overall. The most common side effects are hematologic, 22% (leucopenia and thrombocytopenia); skin rash, 7%; gastrointestinal, 6% (diarrhea, anorexia, nausea, vomiting); and hepatotoxicity. The major problem with 5-flurocytosine is the occurrence of resistant strains. Fungal drug sensitivities should be used to guide and monitor therapy. Serum levels should be followed in these patients with an attempt to keep them between 25 and 50 μg/mL or a serum level four times the minimum inhibitory concentration of the fungus. Therapy for renal candidiasis with 5-flurocytosine and alkalinization of urine is preferred when the fungi are sensitive to 5-flurocytosine. Treatment is continued until cultures are negative. Therapy combined with amphotericin B may be more effective and may decrease the development of resistant organisms.

Amphotericin B is a polyene antibiotic derived from the fungus *Streptomyces nodosus*. It affects fungal cell wall permeability. It is a toxic medication that must be given intravenously for at least 4 to 6 weeks for treatment of systemic candidiasis. Frequently a much longer course of therapy is required. The side effects are frequent, severe, and varied. An initial test dose of 1 mg in 20 mL 5% aqueous dextrose solution over 10 to 20 minutes with follow-up of temperature and blood pressure over 30 minutes for 4 hours is recommended. Afterward, an initial dose of 0.25 mg/kg is given intravenously over 2 to 4 hours. The dose is advanced to 0.5 mg/kg daily by the fifth day. Convulsions, anaphylaxis, hypotension, ventricular fibrillation, or cardiac arrest can be seen with rapid administrations. Other side effects include phlebitis, fever, nausea, vomiting, abdominal pain, nephrotoxicity, anemia, and electrolyte imbalance. Some of these side effects may be partially controlled by premedication with sedatives and antihistamines. If renal insufficiency develops, therapy should be temporarily discontinued.

Multiple agents, parenteral therapy, and surgical drainage or irrigation procedures are often necessary in renal infections. An example would be combined therapy of oral 5-flurocytosine with amphotericin B irrigations and parenteral amphotericin B to treat candidal pyelonephritis. If ureteral obstruction occurs, urinary diversion is required. For patients with large fungal coagulums, primary removal of the coagulum by either operative or endoscopic techniques may be required in addition to the antifungal therapy.

Oral ketoconazole is well tolerated and has little toxicity even after prolonged administration. However, experience with its use in urinary fungal infection is limited. An overall response rate of 50% to 60% has been reported, but it sometimes requires extended periods of therapy of more than 2 years.

Note: Since the submission of this manuscript, a newer class of triazole antifungal agents, fluconazole, has been released by the FDA for the treatment of systemic candidal infections, including urinary tract infections. This agent represents a major advance in the management of candidal urinary tract infections because of low incidence of toxicity and excellent in vitro activity against *Candida* species. It can be administered either orally or intravenously. The recommended dose for systemic candidiasis is a loading dose of 400 mg followed by a daily dose of 200 mg as a single dose each day for one month. Two weeks of therapy are recommended for uncomplicated bladder infections.

SUMMARY

Irritative voiding symptoms, pyuria, flank pain, fever, and elevated WBC count suggests candidal upper UTI. Antifungal therapy is required for these invasive infections. Multiple agents, parenteral therapy, and surgical drainage procedures are often necessary with candidal renal infections. Therapy should be continued for 4 weeks or longer until cultures are rendered negative.

REFERENCE

1. Wise GJ, Kozinn PJ, Goldberg P: Amphotericin B as a urologic irrigant in the management of noninvasive candiduria. *J Urol* 1982; 128:82–84.

ADDITIONAL READINGS

Frye KR, Donovan JM, Drach GW: *Torulopsis glabrata* urinary infections: A review. *J Urol* 1988; 139:1245–1249.

Graybill JR, Galgiani JN, Jorgensen JH, et al: Ketoconazole therapy for fungal urinary tract infections. *J Urol* 1983; 129:68–70.
Kozinn PJ, Taschdjian CL, Goldberg PK, et al: Advances in the diagnosis of renal candidiasis. *J Urol* 1978; 119:184–187.
Michigan S: Genitourinary fungal infections. *J Urol* 1976; 116:390–397.
Sanford JP: *Guide to Antimicrobial Therapy 1989*. West Bethesda, Md, Antimicrobial Therapy, 1989, pp 65–69.
Suits T, Wise GJ, Walters B: Candidal antigenemia: A prognostic determinant. *J Urol* 1989; 141:1381–1384.
Wise GJ, Goldberg P, Kozinn PJ: Genitourinary candidiasis: Diagnosis and treatment. *J Urol* 1976; 116:778–780.
Wise GJ, Kozinn PJ, Goldberg P: Flurocytosine in the management of genitourinary candidiasis: 5 years of experience. *J Urol* 1980; 124:70–72.

12

Genitourinary Tuberculosis

George W. Drach, M.D.

A 67-year-old man recovered from a transurethral prostatectomy performed 3 months ago in another community, but he continues to have pyuria that does not respond to standard antibiotics. A urinary culture is performed and is reported as "no growth." Urinalysis on several occasions continues to show 30 to 40 white blood cells/high-power field (HPF) and more than 50 red blood cells/HPF. While you are evaluating the patient, he complains of decreasing urinary stream, and on cystoscopic examination you find a stricture within the inflamed prostatic urethra. Biopsy of this tissue is interpreted as "acute and chronic inflammation with fibrosis." Physical examination is unremarkable except for a boggy, tender prostate, and the right vas is thickened. Intravenous (IV) pyelography reveals only slight calyectasis of the upper pole of the left kidney.

BACKGROUND

Genitourinary (GU) tuberculosis remains prevalent throughout the world, especially in the developing countries and in those areas where acquired immunodeficiency syndrome infection occurs in high numbers. Although the incidence of pulmonary tuberculosis has declined steadily since the discovery of treatment agents in the 1940s, the incidence of extrapulmonary (and GU) tuberculosis remains relatively high. In Australia, extrapulmonary tuberculosis accounted for 8.5% of patients in 1962. By 1984, it accounted for 24.3% of all newly reported cases. Higher incidence groups in North America include migrant workers, Asian immigrants, native Americans, health care workers, and individuals with significant underlying illness or those receiving immunotherapy. It appears in about 5% to 10% of those who have pulmonary tuberculosis, but it is seldom found to exist concomitantly with pulmonary tuberculosis. Most often the bacillemia that follows pulmonary infection seeds the kidney. The pulmonary infection clears spontaneously, and the renal infection appears years later.

Infections of the ureters, bladder, prostate, and vasa occur most often as a result of downstream seeding of tubercle bacilli from the kidney to these organs. On the other hand, direct hematogenous seeding (especially of the prostate) is also possible.

This patient has symptoms and signs that force evaluation for GU tuberculosis. He has persistent, irritative voiding symptoms and sterile pyuria. Radiography reveals minor calyectasis of an upper pole of the kidney, which is classic for granulomatous disease. The stricture of the prostatic urethra and the thickening of the vas produce a total of four objective findings that should make the physician very suspicious of GU tuberculosis. What do we do next?

IMAGING

A chest film is not mentioned in this presentation, but I am sure a chest film would be performed. Some patients with GU tuberculosis will show evidence of past or present pulmonary involvement, but a normal chest film does not exclude GU tuberculosis.

I do not think that further urinary imaging would be useful. The IV pyelogram can define most of the characteristic findings of renal tuberculosis: localized "moth-eaten" calyces, stenosis of the calyceal infundibulum, deposition of spotty calcium in the areas of involvement, and areas of loss of renal anatomy (the so-called autonephrectomy). Ureteral stricture occurs commonly at presentation or during treatment. Additional physical findings may include renal tenderness, prostatic or vasal nodularity, or cutaneous fistulas from kidney, prostate, or vasa.

LABORATORY

I continue to perform tuberculin skin tests on all patients suspected of GU tuberculosis. Normal test results do not eliminate the possibility of active disease, because anergy may exist. Abnormal skin test results certainly indicate exposure to tuberculosis and increase the likelihood of urinary involvement.

Culture of tuberculosis bacilli from urine can be difficult. Most authorities recommend culturing a minimum of three first-voided morning specimens. Some laboratories also perform centrifugation of these specimens. They then culture the sediment and stain it for mycobacteria by fluorescent or other techniques. About 80% to 90% of those proved to have GU tuberculosis will grow the organisms on culture. The others have their disease proved by specific staining of biopsy material or purulent drainage. Although classically the patient has "sterile pyuria," tuberculosis may coexist with routine gram-negative urinary tract infections.

TREATMENT

Let us assume that this patient grows tubercle bacillus from one or more urinary specimens. How do we treat him? Whatever drugs we use, it must be a "multiple drug treatment regimen." Single-drug treatment of tuberculosis does not succeed. Eighty percent of these patients relapse after treatment, whereas less than 10% relapse after a triple-drug treatment regimen. Table 12–1 lists the drugs available for treatment now.

Rifampin and isoniazid (INH) now form the basis for most treatment regimens. In the past, these were combined with ethambutol or pyrazinamide as a triple-drug treatment for at least 2 years. The most common GU treatment program presently used includes rifampin, 600 mg; isoniazid, 300 mg; and etham-

TABLE 12–1.
Agents Used in the Treatment of Tuberculosis

Drug	Usual Dose	Route
Isoniazid	300 mg/day	PO
Ethambutol	25 mg/kg/day	PO
	15 mg/kg/day	PO
Rifampin	600 mg/day	PO
Pyrazinamide	1,000 mg/day	PO
Ethionamide	750–1,000 mg/day	PO
Cycloserine	750–1,000 mg/day	PO
P-aminosalicyclic acid	10–12 g/day	PO
Streptomycin	750–1,000 mg/day	IM

butol, 15 mg/kg, daily for 2 months. The ethambutol is then discontinued and the rifampin and isoniazid continued twice or thrice weekly for an additional 7 months. Pyridoxine (vitamin B_6), 10 to 25 mg/day, is also administered to avoid the occasional peripheral neuropathy related to INH. Therapy therefore covers 9 months. Some experts now propose shorter courses of treatment: 6 or even 4 months. These short courses require more confirmation before they supplant our recommended 9-month treatment program.

Primary surgical treatment of GU tuberculosis was once used extensively. Now one treats with the previously listed medical regimen and expects cure in the majority of cases. Surgery is reserved for those patients who require intervention for intractable pain, persistent abscess or infection, life-threatening hematuria, or persistent fistula. More often, patients require surgical repair of the complications of healing of the tuberculosis: ureteral or (as in our patient) urethral stricture, contracted bladder, or obstructed vasa. Hypertension, probably secondary to renal involvement, occurs in nearly 10% of patients, but nephrectomy is advisable only if the hypertension is proved to be related to elevated renin from the affected kidney.

POSTTREATMENT OBSERVATION

As noted previously, some of the most difficult complications of GU tuberculosis occur after treatment is initiated. Most important, about 10% of patients may not respond to the treatment regimen. To discover failure, they must have continued testing of urinary specimens for tubercle bacillus. Most authorities recommend urinary cultures every 3 to 4 months for at least 2 years.

Complications of therapy related to scar formation can occur very quickly. Imaging of the urinary tract should be done about 2 to 3 weeks after beginning therapy and 3 weeks later. If these reveal significant healing by stenosis of the infundibula or ureter, one can administer 5 mg of prednisone four times daily along with the anti-tuberculosis therapy. Improvement in stenosis can be expected in about 70% of patients. Those who do not improve on this treatment must undergo some type of surgical intervention. If healing is normal, additional imaging should occur at 6 months and yearly thereafter for 2 to 3 years.

CONCLUSION

Our patient did not grow tubercle bacillus from his urinary specimens. Because he had such classic symptoms and signs, he was placed on triple-drug therapy, as mentioned earlier, for 9 months, and had complete resolution of his irritative voiding symptoms and perineal pain. He gained weight and resumed playing golf. In other words, he confirmed the diagnosis of GU tuberculosis by his response to specific anti-TB therapy. This need for treatment without proving mycobacteria occurs in about 5% of patients with GU tuberculosis.

In addition, he developed worsening prostatic urethral stricture disease. Urethral dilations were performed but lasted only 1 week, and he could not tolerate a self-dilation program. He failed to show up for several office visits, and on his return, he had urinary retention and an impassable stricture of the prostatic urethra. Suprapubic cystostomy was performed, and he has decided on this means of survival at this time.

BIBLIOGRAPHY

Cos LR, Cockett AT: Genitourinary tuberculosis revisited. *Urology* 1982; 20:112–117.

Dwyer DE, MacLeod C, Collignon PJ, et al: Extrapulmonary tuberculosis—a continuing problem in Australia. *Aust NZ J Med* 1987; 17:507–511.

Gow JG, Barbosa S: Genitourinary tuberculosis. A study of 1117 cases over a period of 34 years. *Br J Urol* 1984; 56:449–455.

Webster A, Wright DJ: Ziehl-Neelsen staining of urine deposits in the diagnosis of genitourinary tuberculosis [letter]. *J Clin Pathol* 1985; 38:236.

13

Prostatitis

George W. Drach, M.D.

After he has his third episode of urinary tract infection (UTI) in 2 years, this 58-year-old patient requests that you "get to the bottom of [his] problem." Each urinary culture has grown *Enterococcus*. Urinary maximum flow rate varies from 22 mL/second while healthy to 14 mL/second during bouts of infection. He has diabetes and also has mild aortic valvular stenosis. Divided urinary specimens for culture while the patient is receiving no therapy are as follows: initial voided (VB_1), or urethral, specimen, 100 colonies of *Enterococcus*/mL; VB_2, or bladder, specimen (midstream), 0 colonies of bacteria/mL; expressed prostatic secretions (EPS), 1,500 colonies of *Enterococcus*/mL; and postprostatic massage (VB_3) specimen, 1,000 colonies of *Enterococcus*/mL. He has no known drug allergies.

Some points in this patient's story favor prostatitis as the cause of his recurrent UTIs: multiple infections with the same germ, decreases in urinary flow rate during infectious episodes, and localization of his infection to the prostate in divided culture studies.

But let us take this patient's problem step by step. Any man with relapsing UTIs must be evaluated for prostatitis. First, examination of the external genitalia and prostate are required. Is the penis normal? Is the meatus adequate? Meatal stenosis can contribute to persistent prostatitis, as can urethral stricture. Has the patient any history of or evidence of epididymitis? Again, this can be a complication of chronic prostatitis.

On examination the prostate of a patient with chronic prostatitis may be relatively pain free and may feel normal. I seldom can make the diagnosis by examination alone. Examination of the expressed prostatic fluid is the most important part of confirming the diagnosis. Before the prostatic massage, the patient collects a VB_1 specimen (about 10 mL) after cleansing the meatus. A VB_2 specimen follows immediately. These are placed in the office laboratory, and urinalysis is performed on the VB_2 specimen. This patient's urinalysis was normal except for a trace of urine glucose.

After performing the prostatic examination, one massages the prostate from lateral to medial on the right lobe and on the left. Finally, one strips centrally from superior to inferior to start the journey of the fluid down the urethra. Only two to three drops result, so these must be harvested carefully into a wide-mouthed collection jar that is not contaminated by the penis, hair, and so forth. I find that having the patient cough may improve transport of prostatic fluid along the urethra.

One of the precious drops is placed under a coverslip on a clean glass slide. Individuals with fewer than 10 white blood cells (WBCs)/high-power field (HPF) most likely do not have prostatitis. Those with more than 20 WBCs/HPF have some prostatic inflammation and, therefore, prostatitis. Those with between 10 and 20 WBCs/HPF may or may not be afflicted. This patient had more than 30 WBCs/HPF and, as we are told, bacteria in the prostatic fluid. The 2 or more drops of EPS are sent to the laboratory along with the VB_1 and VB_2 specimens for differential quantitative culture. If you cannot get any EPS, collect the first 10 mL of urine voided after the prostatic massage (VB_3) and submit it as the postmassage urine specimen.

How does one interpret the bacterial counts in the divided urinary specimens? Bacterial prostatitis is diagnosed when the number of bacteria in the expressed prostatic fluid or VB_3 specimen exceed those of the VB_1 and VB_2 specimens by a factor of at least 10 (1 log). This patient's values for expressed prostatic secretions are 15 times greater than the VB_1 specimen. The VB_3 specimen exceeds the VB_1 specimen by a factor of 10. The VB_2 specimen is sterile. Hence, the criteria for diagnosis of bacterial prostatitis are met.

When bacteria are recovered from prostatic fluid, one should ask the laboratory to perform drug sensitivity studies. Drugs that may be optimal for treating the infecting bacterium may not be useful in patients with prostatitis. Many standard antibiotics such as ampicillin or tetracycline do not have the characteristics needed to cross the blood-prostate barrier. Only those listed in Table 13–1 have demonstrated usefulness in therapy of prostatitis. These need to be compared with the sensitivity results to decide on the most efficacious drug.

This patient has another risk factor that must be considered along with prostatitis: cardiac valvular disease. Subacute bacterial endocarditis caused by bacteria identical to those found in prostatitis is not unusual, so there is a strong reason to treat this patient carefully and definitively. Physical examination and echocardiography were performed and did not indicate any valvular involvement in this patient, however. Several blood cultures were unremarkable.

Duration of therapy for prostatitis exceeds that for UTIs. Minimum duration of treatment for this patient would be 6 weeks. He should be reexamined on a routine basis about 1 month after cessation of therapy, and if his infection recurs, he should be treated for another 6 weeks. A third course of treatment may be necessary. Finally, if one cannot rid the prostate of the infection, it may be advisable to place the patient on suppressive antibiotic therapy so that he can avoid repeated UTIs.

This discussion does not include those patients who have nonbacterial prostatitis. They have purulent prostatic fluid but sterile cultures. Nor are patients with prostatodynia reviewed, because they have only neuromuscular discomfort of the prostate and perineum and no evidence of prostatic infection. More information on such afflictions can be found in the references.

BIBLIOGRAPHY

Clements R, Griffiths GJ, Peeling WB, et al: Transrectal ultrasound in monitoring response to treatment of prostatic diseases. *Urol Clin North Am* 1989; 16(4):735–740.

TABLE 13–1.
Oral Antimicrobial Agents Used to Treat Prostatitis

Carbenicillin indanyl sodium
Chloramphenicol
Erythromycin
Fluoroquinolones
Ciprofloxacin
Norfloxacin
Long-acting tetracyclines
Doxycycline
Minocycline
Trimethoprim (often with sulfamethoxazole)

Drach GW: Prostatitis, man's hidden infection. *Urol Clin North Am* 1975; 2:499–520.
Krieger JN, McGonagle LA: Diagnostic considerations and interpretation of microbiological findings for evaluation of chronic prostatitis. *J Clin Microbiol* 1989; 27:2240–2244.
Meares EM Jr, Stamey TA: Bacteriologic localization patterns in bacterial prostatitis and urethritis. *Invest Urol* 1968;5:492–518.
Shortliffe LMD, Wehner N, Stamey TA: Use of solid-phase radioimmunoassay and formalin-fixed whole bacterial antigen in the detection of antigen-specific immunoglobulin in prostatic fluid. *J Clin Invest* 1981; 67:790–799.

14

Immune Aspects of Prostatitis

Linda M. Dairiki Shortliffe, M.D.

You examine a 36-year-old man with recurrent dysuria, frequency, and urgency in the absence of detectable urinary tract infection (UTI). He states that he has been told that he has prostatitis. Prostatic fluid obtained from massage has 30 white blood cells (WBCs)/high-power field (HPF). The only organism recovered from cultures of divided urinary and prostatic specimens is *Escherichia coli,* with 1,200 colonies found only in the expressed prostatic secretions. All of the serum titers of IgA, IgG, and IgM to the organism are low. The patient is concerned because his internist believes that he will never get rid of the prostatitis because of a "lack of antibody response."

It is clear that prostatitis is not a single disease. Prostatic inflammation characterized by elevated numbers of leukocytes in the prostatic fluid (>10 WBCs HPF) may be found in both bacterial and nonbacterial prostatitis. In bacterial prostatitis lower urinary tract bacterial localization cultures (divided urinary and prostatic specimens: the initial voided 5–10 mL [VB_1], the midstream urine [VB_2], the expressed prostatic fluid, and the first 5 to 10 mL voided after prostatic massage [VB_3]) show bacteria in the prostatic fluid and VB_3 specimen, whereas in nonbacterial prostatitis no such localization appears to be present. Often, however, determining which men have bacterial prostatitis may be difficult or impossible, because cultures of the prostatic fluid may be inadequate or uninterpretable resulting from previous antimicrobial treatment, bacteriuria, or poor specimen collections. In some instances of suspected bacterial prostatitis, prostatic fluid may be unobtainable because surgery, such as transurethral or retropubic prostatectomy, prevents access to the fluid. It is in these situations that prostatic fluid antibodies may be helpful to diagnose or confirm the kind of prostatitis an individual has.

PROSTATIC IMMUNE RESPONSE

The production of immunoglobulins in the serum and at some mucosal surfaces, as the respiratory, gastrointestinal, and genitourinary surfaces, is one measure of the human immune response to invasion by foreign substances (or substances thought to be foreign). Measurement of antibody levels in the prostatic fluid has shown that the prostate is a secretory gland capable of producing a discrete response to bacterial infection that differs from the systemic response produced in the serum. Antibodies to various bacteria or groups of bacteria may be measured in serum or the prostatic fluid by simple radioimmunossays or enzyme-linked immunosorbant assays and have been measured in several research institutions. Although the exact immune response generated by the prostate may depend on the clinical course of the patient, men with bacterial prostatitis have higher levels of prostatic fluid IgA and IgG than men without UTIs or prostatic infections.

These men have specific elevation of prostatic antibodies against infecting Enterobacteriaceae for 12 to 18 months after curative treatment, and these elevated levels persist indefinitely after ineffective treatment. Even if bacteriuria is suppressed by daily antimicrobial therapy, prostatic antibody levels remain elevated; levels decrease toward normal only after cure. This response is, moreover, independent of the systemic immune response to the prostatic infection that can be measured in the serum.

In bacterial prostatitis, serum immunoglobulin levels may or may not be elevated over normal levels (Table 14–1). Levels of serum antibodies often

TABLE 14–1.

Factors Differentiating Prostatic Syndromes

	Microscopic Examination of Prostatic Fluid Per High Power Microscopic Field	Lower Urinary Tract Bacterial Localization	Prostatic Fluid IgA and IgG Antibodies to Bacteria	Serum IgA and IgG Antibodies to Bacteria
Normal uninfected males	$<$10 leukocytes	No localization	Not detected	Normal
Bacterial prostatitis	$>$10 leukocytes	Localizes to prostate	Elevated	Normal or elevated
Nonbacterial prostatitis	$>$10 leukocytes	No localization	Not detected	Normal

will rise acutely during early, acute infection of the prostate but will return to normal or baseline levels as the prostatitis becomes chronic. Serum antibodies representing systemic production frequently will bear no relation to expressed prostatic fluid antibodies generated by the local secretory immune system. Even though bacterial prostatitis may cause local prostatic fluid antibody levels to be elevated, the mere presence of antibodies directed against infecting bacteria does not appear to confer spontaneous remission of the bacterial infection or prevent future reinfection of the prostate with different organisms. Using prostatic antibodies, researchers have documented that men who might have been diagnosed to have a persistent *E. coli* prostatitis actually had been cured of infection and became reinfected with a different type of *E. coli*.

CLINICAL USE OF PROSTATIC ANTIBODIES

When men treated for a bacterial UTI get recurrent UTIs with the same organism, it usually is not difficult to diagnose a bacterial prostatitis. The prostatic fluid shows a leukocytosis, and lower urinary tract bacterial localization cultures may show bacteria localizing to the prostatic specimen. In these men with bacterial prostatitis, prostatic fluid IgA and IgG levels are generally elevated and levels of specific antibodies directed against the infecting bacteria are elevated and remain elevated for 12 to 18 months. If urinary localization cultures are unobtainable or confusing or antimicrobial therapy has already been started, making recovery of an infecting organism by culture unlikely, elevated levels of prostatic fluid antibodies against common gram-negative organisms will persist if there is bacterial prostatic infection.

Diagnosing bacterial prostatitis in men in whom a prostatic fluid specimen is inadequate or unobtainable is more of a challenge. In these men recurrent UTIs with the same organism may suggest a bacterial prostatitis, but the lower urinary tract localization cultures may not verify this. In these men measuring IgG and IgA antibodies against common gram-negative organisms in the VB_2 and VB_3 specimens may confirm a bacterial prostatitis. The VB_3 specimen contains prostatic fluid from the massage, and therefore the urinary IgG and IgA levels when screened against mixtures of common gram-negative organisms are elevated in bacterial prostatitis.

When a man has had no documented bacterial UTIs or only a few bacterial organisms cultured, the diagnosis of bacterial prostatitis may be suspect. In these men the symptoms may be caused by nonbacterial prostatitis. That is, these patients may have symptoms indistinguishable from those of patients with chronic bacterial prostatitis but lack any episodes of documented bacterial cystitis.

Because these men have often been treated with multiple antimicrobial agents indiscriminately, they may not know whether bacterial organisms were found at the time of their initial complaints or may incorrectly believe they had a UTI. The prostatic fluid shows prostatic inflammation (>10 WBCs/HPF), and lower urinary tract localization cultures reveal no gram-negative organisms that localize to the prostate. In these men prostatic fluid antibodies may be helpful to distinguish between bacterial and nonbacterial prostatic infection. If no prostatic fluid antibodies to gram-negative organisms are detected, bacterial prostatitis is not present.

THE CASE

In the patient described there is no documented history of UTIs, but a lower urinary tract bacterial localization with 1,200 colony-forming units of *E coli* cultured from the prostatic fluid appears to show an *E. coli* localizing to the prostate. Levels of *local prostatic fluid* antibodies to Enterobacteriaceae will be elevated if there is an active bacterial prostatitis and the *E. coli* is not a urethral contaminant. The fact that the level; of *serum antibodies* to the infecting organism are not elevated does not affect the diagnosis of bacterial prostatitis because the local immunoglobulins are stimulated in bacterial prostatitis. This is reflected by elevated levels of antibodies to the infecting organism measured in the prostatic fluid. If antibodies to the gram-negative organisms are detected, the diagnosis of chronic bacterial prostatitis is confirmed and the man should be treated for 8 to 12 weeks with an antimicrobial agent to which the organism is sensitive and preferably an agent that enters the prostate.

BIBLIOGRAPHY

Shortliffe LMD, Elliott K, Sellers RG: Measurement of urinary antibodies to crude bacterial antigen in patients with chronic bacterial prostatitis. *J Urol* 1989; 141:632–636.

Shortliffe LMD, Wehner N: The characterization of bacterial and nonbacterial prostatitis by prostatic immunoglobulins. *Medicine* 1986; 65:399–414.

15

Nonbacterial Prostatitis

Edwin M. Meares, Jr., M.D.

A 36-year-old man consults you because he has complaints of mild dysuria, perineal aching, and some degree of urinary urgency. He has seen three urologists previously. None of them has been able to culture any bacteria from the prostatic fluid, yet he has been told that his prostatic fluid contains "pus." Within the past 2 years he has decreased his sexual activity on the advice of physicians, but this has not helped. He has taken tetracycline, nitrofurantoin, sulfamethoxazole-trimethoprim, and ampicillin for up to 2 weeks without any improvement. You receive reports that the intravenous pyelogram, cystoscopy, and voiding cystourethrogram are interpreted as normal. He is not taking any medications now, and he denies allergies. Your examination indicates normal abdomen and genitalia. Rectal examination is unremarkable except for a boggy, 25-g prostate. Microscopic examination of the expressed prostatic fluid shows 30 to 40 white blood cells/high-power field and numerous fat-containing cells. Cultures of urethral urine, midstream urine, and prostatic secretions show "no growth."

Whereas prostatitis syndromes are exceedingly common, little is known about the true incidence of prostatitis. Lipsky[1] recently reviewed the topic of urinary tract infections (UTIs) in men and cited a National Health Center for Health Statistics study indicating that during 1977 and 1978 there were 76 office visits annually per 1,000 men for genitourinary tract problems. About 25% of these visits were for prostatitis (all types).

The most common types of currently recognized prostatitis syndromes include acute and chronic bacterial prostatitis (CBP), nonbacterial prostatitis (NBP), and prostatodynia (PD). Bacterial prostatitis is a prostatic infection caused primarily by gram-negative enteric organisms but occasionally by gram-positive bacteria, especially enterococci. It is associated with positive prostatic fluid cultures, purulent prostatic secretions, and relapsing recurrent UTIs caused by persistence of the pathogen within the prostate. The patient with NBP has symptoms of prostatitis and excessive inflammatory cells in the prostatic fluid but typically has negative prostatic fluid cultures and no history of recurrent UTI. Patients with PD characteristically have variable irritative and obstructive voiding dysfunction, but mainly complaints of pain and discomfort perceived variably throughout the distribution of a male swimming trunk—a pelvic pain syndrome. These patients not only have negative cultures and histories of UTI but also typically have normal prostatic expressate.

In evaluating the patient with prostatitis, the clinician must realize that most cases of prostatitis are not caused by a bacterial infection. Indeed, Brunner et al.[2] evaluated 597 men attending a special prostatitis clinic in Germany and found that 5% had bacterial prostatitis, 64% had NBP, and 31% had PD.

CLINICAL MANIFESTATIONS

This case history presents a typical clinical picture of NBP. The genitourinary tract symptoms suggest a prostatitis syndrome, and the prostatic expressate shows excessive numbers of leukocytes and fat-laden cells. Most important, however, are repeated cultures that fail to localize a bacterial pathogen to the prostate and a negative history of associated UTIs. It is therefore not surprising that he has responded poorly to therapy using various antimicrobial agents. This man has NBP, not CBP. Antimicrobial agents thus should not be used to treat his condition.

PATHOGENESIS

Infectious Agents

Controversy continues about the possible role of gram-positive organisms as causative agents in proastatitis. It is established that strains of *Enterococcus faecalis* and *Staphylococcus aureus* do occasionally cause bacterial prostatitis and relapsing recurrent associated UTI. The controversy relates to other gram-positive organisms, which sometimes are localized by culture to the prostatic expressate. Patients with these organisms do not have associated UTI, seldom have the same organisms on repeat localization cultures, show no immune response to these organisms in their prostatic fluid, and generally respond poorly to antimicrobial therapy.[3] It therefore appears that gram-positive bacteria other than *E. faecalis* and *S. aureus* are not important causative agents in prostatitis.

Many clinicians believe that most cases of apparent NBP actually are prostatic infections caused by *Chlamydia trachomatis* or *Ureaplasma urealyticum*. Because most cases of nongonococcal urethritis are caused by these organisms, it is tempting to assume that they can readily infect the prostate. Furthermore, *C. trachomatis* is the most common cause of acute epididymitis in heterosexually active men younger than 35 years. However, prostatic fluid cultures do not grow *C. trachomatis,* and no immune response to this organism can be demonstrated in the prostatic fluid of most men who have NBP. The findings are the same for ureaplasmas. Current scientific evidence therefore negates these organisms as important causes of prostatitis.

Intraprostatic Urinary Reflux

Urinary reflux into prostatic ducts and the ejaculatory duct system may be a key factor in the pathogenesis of all prostatitis syndromes. Prostatic stones, exceedingly common in middle aged and older men, often are composed of substances found in urine but not in prostatic secretions. Intraprostatic urinary reflux is therefore implicated in the formation of these calculi. In 1982, Kirby et al.[4] proved intraprostatic urinary reflux clinically by instilling a carbon-particle solution into the bladders of ten men immediately before transurethral prostatectomy (each man then voided before surgery) and of five men who had carefully documented NBP. Seven of the 10 men who underwent surgery had carbon particles within the prostatic ducts and acini of their resected tissue. Likewise, all five men with nonbacterial prostatitis had numerous macrophages studded with intracellular carbon particles in their prostatic expressates 72 hours later. At times, intraprostatic urinary reflux is so severe that it can be demonstrated by voiding cystourethrography.

It is thought that intraprostatic urinary reflux occurs intermittently, but commonly, and serves as an important mechanism for bacteria to gain access to the prostate. Furthermore, the reflux of sterile urine, resulting in a "chemical" prostatitis, may be the cause of nonbacterial forms of prostatitis. In addition, because urine normally contains substances that are known to be inmunogenic (e.g., Tamm-Horsfall protein), the question of an autoimmune etiology of NBP seems plausible.

URODYNAMIC STUDIES

Clinical and videourodynamic studies of my patients with NBP, especially those with prostatodynia, demonstrate that most have "spastic" dysfunction of the bladder neck and prostatic urethra—the internal urinary sphincter. Principal findings include a depressed urinary flow rate, incomplete opening or relaxation of the bladder neck and prostatic urethra to a point just proximal to the external urinary sphincter, and abnormally high maximum urethral closure pressure at rest. Typically, the external urinary sphincter relaxes normally during voiding, and uninhibited bladder contractions are unusual. Because these patients are otherwise normal neurologically, an acquired form of bladder–internal sphincter dyssynergia—a bladder neck–urethral spasm syndrome—appears responsible for the clinical syndrome. My postulate concerning the basis for symptoms in these patients is that smooth muscle spasm of the bladder neck and prostatic urethra causes elevated pressure in the prostatic urethra, leading to intraprostatic and ejaculatory duct urinary reflux and an associated chemical prostatitis, seminal vesiculitis, and even epididymitis. Some patients may even develop a form of autoimmune reaction to urinary constituents.

TREATMENT

Because the cause of NBP is uncertain, a cure is seldom achieved; indeed, therapy consists mainly of measures to relieve or control symptoms. If one suspects that ureaplasmas or *C. trachomatis* may be responsible for the prostatitis, a clinical trial using minocycline, doxycycline, or erythromycin in full dosage for 2 to 4 weeks is a reasonable approach. Unless the response is definitely favorable, however, the additional use of antimicrobial agents is unwarranted.

Once the diagnosis of NBP is established, my practice is to have a frank discussion with the patient about his condition. I emphasize that he has no infectious or contagious disease that will lead to cancer or other serious complications. I compare NBP to other noninfectious conditions, such as bursitis or arthritis—inflammatory processes that cause chronic or intermittent symptoms of variable intensity but that are not caused by infection. Normal sexual activity and exercise are encouraged, and no dietary changes are recommended unless the patient notices that alcoholic beverages or certain foods definitely provoke symptoms. Hot sitz baths afford temporary relief and are encouraged. I recommend periodic prostatic massage only in men who have "congested" prostates associated with infrequent sexual activity.

Several different types of medication are often effective in achieving symptomatic relief. Irritative voiding dysfunction may respond to the use of anticholinergic agents (e.g., 5 mg of oxybutynin chloride taken orally three times daily). Pain and discomfort usually improve when antiinflammatory drugs are prescribed (e.g., 600 mg of ibuprofen taken orally four times daily). Oral zinc preparations and megavitamins have no proved efficacy in the treatment of prostatitis. Prostatectomy or other surgical procedures, such as prostatotomy, are seldom indicated in management.

Regardless of the microscopic appearance of the prostatic expressate, most of my patients with NBP, similar to patients with PD, appear to have a bladder neck–urethral spasm syndrome and respond best to treatment using an α-adrenergic-blocking agent. Because the bladder neck and prostate are rich in α-adrenergic receptors, whereas the detrusor has mainly β-adrenergic receptors, the α-blocking agents are thought to work selectively to reduce "functional" obstruction at the bladder neck and prostate level. Symptomatic improvement usually is attained in most patients, provided they take enough medication. Adverse side effects (e.g., postural hypotension, vertigo, palpitations, headaches, fatigue) occur in some patients at medication levels below that required to effectively treat the prostatitis syndrome. Because I initially prescribe the lowest possible dosage and increase it gradually, most of my patients tolerate the α-blockers well with minimal side effects. My preference is to prescribe 1 mg of prazosin taken orally daily at bedtime for 7 days, followed by 1 mg twice daily for 7 days, followed by 2 mg twice daily for 4 weeks. Most patients tolerate this dosage well and experience improvement in symptoms. The goal is to find a proper dosage that affords good relief and insignificant adverse side effects. Some patients cannot take 2 mg twice daily because of adverse side effects; some patients require even higher doses to gain relief (and remarkably suffer no adverse side effects). Those patients who achieve relief with parazosin invariably become symptomatic again soon after the medication is withdrawn. For this reason, most patients require indefinite therapy.

Some patients with NBP and PD have a significant component of tension myalgia of the pelvic floor muscles and respond best to therapy using prazosin plus 5 mg of diazepam taken orally three times daily. Stress is an important factor in nonbacterial prostatitis syndromes. Whether stress causes NBP and PD or is an effect is often difficult to sort out. Certainly those patients with prostatitis who have high levels of stress should be referred to an interested psychologist or psychiatrist for stress management.

REFERENCES

1. Lipsky BA: Urinary tract infections in men: Epidemiology, pathophysiology, diagnosis, and treatment. *Ann Intern Med* 1989; 110:138–150.

2. Brunner H, Weidner W, Schiefer HG: Studies on the role of *Ureaplasma urealyticum* and *Mycoplasma hominis* in prostatitis. *J Infect Dis* 1983; 147:807–813.
3. Meares EM Jr: Acute and chronic prostatitis: Diagnosis and treatment. *Infect Dis Clin North Am* 1987; 1:855–873.
4. Kirby RS, Lowe D, Bultitude MI, et al: Intra-prostatic urinary reflux: An aetiological factor in abacterial prostatitis. *Br J Urol* 1982; 54:729–731.

16

Acute Prostatitis and Prostatic Abscess

Michael K. Brawer, M.D.

Your emergency room calls you to evaluate a 54-year-old man who has urinary retention, temperature of 39.5°C, and a markedly tender prostate on examination. You place a no. 16 French Foley catheter, and your specimen for urinalysis shows numerous white blood cells per high-power field and probable gram-negative bacteria.

DIAGNOSTIC WORK-UP

This patient appears by history to have acute bacterial prostatisis. Other disease entities that might have similar signs and symptoms would include prostatic infarction, bladder outlet obstruction secondary to vesical calculus or benign prostatic hyperplasia with secondary bacterial cystitis, pyelonephritis with cystitis, and acute proctitis or perirectal abscess. These latter entities would be decidedly less common than acute prostatitis, given this clinical scenario.

When this patient is seen, the history should be carefully reviewed. General medical condition, particularly the patient's cardiovascular, pulmonary, and renal status, is important to ascertain so that an assessment can be made regarding his ability to cope with the prostatitis and probable sepsis. Any history suggestive of an immunocompromised status must be determined. Therefore, a history of diabetes mellitus, human immunodeficiency virus infection, or cancer should be ascertained.

Eliciting a history of past urologic problems is of great importance. Past genitourinary instrumentation, including previous prostatectomy or prostate needle biopsy, is important, as is a history of urolithiasis or urinary tract infection. Recent antibiotic exposure or hospitalization should be determined.

In addition to a general physical examination careful rectal examination should be repeated by the urologist. Care should be taken to avoid prostatic massage or vigorous examination in this setting. Attempt at lower urinary tract bacterial localization[1] is pointless because of the obvious infection of the urine (positive VB_2 results), as well as being contraindicated because of the risk of inducing sepsis. In the acute setting, the physician must perform only a prostatic examination to establish a baseline for subsequent follow-up examination and to rule out fluctuance suggestive of prostatic abcess. One must be alert to associated rectal pathologic conditions, such as perirectal abscess. Laboratory investigations should include careful examination of the spun urinary sediment and a complete blood cell count, electrolytc values, blood urea nitrogen value, creatinine, and serum glucose level. Before the initiation of antimicrobial therapy, paired blood cultures for both anaerobic and aerobic bacteria and specimens for urine culture must be obtained.

IMAGING

I believe that upper urinary tract imaging studies are important in this setting. Generally, I would recommend a flat-plate x-ray film of the abdomen (kidneys, ureters, and bladder) to determine possible radiopaque calculi and renal ultrasound to rule out hydroureteronephrosis. Alternatively, an intravenous (IV) urogram may be obtained.

The role for prostate imaging in this setting is controversial. Changes on the IV urogram are often nonspecific, and accurate imaging of the prostate requires either computed tomography (CT), magnetic resonance imaging (MRI), or transrectal prostate ultrasonography. We[2] have had excellent experience with CT in the evaluation of prostatic abscess, as initially suggested by Dennis and Donohue[3] (Fig 16–1). Undoubtedly, MRI can provide excellent imaging in this setting, although I have no personal experience.

Transrectal ultrasound is an ideal method for imaging the prostate of men with prostatitis. This modality is rapidly becoming the urologist's mainstay for evaluating the prostate in a variety of disease processes. The ultrasonographic appearance of chronic prostatitis has been well studied and has been recently reviewed by Doble and Carter.[4] These authors noted a variety of ultrasonographic patterns in men with documented clinical prostatitis, including varying gland echogenicity, echolucent zones, capsular irregularity and thickening, ejaculatory duct calcifications, and periurethral irregularity. They refuted the specificity of the so-called halo sign, first described by Griffiths et al.[5] This is a low-amplitude area surrounding a slightly more echogenic region within the peripheral zone.

Less information is available about the ultrasonographic appearance of acute prostatitis. In general, prostatic enlargement with increased anteroposterior diameter, giving a more rounded configuration of the gland, with a symmetric capsule is present. There may be areas of relative hypoechogenicity, pri-

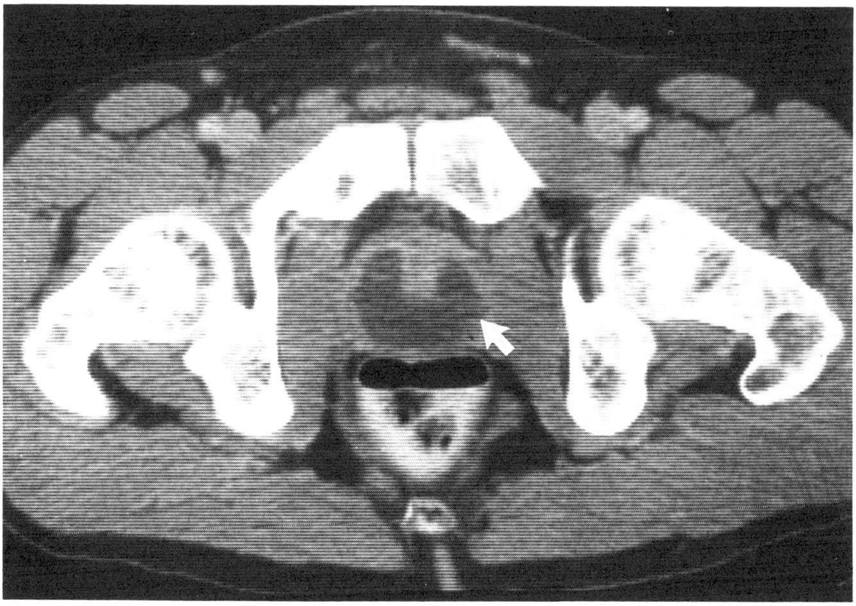

FIG 16–1.
Computed tomography of large prostatic abscess *(arrow)*.

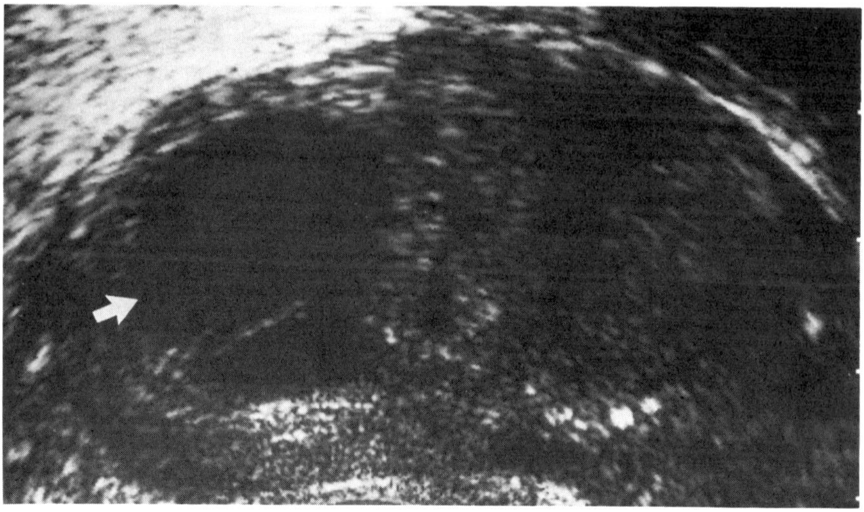

FIG 16–2.
Transrectal ultrasound of a patient with a prostatic abscess. Note large echopenic region in right side of prostate *(arrow)*.

marily in the peripheral zone. These changes may resolve after effective treatment.[5–7]

The ultrasonographic appearance of prostatic abscess is similar to that noted in abscess formation in other organs, namely, relative hypoechogenicity with increased through transmission of the sound waves, irregular internal echoes, and indistinct borders within the surrounding parenchyma.

Prostate ultrasonography can be used in combination with transperineal aspiration of suspected prostatic abscesses to confirm its presence, as well as to obtain specimens for bacteriologic culture. Transrectal aspiration is ineffective because normal rectal flora represent the usual pathogens for prostatic abscess and would result in an uninterpretable culture spectrum.

I have had excellent results with transrectal ultrasound in the evaluation of acute prostatitis and prostatic abscess (Fig 16–2). The rather significant prostatic manipulation that may occur with transrectal ultrasonography suggests that before the performance of this examination, the patient should be covered with appropriate antimicrobial agents.

TREATMENT

The treatment of acute bacterial prostatitis is fairly straightforward. I recommend hospitalization for virtually all patients. Stamey[8] and others have reported that the acutely inflamed prostate allows penetration of most common antimicrobial agents, including oral drugs, into the prostate. However, patient toxicity and the risk of sepsis and shock mandate hospitalization.

Initiation of antimicrobial therapy should commence immediately after blood and urine specimens are obtained for culture. I generally begin with an aminoglycoside and a β-lactam agent, usually ampicillin. Alternatively, one of the newer quinolones might be selected. These are currently available in parenteral form. An alternative approach would be the IV administration of trimethoprin-sulfamethoxazole. These agents are administered until there is resolution of the patient's toxic status. Following this, I recommend long-term antimicrobial therapy. Agents with proved prostatic bactericidal efficacy (usually either trimethoprin-sulfamethoxazole or carbenicillin) should be employed. The oral forms of quinolone with their broad-spectrum, low rate of resistance development and relatively high tissue bioavailability may have excellent utility in this setting.[9]

The optimum treatment of acute prostatitis includes urinary diversion. I believe that a urethral catheter is contraindicated because of the patient discomfort and, more important, because of the potential problem of a foreign body further compromising prostatic duct drainage. Rather, I perform a punch suprapubic cystostomy in these patients. General supportive care includes the IV administration of fluids, bed rest, analgesics, and local therapy, such as sitz baths and stool softeners.

The duration of antimicrobial therapy is controversial. The management of chronic bacterial prostatitis is discussed in Chapter 13. Generally, I administer 30 days of appropriate oral antimicrobial therapy, and 1 week after cessation of therapy, I perform lower urinary tract localization studies as described by Meares and Stamey.[1] Persistent infection is treated for an additional 6 weeks, followed again by bacterial localization testing. Fowler[10] has described a case where poor patient compliance resulted in failure to sterilize the prostate, with resulting acute epididymo-orchitis and subsequent orchidectomy.

CASE REPORT STATUS UPDATE

One week after parenteral institution of ampicillin and gentamicin, to which the *Escherichia coli* isolated from his urine and blood was sensitive, this patient continues to have spiking fever and leucocytosis.

Potential complications of acute bacterial prostatitis include septicemia and resulting shock, as well as pyelonephritis, epididymo-orchitis, and the development of chronic bacterial prostatitis. In addition, prostatic abscess formation may occur.

Prostatic abscess is decreasing in incidence largely because of declining gonococcal urethritis and associated stricture disease. Fairly recent reviews have recorded a prostatic abscess incidence of between 0.5% and 2.5% of all patients admitted to hospital for prostatic disease.[11, 12] Despite the low incidence, the mortality remains high—21% to 88%.[12, 13] The most important factor in the diagnosis of prostatic abscess is awareness of its potential. Harbingers include fluctuance noted on rectal examination, a prolonged course after institution of appropriated antibiotics for the treatment of acute prostatitis, or isolation of unusual pathogens.

We[2] recently reported a case of prostatic abscess caused by anaerobic bacteria. This man had a 10-year history of irritable voiding symptoms. An anaerobic process was considered following an episode of anaerobic septicemia after cystoscopic examination. Computed tomography scan confirmed the diagnosis of prostatic abscess (see Fig 16–1), which was treated with transurethral resection and prolonged antimicrobial therapy. Bacterial localization, as well as perineal aspiration of the abscess, confirmed the anaerobic etiology. The imaging modalities noted earlier can be useful in diagnosing a prostatic abscess. However, despite no abscess being present on the initial evaluation, if the clinical course is prolonged, I recommend repeat transrectal ultrasound to rule out abscess formation.

The treatment of prostatic abscess includes all of the measures described earlier in the management of acute bacterial prostatitis and appropriate drainage. Traditionally, transurethral resection, first described by Timberlake,[14] has been employed. Alternatively, drainage can be achieved by transperineal or transrectal incision. Percutaneous perineal drainage under ultrasound guidance would seem to be a possible technique, but I personally have no experience and am unaware of any such reports. Before institution of the drainage procedure, the patient should receive appropriate antibiotics.

Whatever drainage technique is used, I recommend evaluation of the adequacy of the procedure by transrectal ultrasound to obviate presence of persistent fluid collections. Otherwise, the follow-up of patients with prostatic abscess is the same as that described for acute bacteria prostatitis.

SUMMARY

I believe that acute bacterial prostatitis represents a potential urologic emergency. Patients require hospitalization and appropriate supportive measures in addition to institution of broad-spectrum antimicrobial therapy. Evaluation of potential prostatic abscess should include prostate imaging and drainage as indicated. Transrectal ultrasound provides an excellent method of evaluating these patients. Long-term careful bacteriologic follow-up is necessary to avoid the sequel of persistent infections.

Acknowledgment

Supported in part by a Veterans Administration Merit Review Award.

REFERENCES

1. Meares EM, Stamey TA: Bacteriologic localization patterns in bacterial prostatitis and urethritis. *Invest Urol* 1968; 5:492–518.
2. Brawer MK, Stamey TA: Prostatic abscess owing to anaerobic bacteria. *J Urol* 1987; 138:1254–1255.
3. Dennis MA, Donohue RE: Computed tomography of prostatic abscess. *J Comp Assist Tomogr* 1985; 9:201–203.
4. Doble A, Carter S: Ultrasonographic finding in prostatitis. *Urol Clin North Am* 1989; 16:763–772.
5. Griffiths CJ, Crooks AJR, Roberts EE, et al: Ultrasonic appearances associated with prostatic inflammation: A preliminary study. *Clin Radiol* 1984; 35:343–345.
6. Peeling WB, Griffiths GJ: Imaging of the prostate by ultrasound. *J Urol* 1984; 132:217–224.
7. Spirnack JP, Resnick MI: Transrectal ultrasonography. *Urology* 1984; 23:461–467.
8. Stamey TA: *Pathogenesis and Treatment of Urinary Tract Infections*. Baltimore, Williams & Wilkins Co, 1980.
9. Barry AL, Jones RN, Thornsberry, C et al: Antibacterial activities of ciprofloxacin, norfloxacin, oxolinic acid, cinoxacin, and nalidixic acid. *Antimicrob Agents Chemother* 1984; 25:633–637.
10. Fowler JE: Prostatitis, in Gillenwater JY, Grayhack JT, Howards SS, et al (eds): *Adult and Pediatric Urology*. Chicago, Year Book Medical Publishers, 1987, pp 1220–1244.
11. Dajani AM, O'Flynn JD: Prostatic abscess. A report of 25 cases. *Br J Urol* 1968; 40:736–739.
12. Trapnell J, Roberts M: Prostatic abscess. *Br J Surg* 1970; 57:565–568.
13. Pai MG, Bhat HS: Prostatic abscess. *J Urol* 1972; 108:599–600.
14. Timberlake G: An electro-prostatome; relief of prostatic abscesses and acute obstructive prostatitis by transurethral prostatotomy. *J Urol* 1938; 40:343–345.
15. Kadman D, Ling D, Lee JKT: Percutaneous drainage of prostatic abscesses. *J Urol* 1986; 135:1259.

17

Acute Epididymitis

Richard E. Berger, M.D.

Dr. Brown, your colleague in family practice, asks you to evaluate this 28-year-old seaman who developed a painful swollen right testicle this morning. The patient, on your questioning, denies any prior similar episodes. He was treated intramuscularly with penicillin 3 months ago for urethral "drip" but denies all other genitourinary disease or symptoms. On examination he has a tender, swollen right scrotum and testicle (length 10 cm with longitudinal position). The mass does not transilluminate. The right cord is slightly tender. The left scrotal contents are normal, and prostatic examination is unremarkable.

Acute epididymitis is a common condition that occurs in males of all ages. It is a major cause of disability and morbidity. The proper diagnosis and treatment of epididymitis can considerably decrease complications and the length of time needed for recovery.

In children epididymitis is most commonly related to bacteriuria and infection of the urinary tract. The infection from the urine spreads to the ejaculatory ducts down the vas deferens and into the epididymitis. In children epididymitis is commonly associated with structural urinary abnormalities, which are predisposed to bacteriuria. Fortunately epididymitis is relatively uncommon in children.[1]

In heterosexual teenagers and men less than 35 years old, bacteriuria is relatively uncommon and epididymitis related to bacteriuria is uncommon. However, infection of the urethra with sexually transmitted pathogens is quite common. The most common causes of epididymitis in heterosexual men less than 35 years of age are the sexually transmitted pathogens that cause urethritis, *Nesseria gonorrhoeae* and *Chlamydia trachomatis*. Young homosexual men who practice unprotected anal intercourse may more often have epididymitis caused by bacteriuria. Numerous studies throughout the world are now showing that approximately two thirds of the cases of epididymitis in young men are caused by these sexually transmitted pathogens.[2–3]

In men more than age 35 years sexually transmitted disease becomes less common. However, acquired structural abnormalities of the urinary tract again predispose men to bacteriuria. Therefore, after age 35 years the most common cause of epididymitis is again related to bacteriuria.

The accurate initial determination of treatment for epididymitis, as well as its differentiation from other noninfectious diseases, is necessary to properly evaluate and treat men with acute scrotal pain. It is extremely important that the different causes of epididymitis be diagnosed and treated according to their antibiotic susceptibilities.

DIFFERENTIAL DIAGNOSIS

The acute onset of scrotal pain does not always indicate the diagnosis of epididymitis. In preadolescent boys where epididymitis is relatively uncommon, torsion of the testicle is the most likely diagnosis. In men less than the age of 35 years, torsion and epididymitis are both common entities, and differentiation between the two is crucial. In men more than the age of 35 years, torsion again becomes relatively uncommon, and epididymitis is the most common entity. Other entities such as an acutely thrombosed varicocele, incarcerated hernia, testicular tumor, and trauma must be methodically eliminated in the evaluation of epididymitis.

EVALUATION

The onset of acute epididymitis is often gradual occurring over a period of several hours or even days. However, the onset may also be quite sudden and may occur abruptly during heavy lifting. The sudden onset during heavy lifting may be related to the forcing of infected contents of the ejaculatory ducts or seminal vesicles down the vas deferens, causing acute pain and inflammation. Although testicular tumors are classically painless, at least 25% of men with testicular cancer have scrotal pain. A tumor located under the epididymis may feel exactly like an indurated epididymis. Men with sexually transmitted epididymitis always have a history of sexual contact in the past. This contact may have been 2 or even 6 months before the onset of epididymitis whether it is caused by gonorrhea or chlamydia. [4] Urinary symptoms will be noted in some patients but may be absent with either sexually transmitted epididymitis or epididymitis related to bacteriuria. Some men with urethritis will notice a urethral discharge. There may be a history of treatment for gonococcal urethritis but without tetracycline or doxycycline treatment to cover the concomitant chlamydia infection, which occurs in 25% to 30% of men with gonococcal urethritis. The chlamydia then remains and later causes postgonococcal urethritis or epididymitis.

Physical examination of men with urethritis is an extremely important part of the evaluation. Early in the course of epididymitis the tail of the epididymis is almost always the first portion involved. The tender indurated swelling at the tail of the epididymis gradually progresses to involve the entire epididymis and ultimately the testicle. A reactive hydrocele then often develops, obscuring all landmarks and making the differential from other acute scrotal entities almost impossible by physical examination alone. It is important to note that almost 15% of cases of acute torsion have initially more swelling of the epididymis than the testicles and therefore can be readily confused with acute epididymitis. In epididymitis the testicle often hangs in its normal position, although it may be reflexly drawn up. In torsion the testicle is almost always high riding. The spermatic cord is always involved and tender and swollen in acute epididymitis and is intimately involved in the inflammatory process. In contrast, in early torsion the testicular cord is not involved and usually is not tender. Testicular tumors occurring in the area of the testicle underneath the epididymis may feel exactly like epididymitis. Furthermore, tenderness can be a consistent finding in the presentation of tumors. In torsion of the testicle, examination of the opposite side may reveal an anterior epididymis, suggesting a partial torsion on the opposite side as well. Prehn's sign, which involves the alleviation of pain on elevating the testicle with epididymitis, is usually not helpful in the clinical evaluation of the patient with scrotal pain. In some instances where physical examination is so painful that it cannot be conducted adequately, a nerve block of the spermatic cord at the external ring with 1% lidocaine (Xylocaine) will probably give the patient relief of his pain but also allow the physician to adequately evaluate him.

The urethra should also be examined for discharge. Because it is uncommon (although torsion with epididymitis occurs simultaneously), the presence of urethritis with urethral discharge is an excellent clue to the cause of the epididymitis and therefore its proper treatment.

The initial laboratory evaluation of a man with epididymitis should always begin with a urethral swab for Gram stain and culture. The presence of 5 or more leukocytes/high-power field indicates urethritis. Gram-negative intracellular diplococci indicate a gonococcal etiology in approximately 95% of cases. If there is no urethritis present, the diagnosis of sexually transmitted urethritis is suspect. It must be noted, however, that the urethra should be swabbed after the patient has been continent of urine for at least 2 (and preferably 4) hours. Unfortunately, patients are often asked to urinate on arrival in the emergency room, and the process of urination washes away the evidence of urethritis and can even make the Gram stains negative. Urethritis also can be diagnosed by looking at the first 10 mL of voided urine before a midstream urine specimen is obtained. The presence of 10 white blood cells/mL in the urethral specimen indicates urethritis in the absence of bacteriuria. A midstream urine specimen should then also be examined and the presence of bacteriuria noted. One bacterium per high-power field indicates greater than 10^5 bacteria/mL of urine. In the absence of any indication of urethral or urinary tract infection, the diagnosis of epididymitis should be highly suspect. Other entities such as torsion of the testicle, testicular tumor, or incarcerated inguinal hernia must be strongly considered.

USE OF DOPPLER ULTRASOUND, GRAY SCALE ULTRASOUND, AND TESTICULAR SCANS

If one makes the diagnosis of torsion in the emergency room, it behooves the physician to get the patient to the operating room to perform detorsion as soon as possible. In a child, a history of acute testicular pain should be presumed to be a torsion and exploration undertaken. In a child, adolescent, or young adult with an initial diagnosis of torsion, confirmatory diagnostic imaging studies should be performed only if it does not delay operative detorsion. On the other hand, in a young man diagnosed as having epididymitis, diagnostic studies should be undertaken to further objectively rule out torsion of the testicle. The wrong diagnosis of epididymitis could cause the loss of a testicle. The use of Doppler ultrasound may be helpful in emergency setting to confirm the diagnosis of torsion. Decreased blood flow over the affected testicle when compared with the contralateral testicle indicates a high likelihood of torsion, and exploration should still be undertaken. On the other hand, increased blood flow on the affected side is confirmatory for epididymitis. If one finds increased blood flow, however, it is possible that it may be caused by inflamed scrotal secondary to testicular torsion. Therefore, cord compression at the external ring should be undertaken simultaneously. If the increased signal disappears with cord compression, it is indeed coming from the testicle. On the other hand, if the increased signal does not go away with cord compression, it must be coming from the scrotal vessels. Torsion may still be present. If readily available, radionuclide renal scanning is one of the most reliable methods with which to confirm the diagnosis of epididymitis.[5] Increased blood flow to the testicle is confirmatory for epididymitis. Gray scale ultrasound imaging is occasionally useful to show that a mass is indeed in the testicle. Abnormal echoes in the testicle are, however, common in both torsion and epididymitis. Gray scale ultrasound is very useful if a reactionary hydrocele is present preventing adequate testicular palpation and one wishes to confirm the normality of the underlying testicle. However, many times in epididymitis the underlying testicle will show abnormal echoes confusing the diagnosis.

TREATMENT

Treatment of epididymitis may be divided into supportive and etiology-specific care. Bed rest with scrotal elevation should be prescribed for all patients. This will allow the best drainage of the lymphatics of the scrotum and will greatly hasten recovery. Preferably the patient should continue bed rest until pain subsides.

If the patient has bacteriuria, he should be treated with a broad-spectrum antibiotic that will cover all organisms possibly causing the infection. If the man is septic, bed rest and intravenous (IV) multiple antibiotic coverage should be prescribed until results have returned. If the patient is not ill or is minimally symptomatic, antibiotic coverage with a quinolone antibiotic is appropriate. Ampicillin or tetracycline therapy alone should never be used as initial therapy because a large number of community-acquired organisms are now resistant to these antibiotics.

If the patient has urethritis-associated epididymitis, he should be treated intramuscularly with 250 mg of ceftriaxone to cover gonorrhea and then treated for an additional 10 days with 100 mg of doxycycline two times daily to cover chlamydia. Sexual partners should be treated with the same regimen.

FOLLOW-UP

All patients should be seen in follow-up approximately 1 week after administration of antibiotic therapy to determine response to therapy. If considerable improvement is not present, the patient should be warned that he should remain supine with the scrotum elevated to receive maximum rate of recovery. Patients with bacteriuria should be scheduled for IV urogram to rule out structural urinary pathologic conditions. Epididymitis usually resolves slowly: however, pain should be absent within 2 weeks. Swelling with the epididymitis often remains for a longer time. If the swelling does not resolve, consideration should be given to scrotal exploration to rule out testicular tumors.

REFERENCES

1. Anderson PA, Giacomantonio JM, Schwarz RD: Acute scrotal pain in children: Prospective study of diagnosis and management. *Can J Surg* 1989; 32:29–32. (published erratum appears in *Can J Surg* 1989; 32:158.)
2. Berger RE, Alexander ER, Harnisch JP, et al: Etiology, manifestations and therapy of acute epididymitis: prospective study of 50 cases. *J Urol* 1979; 121:750–754.
3. Berger RE, Kessler D, Holmes KK: Etiology and manifestations of epididymitis in young men: Correlations with sexual orientation. *J Infect Dis* 1987; 155:1341–1343.
4. Watson RA: Gonorrhea and acute epididymitis. *Milit Med* 1979; 144:785–787.
5. Vordermark JS II, Buck AS, Brown SR, et al: The testicular scan. Use in diagnosis and management of acute epididymitis. JAMA 1981; 245:2512–2514.

18

Gonorrhea

William O. Harrison, M.D.

A 23-year-old homosexual man was treated for culture-proved gonococcal urethritis with 4.8 million units of procaine penicillin intramuscularly, accompanied by 2 g of probenecid orally. Two weeks after this treatment, he returned to his primary care physician with recurrent symptoms of dysuria and a yellowish urethral discharge. He states that his only sexual encounter over the last 6 months was one episode of anal intercourse before the initial onset of urethritis. He is distressed about the recurrence, and his physician refers him for consultation. Your Gram stain of the urethral discharge shows multiple polymorphonuclear neutrophils (PMNs) with scattered gram-negative intracellular diplococci.

INITIAL EVALUATION AND HISTORY TAKING

It is vital to obtain an adequate sexual history when one is treating sexually transmitted diseases (STDs) and other sexual problems. In most medical schools, students are never taught how to obtain a sexual history, and the development of good technique is left to chance.[1] To obtain a good history, one must be comfortable with both questions asked and answers given. Most physicians, when dealing with homosexuals, tend either to not ask appropriate questions or to skim over answers quickly, without listening carefully. In the present case, several more facts need to be obtained.[2]

The patient must be questioned about sexual activity other than penetrating intercourse. Has there been external sex play, including mutual masturbation? Has there been use of so-called sex toys, including dildos or butt plugs? In the one episode of anal intercourse was the patient the receptive or insertive partner? Was the partner well known to the patient or a casual contact? Was the initial infection acquired in a major metropolitan area of the United States, a smaller city, or overseas? Had the partner recently been out of the United States? Has the patient had earlier infections with STDs? Has the patient had serology testing for human immunodeficiency virus (HIV). If so, was it positive? The answers to these questions will guide the clinician in determining whether the present symptoms are the result of reinfection or failure of the initial treatment. They will also help to determine whether other STDs may be present or a possibility.

PHYSICAL EXAMINATION

A thorough physical evaluation must be performed. It is not enough to merely view the penile tip with its purulent urethral discharge. Ideally the patient should be completely disrobed so that rashes, hemorrhagic pustules, Kaposi's sarcoma, ectoparasites, and other manifestations of various STDs can be visualized if present. The genitalia must be examined for evidence of chancre, ulcer, condylomata, adenopathy, and lesions of the testes, scrotum, penile shaft, glans, and foreskin, in addition to the discharge. Depending on the body areas indicated as sites of sexual activity, examination of the anal canal, rectum, and oropharynx are necessary. In many cases the physical evidence of various STDs is either overlooked or ignored by the patient; it is the clinician's responsibility to discover these and discuss them with the patient. This added examination takes a little more time than a brief "short-arm inspection." Clinicians in a busy Southern California STD clinic were able to expand their examinations to include these suggestions and still see the same number of patients during regular clinic hours (W.O. Harrison, unpublished data, 1990).

LABORATORY EVALUATION

During or at the conclusion of the physical examination, specimens appropriate to the presumed diagnoses must be obtained. In this case, let us assume that no further physical findings except for purulent urethral discharge are noted, and the history suggests no additional STDs. The diagnosis of gonorrhea should be confirmed by demonstration of the causative organisms by both microscopy and culture. Because the history suggests failure of the original treatment program, culture becomes mandatory to obtain the antibiotic susceptibility pattern of the offending organism.

The visualization of intracellular Gram-negative diplococci by microscopic examination of the patient's urethral discharge strongly suggests but does not prove a diagnosis of gonorrhea. A related pathogen, *Neisseria meningitidis,* has been isolated as the sole agent from patients with symptomatic genital infections.[3] In a patient such as this one, urethral culture is mandatory, both for accurate identification and for antibiotic susceptibility testing. If the sexual history notes contact at anus or oropharynx, these sites must be cultured as well, even in the absence of symptoms. Gonococci of differing antibiotic sensitivities can be isolated from separate locations in the body, leading to treatment failures if not identified and then followed up.

When specimens are obtained, it is not sufficient to merely express a drop of pus from the urethral meatus and touch it to a slide. Specimens must be obtained from within the urethra by means of a calcium alginate urethral swab. The swab should be inserted 1 to 2 cm into the urethra and rotated to obtain a good specimen. The material obtained should then be transferred directly to an appropriate culture plate containing specific nutrient media and carried to the laboratory for incubation in a carbon dioxide incubator.[4] If this is not possible, a number of self-contained transport and nutrient systems such as the JEMBEC plate,[5] the BioBag (Marion Scientific, Kansas City, Mo.), or the Gono-Pak (Nasco, Modesto, Calif.) provide both nutrient media and a CO_2-rich atmosphere while the specimen is being transported to the laboratory.

While awaiting the results of cultures, one can make a presumptive diagnosis by means of the Gram stain. When properly prepared and examined by a competent technician (or clinician), the Gram stain is both highly sensitive and specific.[6] Treatment can be administered for the presumptive diagnosis of gonorrhea provided by a Gram-stained specimen of urethral secretions. The presence on microscopic examination of such a specimen of even a single PMN with intracellular gram-negative diplococci provides adequate justification for treatment.

If the Gram stain shows PMNs and mixed bacteria without intracellular gram-negative diplococci, a diagnosis of nongonococcal urethritis or, as in the present case, postgonococcal urethritis, can be made. Because the specimen in the present case did reveal intracellular gram-negative diplococci, the criteria for a presumptive diagnosis of gonorrhea have been met.

SELECTION OF APPROPRIATE THERAPY

The failure of an antibiotic regimen to cure gonorrhea is not a new phenomenon. When sulfanilamide was introduced in the mid-1930s, it quickly became the treatment of choice for gonorrhea. By 1944, however, at least one third of patients given sulfa failed treatment.[7] Penicillin rapidly supplanted sulfa and for the next 45 years was the standard therapy for uncomplicated gonococcal infections. Relative resistance to penicillin began to appear in the mid-1950s, but because of the excellent therapeutic/toxicity ratio of the drug, it continued to be used, albeit in increasingly higher doses.[8] Tetracycline and erythromycin, used with patients who were allergic to penicillin, also showed gradually increasing patterns of resistance by the gonococcus.

In 1975, however, the first cases of completely penicillin-resistant gonococcal urethritis were noted at a U.S. Navy base in the Philippines.[9] In previous years increasing resistance to penicillin had been noted in Southeast Asia,[10] but these new infections failed to respond to as much as 9.6 million units of procaine penicillin G. Soon thereafter, the occurrence of highly resistant strains of gonorrhea was noted in England[11] and the United States.[12] The mechanism by which these isolates had become resistant to penicillin was by the incorporation of a cytoplasmic packet of DNA called a plasmid, or R factor, which coded for the production of TEM β-lactamase.[13] This enzyme opens the β-lactam ring of the penicillin molecule, thus rendering it ineffective. Because this β-lactamase is also known as penicillinase, these strains of gonococci soon became known as penicillinase-producing *Neisseria gonorrhoeae* (PPNG).

Although the origin of PPNG remains obscure, the widespread dissemination of these strains throughout the world has been well documented.[14–15] In many parts of the world, notably the Pacific Rim countries and Africa, they are in the majority.[16] In the United States the incidence increased slowly between 1976 and 1980; the majority of these infections were a result of exposure in or transmission from endemic areas. In 1984, however, endemic transmission within the United States increased strikingly.[17] By 1988, these resistant strains accounted for more than 4% of all reported gonococcal cases, a total of more than 40,000 cases per year.[18] Endemic foci within the United States include Miami, New York, Los Angeles, Seattle, and Denver,[9] with sporadic outbreaks occurring in other circumscribed areas.

More recently, gonococci both penicillinase producing and chromosomally resistant to spectinomycin have been isolated in Korea.[19] Spectinomycin-resistant isolates of gonococci have been documented in very small numbers since the beginning of the use of this drug,[20] but only recently have these resistance factors joined. Such multiply-resistant strains have also been reported from the Philippines and from England.[21]

In addition to these changes in antibiotic susceptibility, in 1983 an outbreak of cases of resistant gonorrhea was reported from North Carolina. This outbreak was caused by a strain of gonococcus that was highly resistant to penicillin but that did not produce β-lactamase.[22] The resistance in these bacteria is produced by a combination of chromosomally mediated factors and is not as readily identified as is β-lactamase. By 1985, reports were noted of highly tetracycline-resistant *N. gonorrhoeae* (TRNG), this time on the basis of a plasmid that produced high-level tetracycline resistance.[23] Thus, the standard first-line antibiotics for treatment of uncomplicated gonorrhea have all seen significant resistance develop over the past decade. Because the patient in this case was treated with the traditional antibiotic for urethritis (penicillin), it is not surprising that the treatment failed.

TREATMENT REGIMENS FOR GONORRHEA IN AN ERA OF RESISTANCE

In determining which antibiotic to use for treatment of uncomplicated gonococcal urethritis, one must take certain factors into account in addition to the sensitivity patterns of the bacteria. Studies have shown that to be effective, serum levels of an antibiotic must reach at least three times the minimal inhibitory concentration of the organism for at least 8 hours or more.[24] Single-dose therapy is preferred because of problems with patient compliance. The likelihood of coinfection with other STDs must always be considered.

The most recent treatment guidelines from the Centers for Disease Control reflect all of the previous considerations. The treatment of uncomplicated genital gonorrhea is 250 mg of ceftriaxone given intramuscularly in a single dose plus 100 mg of doxycycline taken orally twice daily for 7 days.[25] Ceftriaxone is highly effective against all strains of gonococci and at any site of infection,[26] is easily administered as a single dose, and is well tolerated by most patients. In addition, ceftriaxone is highly effective in treating chancroid[27] and has shown some efficacy against incubating syphilis, a frequent concurrent STD.[28] Doxycycline is added to eradicate concomitant infection with *Chlamydia trachomatis*.

Alternative antibiotics are readily available.[29] Table 18–1 lists several parenteral and oral medications that have been shown to be highly effective against resistant gonococci but that are being held in reserve against the development of ceftriaxone resistance or have not yet been approved by the Food and Drug Administration for such use.

TABLE 18–1.
Antibiotics Effective Against PPNG, CMRNG,* and TRNG

Cefoxitin	2 g intramuscularly plus 1 g orally of probenecid
Cefotaxime	1 g intramuscularly
Ceftizoxime	1 g intramuscularly
Cefaclor	500 mg orally four times daily for 5 days
Moxalactam	1 g intramuscularly
Norfloxacin	1.2 g in two doses 6 hours apart
Sulfamethoxazole-trimethoprim	Nine single-strength tablets in a single daily dose for 3 days

**CMRNG = chromosomally mediated resistance to N. gonorrhoeae.*

Additional testing that should be done with this patient and all patients with gonorrhea include a serologic test for syphilis and testing for HIV infection, as well as the offer of confidential counseling.

FOLLOW-UP

Treatment failure after using the combined ceftriaxone-doxycycline regimen is rare; nevertheless, a follow-up culture ("test of cure") is recommended. Such cultures should not be obtained until 1 week after the completion of doxycycline therapy. All sites known to be infected before therapy should be recultured. Sexual partners of the patient during the preceding month should be examined, have cultures taken, and should be treated presumptively ("epidemiologic treatment").

PREVENTION

Despite 20 years of attention and great outlay of research funding, gonorrhea continues to be a major public health problem. The use of condoms and other barrier contraceptives reduces the incidence of gonorrhea but still carries a 10% to 15% failure rate.[30] Prophylaxis, either before or after sexual contact, is effective when used on a small scale, but eventually it leads to the development of antibiotic resistance.[31] Several attempts have been made to develop a gonococcal vaccine, but these have so far been unsuccessful. Although education has been of little value in reaching populations at risk in the past, fear of acquired immunodeficiency syndrome has possibly resulted in a reduction in incidence of gonorrhea recently.[32] It may be that a combination of conscience, counseling, and condoms will result in the disappearance of gonorrhea as a major source of morbidity.

REFERENCES

1. Lewis CE: Taking a sexual history. *West J Med* 1987; 147:165.
2. Ostrow DG: Homosexual behavior and sexually transmitted diseases, in KK Holmes, et al (eds): *Sexually Transmitted Diseases,* ed 2, New York, McGraw-Hill Book Co, 1989, pp 63–65.
3. Hook EW III, Handsfield HH: Gonococcal infections in the adult, in KK Holmes, et al (eds): *Sexually Transmitted Diseases,* ed 2, New York, McGraw-Hill Book Co, 1989, pp 156–157.
4. Mordello JA, et al: *Neisseria and Branhamella,* in EG Lennette, et al (eds): *Manual of Clinical Microbiology,* ed 4, Washington, DC, American Society for Microbiology, 1985, p 176.
5. Martin JE, Jackson RL: A biological environment chamber for culture of *Neisseria gonorrhoeae. J Am Vener Dis Assoc* 1975; 2:28.
6. Kellogg DS, et al: Laboratory diagnosis of gonorrhea, in S Marcus, JC Sherris (eds): *Cumitech 4,* Washington, DC, American Society for Microbiology, 1976.
7. Kampmeier RH: Introduction of sulfonamide therapy for gonorrhea. *Sex Transm Dis* 1983; 10:81.
8. Martin JE, et al: Comparative study of gonococcal susceptibility to penicillin in the United States, 1955–1969. *J Infect Dis* 1970; 122:459.
9. Harrison WO: Antibiotic resistant gonorrhea. *Cutis* 1984; 33:81.
10. Holmes KK, et al: Treatment of "penicillin-resistant" gonorrhea in military personnel in Southeast Asia: A cooperative evaluation of tetracycline and of penicillin plus probenecid in 1263 men. *Milit Med* 1968; 133:642.
11. Phillips I: Beta-lactamase-producing penicillin-resistant gonococcus. *Lancet* 1976; 2:656.
12. Ashford WA, Golash RG, Hemming VG: Penicillinase-producing *N. gonorrhoeae. Lancet* 1976; 2:657.
13. Elwell LP, et al: Plasmid-mediated beta-lactamase production in *Neisseria gonorrhoeae. Antimicrob Agents Chemother* 1977; 11:528.
14. Centers for Disease Control: Follow-up on antibiotic-resistant *N. gonorrhoeae. MMWR* 1977; 26:65.
15. Centers for Disease Control: Penicillinase-producing *N. gonorrhoeae*—United States, worldwide. *MMWR* 1979; 28:85.
16. Perine PL, et al: Epidemiology and treatment of penicillinase-producing *Neisseria gonorrhoeae. Sex Transm Dis* 1979; 6(suppl):152.

17. Centers for Disease Control: Penicillinase-producing *N. gonorrhoeae*—United States, 1986. *MMWR* 1987; 36:107.
18. Zenilman JM et al: Penicillinase-producing *Neisseria gonorrhoeae* in Dade County, Florida. *Sex Transm Dis* 1988; 15:45.
19. Jones O, Strohmeyer G, Brockett J, et al: Spectinomycin-resistant penicillinase-producing *Neisseria gonorrhoeae*. *MMWR* 1983; 32:51.
20. Reyn A, Schmidt H, Trier M, et al: Spectinomycin hydrochloride in the treatment of gonorrhea: Observation of resistant strains of *Neisseria gonorrhoeae*. *Br J Vener Dis* 1973; 49:54.
21. Patefield AJ, Westbrook WC, Johnston NA: Spectinomycin-resistant *Neisseria gonorrhoeae*—worldwide. *MMWR* 1982; 31:632.
22. Faruki H, et al: A community-based outbreak of infection with penicillin-resistant *Neisseria gonorrhoeae* not producing penicillinase (chromosomally-mediated resistance). *N Engl J Med* 1985; 313:607.
23. Centers for Disease Control: Tetracycline-resistant *Neisseria gonorrhoeae*—Georgia, Pennsylvania, New Hampshire. *MMWR* 1985; 34:563.
24. Jaffe HW, et al: Pharmacokinetic determinants of penicillin cure of gonococcal urethritis. *Antimicrob Agents Chemother* 1979; 15:587.
25. Centers for Disease Control: 1989 Sexually transmitted diseases treatment guidelines. *MMWR* 1989; 38:S21–S24.
26. Zajdowicz TR, Sanchez PL, Harrison WO: A comparison of ceftriaxone with cefoxitin in the treatment of penicillin-resistant gonococcal urethritis. *Br J Vener Dis* 1983; 59:176–178.
27. Bowmer MI, et al: Single-dose ceftriaxone for chancroid. *Antimicrob Agents Chemother* 1987; 31:67.
28. Centers for Disease Control: 1989 sexually transmitted diseases treatment guidelines. *MMWR* 1989; 38:S7, S23.
29. Harrison WO: Gonorrhea, Felman YM (ed): in *Sexually Transmitted Diseases* New York, Churchill Livingstone, 1986, p 57.
30. Hooper RR, et al: Cohort study of venereal diseases: I. Risk of transmission from infected women to men. *Am J Epidemiol* 1978; 107:235.
31. Harrison WO, et al: A trial of minocycline given after exposure to prevent gonorrhea. *N Engl J Med* 1979; 300:1074–1077.
32. Harrison WO, Whitten GB III: Reduction of urethritis following intensive education concerning AIDS risk. Proceedings of the Fourth International Conference on AIDS, Stockholm, World Health Organization, 1988, abstract no 5150.

19

Nongonococcal Urethritis

William R. Bowie, M.D.

You consult with the staff of the student health service at a nearby college. A number of young men have developed opalescent, thin urethral discharge 2 to 3 weeks after treatment for culture-proved *Neisseria gonorrhoeae* infection. Microscopic evaluation fails to reveal diplococci or other bacteria, and there are scant numbers of white blood cells (WBCs). Several of the men have been diagnosed as having nongonococcal urethritis and treated with tetracycline for 1 week without success.

BACKGROUND COMMENTS

Typical Presentation of Urethritis

Characteristic presenting symptoms of urethritis include urethral discharge, burning on urination, and an itch in the urethra. The only typical finding on examination is a urethral discharge that may be present spontaneously or may require milking of the urethra, even when the man is evaluated under optimal conditions. The characteristic laboratory finding is increased numbers of polymorphonuclear leukocytes in urethral secretions.

Etiology of Urethritis

Urethritis is classically divided into gonococcal and nongonococcal urethritis. Gonococcal urethritis or gonorrhea is diagnosed when infection with *N. gonorrhoeae* is suspected by the Gram stain appearance of urethral secretions or when it is specifically identified, usually by culture. However, concurrent urethral infection with *Chlamydia trachomatis* is present in 15% to 25% of heterosexual men with gonorrhea and 5% of homosexual men with gonorrhea.

Nongonococcal urethritis is diagnosed when urethritis is present but gonococci are not detected. With acute presentation of an untreated episode of nongonococcal urethritis, *C. trachomatis* can be isolated from 25% to 40% of men, *Ureaplasma urealyticum* from 40% to 50% (often with *C. trachomatis*), and neither organism from 20% to 30%.

A variant of nongonococcal urethritis is postgonococcal urethritis or urethritis noted after treatment of gonorrhea with a regimen that eradicates *N. gonorrhoeae* but does not eradicate concurrent infection with other pathogens. The most frequent cause of documented postgonococcal urethritis is *C. trachomatis*.

Standard Treatment

Recommended treatment for gonorrhea has undergone significant changes in the past decade. These changes have arisen because of recognition of the importance and frequency of concurrent infection with *C. trachomatis* and the development of several types of antimicrobial resistance in *N. gonorrhoeae*. These include high-level resistance to penicillin on the basis of plasmid-mediated resistance (β-lactamase-producing strains), chromosomally mediated resistance to penicillin, high-level plasmid-mediated resistance to tetracyclines, frequent resistance to older antimicrobials like erythromycin, and occasional resistance to other antimicrobials such as spectinomycin.

Thus, current recommendations for treatment of uncomplicated gonococcal urethritis requires use of a single-dose regimen active against *N. gonorrhoeae* and 7 days of a regimen active against *C. trachomatis.*[1] The currently promoted optimal single-dose regimen is 250 mg of ceftriaxone given intramuscularly. Although less well evaluated, single-dose treatment with 500 mg of ciprofloxacin taken orally is likely to be a very satisfactory alternative. Numerous other options are available, including penicillins in areas where penicillin susceptibility remains very prevalent and there are no clinical concerns (e.g., recent travel to an area endemic for resistant isolates, which include many large North American cities, as well as distant places).

The recommended regimens active against *C. trachomatis* are the same as those for nongonococcal urethritis. Tetracyclines are preferred, with a 7-day regimen of either 100 mg of doxycycline taken orally twice daily or 500 mg of tetracycline taken orally four times daily. Alternatively, a 7-day regimen of erythromycin in doses equivalent to a 500-mg erythromycin base taken orally four times daily.

Anticipated Response to Treatment

When patients are compliant with taking medication and they do not resume sexual activity, with use of the recommended regimens microbiologic failure to eradicate *N. gonorrhoeae* and *C. trachomatis* is exceedingly infrequent. Postgonococcal urethritis is unusual.

The clinical outcome with nongonococcal urethritis is less impressive, even though *C. trachomatis* is almost always eradicated. At least 95% of men show some or complete resolution of symptoms by the end of the week of treatment, but by 6 weeks after the end of treatment, up to 40% may show persistent or recurrent urethritis using the criteria of increased numbers of polymorphonuclear leukocytes in urethral secretions.[2] Approximately one half of these men will have symptoms. In the small group of men with proved nongonococcal urethritis initially who show minimal or no response, a proportion have genital herpes in the urethra, a proportion are infected with *Trichomonas vaginalis,* and about one half have tetracycline-resistant *U. urealyticum.* In the larger group of men with an initial response but subsequent recurrent or incomplete response, 10% to 20% have *U. urealyticum* isolated, but in the majority no potential pathogen is recovered.

When men are not compliant with taking medication or have sexual intercourse with new or untreated partners, a portion will be infected with *N. gonorrhoeae* or *C. trachomatis,* and even more will be infected with *U. urealyticum.*

ANALYSIS OF FACTORS PROVIDED

Initial Diagnosis of Gonorrhea (Presumably Urethral)

There should be little room for false positive culture diagnosis of infection with *N. gonorrhoeae,* but because gonococcal urethritis is not frequent in most student health service populations, the possibility of a false positive diagnosis should at least be considered.

Initial Treatment of the Gonorrhea

The initial treatment of the gonorrhea was not stated. It should be clarified. As well, because *N. gonorrhoeae* was initially isolated, the susceptibility of isolates to at least penicillin should be known. The likelihood of failure to eradicate *N. gonorrhoeae* and possible concurrent infection with *C. trachomatis* will depend highly on the regimen used.

Presence of Discharge After Initial Treatment

The fact that patients had discharge after initial treatment is a crucial aspect. As noted earlier, the key questions are the history, the examination, and the laboratory studies. We are not told whether the men were examined under optimal or suboptimal conditions. We are also not told about compliance with medication and resumption of sexual intercourse.

The presence of an "opalescent, thin urethral discharge" is not necessarily abnormal. There is normally meatal moisture, and in addition it sometimes takes awhile for the discharge associated with gonorrhea or nongonococcal urethritis to entirely disappear. From the description given, it is quite possible that the "discharge" might not indicate urethritis. What makes a discharge consistent with urethritis is an increased number of polymorphonuclear leukocytes. We are told that there were "scant numbers of WBCs." I would interpret scant as being less than four polymorphonuclear leukocytes per oil field, the usually accepted breakpoint for the presence of urethritis. Based on the information given, they would not meet diagnostic criteria for nongonococcal or postgonococcal urethritis. Failure to detect gram-negative diplococci makes the already unlikely diagnosis of gonorrhea even more unlikely.

Treatment With Tetracycline

Given the information provided, I would not have treated the men with anything when they were seen 2 to 3 weeks after the initial treatment. However, because they were treated and we do not know what the initial treatment was, a completed course of tetracycline treatment would make persistent infection with

C. trachomatis highly unlikely and would greatly decrease the rate of carriage of *U. urealyticum*.

Lack of Success of Treatment

We are not told how long it was after the tetracycline treatment that they were considered to have failed to respond or by what criteria they were considered to have failed. If the criteria were persistence of the thin discharge and presence of scant numbers of WBCs, their findings would be considered within normal limits. Thus, by objective criteria they would not have failed.

It would be entirely expected that normal findings would not become more normal if these men were on tetracycline therapy.

ADVICE FOR FURTHER EVALUATION AND MANAGEMENT

The initial advice is very simple. Men who have "failed" to respond to tetracycline for presumed postgonococcal urethritis should not receive further therapy but, rather, should be carefully reevaluated. This involves taking a good history to characterize symptoms, compliance with therapy, resumption of sexual intercourse, and, if so, with or without a condom used correctly and with a new partner or an old partner who has or has not been treated.

The physical examination should be performed under optimal conditions when the man has not voided for at least 4 hours and preferably not voided overnight. A thorough genital examination should be performed to detect unusual causes of urethritis such as genital warts, which may suggest urethral warts; painful inguinal lymphadenopathy, which might suggest genital herpes; palpation of the urethra to detect foreign bodies; and urethral discharge.

A swab of intraurethral secretions should be obtained for Gram stain to quantitate the number of polymorphonuclear leukocytes and examination for gram-negative intracellular diplococci. Although results are highly unlikely to be positive in the absence of noncompliance with therapy or resumption of sexual intercourse with an untreated partner and without using a condom, intraurethral specimens should be taken for culture for *N. gonorrhoeae* and *C. trachomatis*. These require inserting an intraurethral swab (special swab on a flexible aluminum shaft) 3 to 4 cm into the urethra. In this situation, cultures are strongly preferred over nonculture techniques for detection of *N. gonorrhoeae* and *C. trachomatis* because of the problem of interpreting false positive results. With a nonculture technique, there is a high likelihood that a "positive" result will, in fact, be false positive.

If available, cultures could also be performed for *U. urealyticum*. These are more likely to be positive (approximately 20%), but a positive culture does not mean that it is causing a problem in a specific individual. To detect *T. vaginalis,* optimally one should obtain cultures of urethral material. Alternatively they may be sought by directly looking at urethral secretions as in a saline preparation or by centrifuging the first 10 mL of urine and looking at the sediment for motile trichomonads.

From the scenario provided it is unlikely that the men will have florid urethritis, and it is probably unlikely that they will even have a polymorphonuclear leukocyte response. Even if they did, unless the Gram stain showed gram-negative intracellular diplococci or test results were positive for *N. gonorrhoeae, C. trachomatis,* or *T. vaginalis,* further antimicrobial therapy would not be indicated at that time and likely would not be required again for this episode.

In this situation there is minimal evidence that further antimicrobial or other medications are beneficial in improving long-term outcome. In the absence of other evidence of prostatitis, evaluation to detect bacterial prostatitis is almost always nonhelpful. Unless there are clinical clues to suggest structural abnormalities of the urethra or intraurethral lesions or urinary flow studies were performed and were abnormal, urethroscopy and cystoscopy are unlikely to show a clinically significant abnormality.[3]

Because many of these men have additional concerns, several points should be discussed. This is especially important for those men who have increased numbers of polymorphonuclear leukocytes and no further antimicrobial therapy is given or further therapy has been given without cure. Men should be informed that:

1. If they were compliant with therapy, and especially if in addition specific microbiologic test results are negative for *N. gonorrhoeae* and *C. trachomatis,* they pose virtually no risk for transmission of causes of urethritis to sexual partners. (They could, of course, still spread other agents such as herpes simplex virus or human immunodeficiency virus.)
2. There is no need for further treatment of partners if the man is in an ongoing monogamous relationship and the partner was initially treated with an appropriate recommended regimen. (Although the focus of this discussion is on men, evaluation and treatment of female partners is an integral part of the management of men with proved or possible infections with *N. gonorrhoeae* or *C. trachomatis.*)
3. Persistence of symptoms in this setting is not an indication that the partner has been "unfaithful" and is reinfecting him.
4. For those with symptoms or increased numbers of polymorphonuclear leukocytes in urethral secretions, even without treatment the expected course is for manifestations to disappear over time.
5. The likelihood of long-term consequences such as infertility are exceedingly unlikely.

6. This problem is not a manifestation of acquired immunodeficiency syndrome (although it could coexist).
7. One episode of urethritis does not provide protection against subsequent episodes.

REFERENCES

1. Centers for Disease Control: 1989 sexually transmitted diseases treatment guidelines. *MMWR* 1989; 38(suppl 8):v-43.
2. Bowie WR, Alexander ER, Stimson JB, et al: Therapy for nongonococcal urethritis: Double-blind randomized comparison of two doses and two durations of minocycline. *Ann Intern Med* 1981; 95:306–311.
3. Krieger JN, Hooton TM, Brust PJ, et al: Evaluation of chronic urethritis: Defining the role for endoscopic procedures. *Arch Intern Med* 1988; 148:703–707.

20

Chlamydial Infection

Andrew W. Bruce, M.D.
Gregor Reid, Ph.D.

A 27-year-old man has come to you after having his second episode of left epididymitis. His internist had treated him for 10 days with ampicillin 2 months ago for the first episode. He improved, but the testicle began hurting and swelling 3 days ago. He is very discouraged. He has had sexual activity with three different women during the past 3 months, and 3 weeks ago he noted only slight morning discharge that lasted for 2 days. He has no other genitourinary history. On examination the left epididymis is enlarged (length 8 cm), firm, and tender at the upper pole. The left testis and cord and the right testis, epididymis, and cord are normal. Urinalysis is unremarkable, but the expressed prostatic secretions after prostatic massage have more than 35 white blood cells (WBCs)/high-power field (HPF). Cultures of urine and prostatic fluid are reported as "no growth."

INCIDENCE OF CHLAMYDIAL INFECTION

In a young patient with evidence of nonbacterial epididymitis, there should be a high suspicion of chlamydial etiology. This is particularly the case in a patient who is sexually active with numerous partners and has a history of recent urethral discharge. Berger et al.[1] reported 85% of patients less than 35 years of age with acute idiopathic epididymitis yielded *Chlamydia trachomatis* on culture. In a series of 18 patients with acute epididymitis involving all ages, our group[2] found a chlamydial incidence of 56% (33% yielded enterobacteria).

Chlamydial infection of the genitourinary system in young sexually active men and women has reached epidemic proportions in North America. Figures from the United States estimate that more than 3 to 4 million new cases of nongonococcal urethritis caused by *C. trachomatis* occur in males each year, along with more than 200,000 cases of epididymitis.[3] In other studies it has been estimated that one in six female teenagers harbor this organism, reflecting the 250,000 patients with chlamydial pelvic inflammatory disease discovered annually.[4–7] Indeed, these epidemiologic studies show that sexually transmitted chlamydial disease is significantly more common than gonococcal and herpes simplex virus infections. An association between prostatitis and chlamydia has also been documented,[2, 8] although the precise incidence at any one clinic is difficult to estimate.

CLINICAL HISTORY AND PHYSICAL EXAMINATION

Significant points include the presence or absence of irritative urinary symptoms, urethral discharge, and the occurrence of acute prostatitis symptoms. All of these may be associated with the primary complaint of scrotal pain and swelling. In the occasional patient there may be associated complaints of joint pains or conjunctivitis, suggestive of Reiter's syndrome.[9]

In addition to careful palpation of the testes, epididymides, and vasa deferentia, the urethral meatus should be inspected and the urethra gently massaged; if discharge is produced, it should be swabbed for microbiologic evaluation. A rectal examination is necessary to assess the consistency of the prostate, the presence or absence of tenderness, and whether the seminal vesicles are palpable. Based on history and signs, a decision may be made to take a prostate fluid swab for chlamydia testing.

Auxillary Examinations

If there is any doubt about the clinical diagnosis, a scrotal ultrasound should be carried out to exclude torsion, testicular neoplasia, and other epididymal pathologic conditions. Transrectal ultrasonography may also be employed to assess prostatic morphology and seminal vesicular size and appearance.

MICROBIOLOGICAL STUDIES

Microscopic Examination of Urethral, Prostatic, and Seminal Fluid

The primary use of microscopic examination is to evaluate WBC counts in urethral urine, expressed prostatic secretion, and seminal fluid specimens. The finding of less than 10 pus cells in urethral, urine, and EPS samples and significant numbers (>20/HPF) of WBCs in the seminal fluid indicates the likely presence of epididymitis. It should be noted, though, that pus cells in prostatic fluid increase after sexual activity and even with sexual excitement.[10]

The localization of infections in the male genitourinary tract is a controversial subject. The use of first voided urethral urine, bladder urine, expressed prostatic secretion after prostatic massage, and subsequent urine sequential cultures was designed to allow localization of infection to the urethra, bladder, and prostate. However, it is unclear if seminal fluid cultures can be used when prostatic fluid specimens are difficult to obtain. In addition, because of asymptomatic urethritis, a patient's urine specimens may not be tenfold lower than the prostatic fluid culture, making diagnosis of prostatitis difficult. In our experience, prostatitis can still be diagnosed clinically in conjunction with symptomatic and asymptomatic urethritis. In the case of chlamydial infection, this is not unusual, because the organisms infecting the prostate invariably have a urethral origin.

For a patient with acute epididymo-orchitis, chlamydial screening is effective by appropriate examination of seminal fluid or serum or aspiration of epididymal fluid.

To confirm chlamydial etiology and pathogenesis, one must rule out *Ureaplasma* and *Mycoplasma* species. Although commercial kits are available for this purpose, most urologists are best served sending specimens off for appropriate culture. Practically, the results take 2 to 3 weeks to achieve, and the organisms are sensitive to a similar spectrum of antimicrobials, as are chlamydia. Where culture facilities are not available, appropriate therapy may be given empirically.

Transportation and Culture Methods for *Chlamydia trachomatis*

An appropriate transport medium for chlamydia is needed and is generally provided by diagnostic laboratories. This medium includes a phosphate buffer to which glucose, fetal calf serum, glutamine, amphotericin B, gentamicin, streptomycin, and vancomycin are added.[8] Combined transport media for viruses and other sexually transmitted disease organisms are being investigated in some laboratories. Specimens of urethral swabs, EPS, seminal fluid, and urine can be used for chlamydial detection. Recent studies have indicated that urine sediments are good specimens for diagnosing *C. trachomatis* infection.[11] Semen is toxic for cell cultures and must first be diluted 1:5 before inoculation.

Culture

Tissue culture techniques are the traditional method used to verify the presence of active *C. trachomatis*. Specimens are inoculated into nonreplicating McCoy or HeLa 229 cells, which are then incubated in a carbon dioxide environment. The organisms multiply inside the cells and at 48 hours are identified as distinct inclusion bodies visible after fixation and staining with Giemsa, iodine, or fluorescinated monoclonal antibodies.

Other methods for identification of chlamydia can be of value, particularly in screening large numbers of specimens.

Immunofluorescent Staining

A direct specimen examination kit is available from various sources. Our experience with the MicroTrak Kit (Syva Diagnostics, Palo Alto, California) has been favorable,[6] although it is cautioned that this kit has received Food and Drug Administration approval for urethral and endocervical specimens only. The specimen is placed on a slide, fixed, then reacted with fluorescein conjugated–monoclonal antibody specific for chlamydia. Under an ultraviolet light source and $\times 100$ oil immersion power, distinct apple green label indicates the presence of immunofluorescent *C. trachomatis* organisms. The finding of one chlamydial elementary body indicates infection. The antibody detects all 15 human serovars of *C. trachomatis* in both the metabolically active reticular and infectious elementary forms.

Enzyme Immunoassays

A number of enzyme immunoassays (EIAs) are available, including the Chlamydiazyme (Abbott Laboratories, North Chicago, Ill.) and IDEIA (Cell-Tech Diagnostics, Slough, UK). These process the specimens in similar ways. In the case of Chlamydiazyme the specimen is added to a reaction tray well containing a treated bead that captures chlamydial antigens, which are detected with rabbit antibody to chlamydia and horseradish peroxidase–conjugated antibody to rabbit immunoglobulin G.[12] After addition of *o*-phenylenediamine substrate, a Quantum II spectrophotometer measures for significant increase in absorbance over controls. The IDEIA test uses a 96-well microtiter plate format and a monoclonal antibody. IDEIA detects chlamydial lipopolysaccharide (LPS), whereas Chlamydiazyme detects several antigenic components, including LPS.

Chlamydial Serology

Various detection systems measure IgG, IgM, and IgA antibodies to *C. trachomatis,* including a commercial test from Savyon diagnostics called IP-Azyme Chlamydia. Clinical studies have shown that the presence of elevated levels of IgG (1:128) and IgA (1:16) may indicate active chlamydial infection. IgA has a half-life of 6 days and may be present only during an active infection, whereas IgG antibody persists for life. It should be noted that although serology testing has been useful for genital tract infections in women,[13] few studies have been conducted to indicate a role for serology testing in men with urinary and genital tract infection. Antigen detection in men by culture, EIA, IF, or DNA probing (which is based on the DNA of the organisms, not serology) assays such as polymerase chain reaction should therefore be employed before serology testing is attempted. The DNA polymerase chain reaction method may well soon replace culture as the gold standard for detecting chlamydia.

It should be clearly stressed that the sensitivity of culture varies between laboratories and is greatly affected by specimen storage, temperature, and choice of swabs that may be toxic to chlamydia.[14] The choice of culture vs. antigen detection will depend on culture availability, expertise of the laboratory, test turn around time, and costs.

CLINICAL AND MICROBIOLOGIC ASSESSMENT OF SEXUAL PARTNERS

Certain principles apply to the assessment of sexual partners:

1. If there is only one partner, he or she should be investigated. This entails examination of urethral and cervical swab specimens.
2. If there are multiple sexual partners, individual examinations may not be possible. Every effort should be made to provide treatment for all at risk.
3. Emphasis should be made on the value of condom protection until all clinical and microbiologic evidence of disease have been eradicated.

TREATMENT OF *Chlamydia trachomatis* INFECTIONS

Choice of Antimicrobial Agent

Chlamydia trachomatis is exquisitely sensitive to the tetracycline group of drugs, and these are the first choice for medication. If the patient is allergic to these drugs, erythromycin[15] or trimethoprim-sulfamethoxazole may prove useful as alternative therapy.[8]

Duration of Therapy

The duration of treatment varies with the pathologic condition. Acute epididymo-orchitis requires a 3- to 4-week course of a tetracycline in full dosage (500 g four times daily). This generally produces a clinical and microbiologic cure.

Acute prostatitis may require a 6- to 8-week course of therapy, whereas acute urethritis usually responds to 7 to 10 days of adequate treatment.

Generally the same principles of therapy apply for sexual partners, with tetracyclines clearing the infection, assuming that they do not remain sexually active without condom protection. The presence of chlamydia in the urethra or cervix of asymptomatic women should be treated with 2 weeks of therapy. On the other hand, if there is symptomatic deep infection (pelvic inflammatory disease), a longer course of therapy or a regimen of more than one antibiotic will be necessary (3–4 weeks). In this situation, a gynecologic consultation should be obtained.

A major problem with treatment is compliance. Individuals with mild or no symptoms often stop taking medications after only 3 or 4 days of a 7- to 10-day course, especially if they see a cessation of urethral discharge. Patients with urethritis must be cautioned against doing this, because the full 7- to 10-day course is necessary to eradicate chlamydia; anything less will result in a recurrence of disease.

Clinical and Microbiological Follow-Up

It is preferable for all infected patients and sexual partners to be followed until they are clinically and microbiologically cleared of disease. In those patients with acute epididymo-orchitis, this involves marked resolution of the scrotal swelling and disappearance of tenderness. Symptomatic sexual partners should be free of symptoms, and repeat microbiologic tests (culture, immunofluorescence, enzyme assays for test of cure) should be carried out. In men with epididymo-orchitis, this should involve examination of seminal fluid. In the female partner, urethral and cervical swabs should be tested.

Acknowledgment

Supported by Physicians Services Incorporated, Toronto, Canada.

REFERENCES

1. Berger RE, Alexander ER, Monda GD, et al: *Chlamydia trachomatis* as a cause of acute "idiopathic" epididymitis. *N Engl J Med* 1978; 298:301.

2. Bruce AW, Chadwick P, Willett WS, et al: The role of chlamydiae in genitourinary disease. *J Urol* 1981; 126:625.
3. Centers for Disease Control: *Chlamydia trachomatis* infections, policy guidelines for prevention and control. *MMWR* 1985; 34:535.
4. Schachter J: Chlamydial infections. *N Engl J Med* 1978; 298:428, 490, 540.
5. Centers for Disease Control: *Chlamydia trachomatis* infections. *MMWR* 1985; 34 (suppl): 535.
6. Sweet RL, Schachter J, Landers DV: Chlamydial infections in obstetrics and gynecology. *Clin Obstet Gynecol* 1983; 26:143.
7. Golden NM, Hammerschlag M, Neuhoff S, et al: Prevalence of *Chlamydia trachomatis* cervical infections in female adolescents. *Am J Dis Child* 1984; 138:562.
8. Bruce AW, Reid G: Prostatitis associated with *Chlamydia trachomatis* in 6 patients. *J Urol* 1989; 142:1006.
9. Calin A: Spondyloarthropathies: An overview, in Calin A (ed): Spondyloarthropathies. Orlando, Fla, Grune & Stratton, 1984, pp 1–8.
10. Jameson RM: Sexual activity and the variations of the white cell content of the prostatic secretion. *Invest Urol* 1967; 5:297.
11. Chernesky M, Castriciano S, Sellors J, et al: Detection of *Chlamydia trachomatis* antigens in urine as an alternative to swabs and cultures. *J Infect Dis* 1990; 161:124.
12. Mahony J, Castriciano S, Sellors J, et al: Diagnosis of *Chlamydia trachomatis* genital infections by cell culture and two enzyme immunoassays detecting different chlamydial antigens. *J Clin Microbiol* 1989; 27:1934.
13. Sellors JW, Mahony JB, Chernesky MA, et al: Tubal factor infertility: An association with prior chlamydial infection and asymptomatic salpingitis. *Fertil Steril* 1988; 49:451.
14. Mahony JB, Chernesky MA: Effects of swab type and storage temperature on the isolation of *Chlamydia trachomatis* from clinical specimens. *J Clin Microbiol* 1985; 22:865.
15. Blenk H, Blenk B, Diemann E: Erythromycin treatment of acute and chronic urethritis, prostatitis and colpitis caused by *Ureaplasma urealyticum* and *Chlamydia trachomatis*. *J Int Med Res* 1980; 8(suppl 2):59–63.

PART TWO

Urinary Stones

21

Acute Stone Episode

George W. Drach, M.D.

You have been called to the emergency room to see this 42-year-old man who developed left renal colic while visiting your city. He has a lengthy history of urolithiasis, but he has failed to follow any treatment regimen. His vital signs are normal, and he is afebrile. Your physical examination reveals significant percussion and palpation tenderness of the left flank. The patient is writhing in pain. Urinalysis indicates many red blood cells per high-power field but is otherwise normal. The x-ray film of the kidneys, ureters, and bladder (KUB) shows at least three left renal calculi, the largest being 1.5 cm (upper pole), and two pelvic stones, 1.4 and 1.2 cm. Two small (3–5 mm) stones sit in the midportion of the right kidney. Analgesics are given, and the patient has an intravenous pyelogram (IVP) performed. It shows delayed function with hydronephrosis behind the 1.2-cm ureteropelvic junction stone. The patient wants you to proceed with whatever treatment is necessary.

Many of our patients with life-long urolithiasis deny their disease and then arrive in the emergency room with one obstructing calculus and evidence of many other nonobstructing calculi. This patient is fortunate that his stones have recurred after 1980, when shock wave lithotripsy was discovered by C. Chaussy (see Chapter 37). But first let us analyze his present needs and propose his immediate management.

I am always cautious when I am called to the emergency room to see a patient "from elsewhere" because of kidney stones. Individuals addicted to drugs may use symptoms and signs of stone disease as a means of obtaining drugs by faking stone disease. To create a high likelihood of true stone disease, I require a minimum of typical colicky pain, some abdominal or flank tenderness, hematuria seen in a reliably collected specimen, and findings consistent with stone within the area of the urinary tract on a KUB film. This patient fulfills these criteria, so I would recommend that he receive immediate pain medication. He may require 10 mg of morphine intramuscularly, followed by 5 mg more in about 30 minutes, before his pain is somewhat relieved. Some patients may require double the usual dosage of narcotics before renal colic can be relieved. After he is comfortable, an IVP (urogram) is obtained to assess the degree of obstruction. Ultrasound imaging or radioisotope scanning would be suitable alternatives to IVP.

This patient did not have any evidence of urinary infection in association with his acute renal colic. If the patient had fever, evidence of sepsis, or pyuria with bacteriuria, relief of his renal obstruction becomes an urgent matter. Broad-spectrum antibiotics and IV fluids should be given immediately. Percutaneous nephrostomy or insertion of a ureteral catheter or stent with the patient under local anesthesia allows drainage and promotes recovery of the kidney. After the patient's condition has improved, specific treatment of the stones follows.

Administration of IV fluids to stone patients is common practice. Certainly persistent vomiting can cause dehydration and require fluid replacement. If no vomiting has occurred, I see no reason for giving fluids intravenously. Most patients can take satisfactory amounts of oral fluids along with analgesics or narcotics, and they can be managed as outpatients. One bit of advice to the patient can be very helpful: They should take their analgesics as soon as the colic threatens to return. Those who wait until the colic is overwhelmingly severe will not be able to control the pain with oral medications alone.

What is the likelihood that his stones will pass? Figure 21–1 summarizes the decision processes associated with deciding whether to obtain (1) a urologic consultation (which had already been decided in this patient) and (2) pathways toward definitive treatment based on stone size.

From Figure 21–1, we see that it is unlikely that his impacted left renal stone will pass spontaneously. The remaining nonimpacted stones will not pass

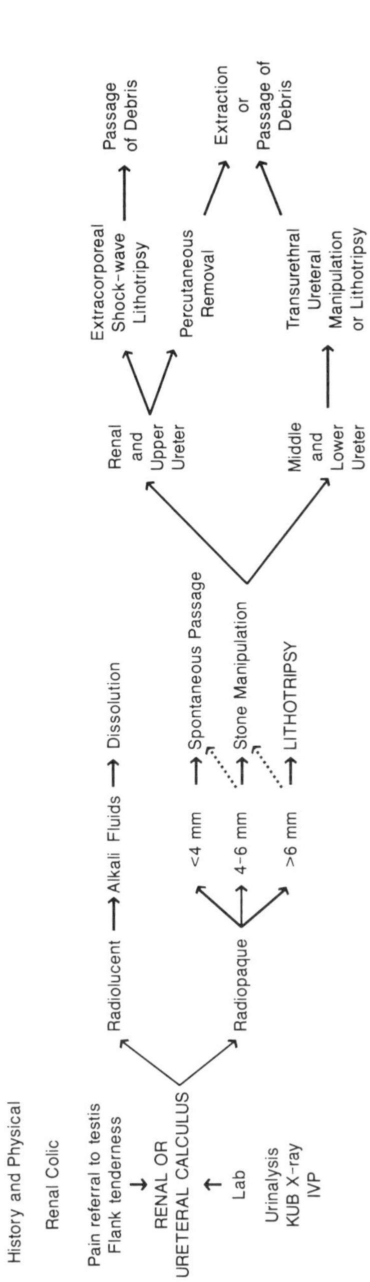

FIG 21–1.
Decision pathways for the acute stone episode.

either. Hence, some procedural treatment must be considered. This patient wanted definitive therapy immediately. If, however, he wanted to delay such treatment, one could offer him insertion of a ureteral stent to relieve obstruction and avoid renal damage. I have certainly done this when the patient had important business to complete within the next few days. I do not like to let stone obstruction go beyond 2 weeks without some type of drainage.

This patient has a total stone burden (sum of linear greatest diameters of stones) of 4.1 cm. Some specialists might suggest percutaneous removal because of this large stone burden. Others would recommend extracorporeal shock wave lithotripsy. Again, in view of the large stone burden, most urologists would insert a ureteral stent peroperatively to try to avoid posttreatment ureteral obstruction by stone fragments (see Chapter 40). In addition, this patient should require more than one treatment to the left kidney, because the large burden of stones might break slowly or incompletely at the first treatment session.

What treatment should be directed at the right renal stones? The 3-mm stone could pass spontaneously (see Fig 21–1), but the 5-mm stone has only a 50% chance of spontaneous passage. Also, the data summarized in Figure 21–1 are accumulated for single stones. Multiple calculi, if they become impacted in the ureter, are less likely to pass spontaneously. For this reason, one should recommend shock wave therapy of the right renal stones also. Should bilateral treatment be done simultaneously? I prefer not to do so. I have had too many problems and complications with patients who had bilateral treatments.

Let us assume that this patient undergoes successful insertion of a left ureteral stent and eliminates all of his left stone burden after two treatments and his right stones after one treatment (done without a stent). His stones are pure calcium oxalate. He is more compliant now and wants some recommendations about prophylactic therapy. He should have a brief metabolic evaluation of some kind either in your office or by one of the commercially available packages. Then you can recommend therapy that will help to avoid recurrences. Present methods of medical therapy can eliminate new stone formation or growth of existing stones 80% to 90% of the time. It would seem worth the effort if I were the patient.

BIBLIOGRAPHY

Coe FL, Boyce WH, Friedman GD, et al: Consensus conference: Prevention and treatment of kidney stones. *J Urol* 1989; 141:804–808.

Drach GW, Dretler S, Fair W, et al: Report of the United States cooperative study of extracorporeal shock wave lithotripsy. *J Urol* 1986; 135:1127–1133.

Pak CYC: Role of medical prevention. *J Urol* 1989; 141:798–801.

22

Uric Acid Stones

F. A. Fried, M.D.

ANALYSIS OF DISEASE PROCESS

Uric acid stones are found in 8% of patients with urolithiasis in the United States[1] and Great Britain.[2] The development of uric acid stones is caused by the lack of the enzyme uricase, which metabolizes uric acid to more soluble allantoin.[3] Uric acid exists in two forms in urine: free uric acid, which is poorly soluble, and salts or urates of sodium and potassium, which are 20 times as soluble. The pK_a of uric acid is 5.75. At this pH, uric acid exists in amounts equal to those of the free acid and the more soluble urates. Patients with a urine pH consistently less than 5.75 will have more of the less soluble free acid in their urine and are therefore at an increased risk for developing uric acid stones.[4]

In addition to the urinary pH, the development of uric acid stones is also related to the amount of uric acid excreted by the kidneys and the urine volume. The average man excretes approximately 400 mg of uric acid daily; women excrete a somewhat lower value.

Uric acid excretion is the result of both endogenous uric acid production and exogenous intake of uric acid, most often attributed to eating large amounts of red meat and foods high in purine content. The 24-hour urine volume is a key factor in prevention of stones of all types.[5, 6] Increasing the urine volume is thought to have two beneficial effects: (1) increased volume produces a more dilute urine with regard to stone-forming agents and would prevent crystallization; and (2) the increased rate of flow through the kidney reduces the amount of time that a free particle resides in the kidney, thereby decreasing the opportunity for it to reach a size great enough for it to become arrested in the collecting ducts of the renal papillae. Of prime importance is the ability of the urine to maintain uric acid in solution. As mentioned earlier, the solubility of uric acid is greatly influenced by the urinary pH. It has been shown that at a pH of 5.0, 1 L of urine can hold about 60 mg of uric acid in solution; however, when the pH is raised to 6.0, 200 mg can be held in solution, and at a pH of 7.0, the amount held in solution jumps to 1,500 mg. The effect of pH on uric acid solubility forms the basis for treatment and prevention of uric acid stones (Figs 22–1 and 22–2).

CLINICAL CASE 1

A 62-year-old woman has had renal colic, followed by passage of a 3- to 4-mm uric acid stone about once yearly for the past 4 years. Her prior evaluations showed normal values for serum electrolytes, blood urea nitrogen, (BUN), creatinine, and uric acid. Urinary uric acid output is 750 mg/day on two occasions. She denies intake of excessive red meats, but she does eat many legumes and nuts. Her only medication is a daily nonsteroidal anti-inflammatory drug for chronic arthritis. Your evaluation confirms normal serum values and hyperuricosuria. Her measure-

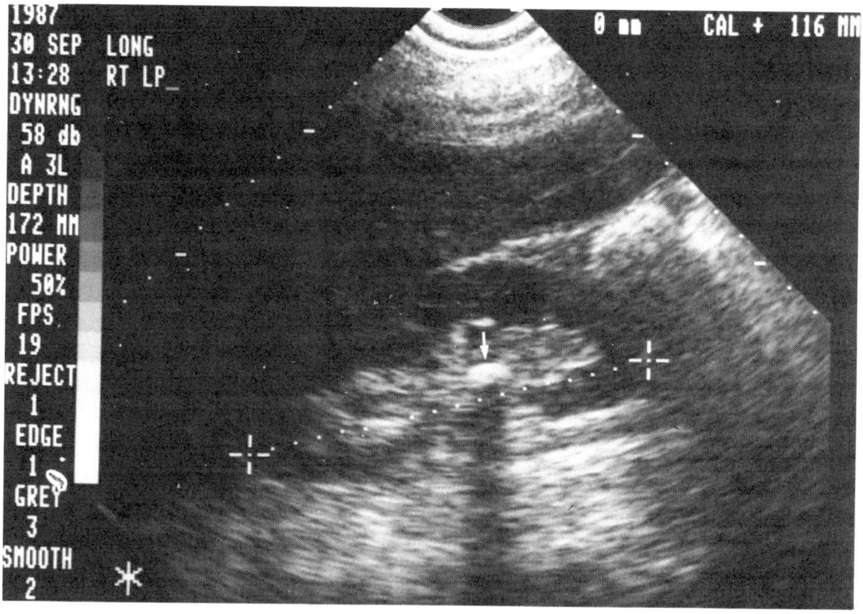

FIG 22–1.
Renal ultrasound demonstrates calculus in right kidney *(arrow)* with characteristic acoustic shadowing.

ment of pH of voided urines for 5 days reveals no value greater than 6.0, and her volume output per day is always less than 1 L. In the past she had been given allopurinol daily but had another stone, so she stopped taking the allopurinol.

Specific Factors

Even though the patient has a normal serum level of uric acid and normal electrolyte levels, several factors contribute to her formation of uric acid stones. First, the 24-hour excretion of uric acid is very high—750 mg. Second, her 24-hour urine volume is consistently less than 1 L. Third, she is taking a nonsteroidal anti-inflammatory agent for management of "arthritis," which may result in increased excretion of uric acid and may also lower the urinary pH. Fourth, she has been found to have a consistently acid urinary pH. Fifth, she may have gout.

Recommendations for Further Evaluation

Intravenous (IV) urography is needed to determine the presence of additional silent uric acid stones and possible renal obstruction. Appropriate skeletal films

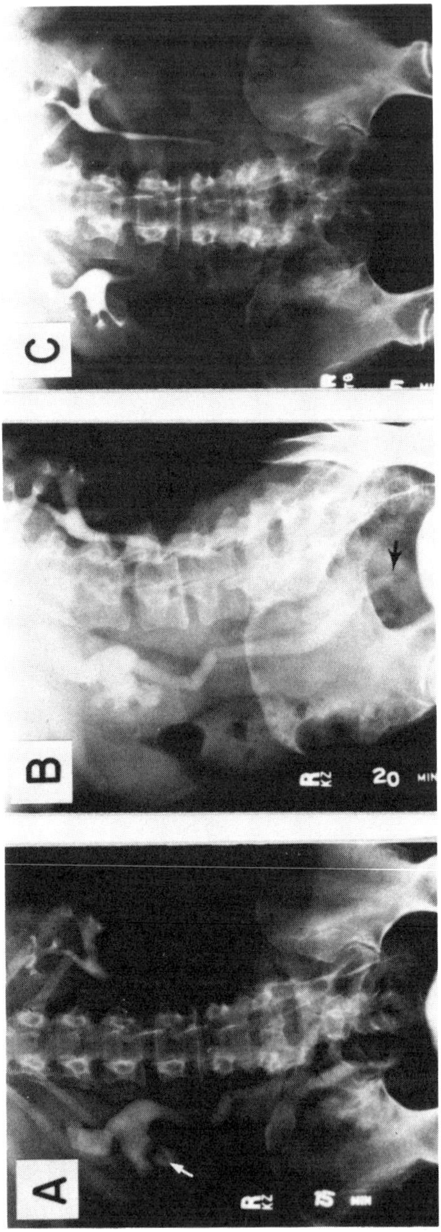

FIG 22–2.
Intravenous pyelogram of patient seen in Figure 22–1. **A,** filling defect seen in lower pole collecting system *(arrow)*. **B,** ureteral obstruction caused by poorly seen lucent defect in the lower ureter *(arrow)*. **C,** IVP after 6 months of alkalization therapy shows resolution of hydronephrosis and collecting system filling defect.

should be obtained to determine the nature of the arthritis. The very high excretion of uric acid suggests the possibility of an underlying myeloproliferative disease, and so at the very least a careful physical examination looking for abnormal lymphadenopathy and splenomegaly should be performed.

Recommendations for Therapy

Increased fluid intake is the cornerstone of any therapeutic program for stone disease and certainly so in this patient who has a 24-hour urine volume of less than 1 L as determined on several occasions. It has been shown that the chances of forming new stones when the 24-hour urine volume is consistently greater than 2 L are much reduced.

This patient is a prime candidate for alkalization therapy. Alkalization is not only of benefit in preventing new stones from developing but also has been shown to be effective in the dissolution of existing uric acid stones. A simple way to achieve alkalization is with the use of sodium bicarbonate, which is available in tablets of 600 mg. My preference is to instruct patients in the use of Nitrazine paper and have them monitor their urine pH for 2 days before starting therapy. Patients are then instructed to take 1.2 g every 4 hours (except nights). A urine pH should be checked immediately before the next dose is taken. If the pH is less than 6.5, they increase the dose by one tablet; if the pH is less than 6.0, they increase the dose by two tablets. Patients quickly learn the proper dose, and usually only minor alterations are needed. If the patient is hypertensive and sodium intake is an issue, alternative agents for alkalization include potassium citrate, which is available as Polycitra-K. Regardless of the agent used, the patient should continue to monitor the urine pH and should be instructed about the signs of metabolic alkalosis, such as hyperventilation.

If the patient cannot tolerate alkalization or if stones continue to be a problem in the face of adequate therapy, further reduction of urine levels of uric acid could be achieved by the use of allopurinol, but I have not found this to be necessary. The patient should understand that stones may continue to pass after treatment has been started and that this does not indicate a failure of therapy but may simply represent stones that have formed before the initiation of therapy.

A low-purine diet will probably not make a significant difference in this patient because her dietary history does not indicate that she consumes large amounts of purines.

CLINICAL CASE 2

This patient is a 59-year-old insulin-dependent diabetic man who has a long history of bladder outlet obstructive symptoms. In the past he has had a pyelolithotomy for a uric acid stone and has since experienced several episodes of flank pain reminiscent of renal colic. His laboratory evaluation reveals normal values for serum electrolytes, creatinine (1.2 mg/dL), BUN (20 mg/dL), and uric acid (8.5 mg/dL). A urine sediment shows more than 100 red blood cells/high-power field. A urine culture is sterile. The 24-hour urine chemistry values are 180 mg of calcium and 700 mg of uric acid. The volume ranges from 800 to 1,100 mL/24 hours. The urine pH has never been found to be more than 5.5, and there are a moderate amount of ketones consistently present. An IV pyelogram (IVP) demonstrates normal upper urinary tracts. The bladder film shows a radiolucent defect consistent with a uric acid stone, as well as a large prostate and poor bladder emptying. His physical examination is noteworthy for lower extremity sensory defects. The prostate is moderately enlarged, but there are no nodules palpable.

Specific Factors

As in the first case, multiple factors are involved in the development of uric acid stones. First, this patient's urine is conducive to uric acid stone growth because of low volume, low pH, and elevated urinary uric acid excretion. In addition, the patient has bladder neck obstructive symptoms, which presumably caused the development of a uric acid bladder stone.

Recommendation for Further Evaluation

Cystoscopy is needed to clarify the bladder-filling defect seen on the IVP, as well as to evaluate the bladder neck area regarding the likelihood of benign prostate hypertrophy. The physical findings in a diabetic patient raise the question of a possible neurogenic bladder, which may be the origin of voiding difficulties and in a relatively young patient should be evaluated with urodynamic studies.

Recommendations for Therapy

Better control of the diabetes is important in that it may help reduce the urinary acidity. A transurethral resection of the prostate should be considered in view of the finding of bladder stone.

Because this patient is hyperuricemic, he should be treated with 300 mg of allopurinol/day. If tighter control of the diabetes results in higher urinary pH, it may not be necessary to add alkalization. However, if there is no appreciable change in the urinary pH, I would also favor alkalization therapy. Finally, there is no substitute for adequate fluid intake. As discussed earlier, the patient should measure his 24-hour urine output and adjust his fluid intake to achieve an output of at least 1.5 to 2 L daily. His diet should be reviewed to determine his adherence to a diabetic diet and the avoidance of foods rich in purines. Active stone-forming patients need to be followed periodically to help them remain on the stone preventive program and to determine that no new stones are developing.

REFERENCES

1. Prien EL Sr, Gershoff SF: Magnesium oxide–pyridoxine therapy for recurrent calcium oxalate calculi. *J Urol* 1974; 112:509.
2. Westbury EJ: Some observations on the quantitative analysis of over 1000 urinary calculi. *Br J Urol* 1974; 46:215.
3. Yu F: Urolithiasis in hyperuricemia and gout. *J Urol* 1981; 126:424.
4. Cifuentes L, Rapado A, Abehsera A, et al: Uric acid lithiasis and gout, in *Urinary Calculi: International Symposium on Renal Stone Research*. Basel, S Karger, 1973, p 115.
5. Drach G: Urolithiasis, in Conn HF (ed): *Current Therapy*. Philadelphia, WB Saunders Co, 1976, p 552.
6. Finlayson B: Symposium on renal lithiasis. Renal lithiasis in review. *Urol Clin North Am* 1974;1:181.

23

Cystine Stones

George W. Drach, M.D.

A 34-year-old man consults you because of problems with continued cystine stone formation even though he follows his regimen of alkalization and high-fluid intake very well. His first stone occurred at age 17 years. Since then he has had an average of two stones per year. Four open surgical operations, two extracorporeal shock wave lithotripsy (ESWL) treatments, and seven ureteral stone removals have been necessary to remove impacted stones. His serum creatinine level is normal, and creatinine clearance is 96 mL/minute (corrected). Urinary cystine excretion averages 1,200 mg/day. D-Penicillamine therapy resulted in development of severe nephrosis even when slow adaption therapy was attempted. Your tests of urinary pH always indicate 8.0, and his measured 24-hour urinary output is 3,800 mL. He is very discouraged about his continued stone formation.

This patient illustrates several important points in the management of recurrent cystine urinary lithiasis. First, he has had multiple procedures for his stones. Although extracorporeal shock wave lithotripsy (ESWL) was attempted, it was poorly successful, and other procedures were needed for removal of calculi. Second, he seems to be conforming to the usual admonitions of high-water intake to increase urinary output. In addition, he must be taking alkali, because it is not possible to achieve a urinary pH of 8.0 unless there is some outside source of alkali. Finally, it is unfortunate that he cannot tolerate D-penicillamine. Most patients with urinary cystine excretions of more than 600 to 800 mg/day will require oral medications to complex urinary cystine if we are to maximize their therapy.

BACKGROUND

Before we propose the treatment program for this patient, let us review the background of cystine urolithiasis. Cystinuria represents a complex inherited defect in renal reabsorption of four amino acids: cystine, ornithine, lysine, and arginine. One easy way to remember them is to combine their first letters into the mnemonic COLA. Overexcretion of cystine results in urinary oversaturation, especially at pH less than 7.8. As mentioned earlier, urine normally does not achieve this high pH, so crystallization of cystine occurs easily. Loss of the other three amino acids has no effect on the urine or on the patient, except perhaps to lead to decreased growth and smaller than average body stature.

Normal persons may excrete as much as 100 mg of urinary cystine each day. Persons who are heterozygous for a single allele of cystinuria do show evidence of hyperexcretion of the four amino acids in their urine, but the expression of the gene is variable. Hence, experts divide this type of heterozygote state into three types. Type I patients have normal amounts of aminoaciduria because the gene is completely recessive. Types II and III are incompletely recessive, and afflicted persons excrete amounts of cystine that vary from 150 to 300 mg/day. These individuals rarely form calculi. The cystinuric patient must excrete more than 600 mg/day before calculi form. These stone-forming patients are either pure homozygotes (e.g., they have alleles I/I, II/II or III/III) or compound heterozygotes with various allele combinations, such as I/III.

Further investigation of the amino acid transport defect in these patients reveals that it exists in the intestinal mucosa and the renal tubular cells. The incidence of clinically evident cystinuria is estimated at about 1 in 20,000 persons. Because urinary stone disease of all types occurs at a rate of about 3 to 4 out of 100 persons, one can see why cystine stone disease represents only a small portion of urolithiasis. It accounts for only 2% to 3% of all stones.

Urine can maintain about 300 to 400 mg of cystine soluble in 1 L of urine, within the normal urinary pH range of 4.5 to 7.0. Another method of estimating solubility predicts that patients can maintain 180 mg soluble per gram of creatinine. However, as mentioned earlier, elevation of the pH to 7.8 or higher almost doubles the solubility of cystine in urine. These observations will lead us to the "cornerstone therapy" of urinary dilution and alkalization.

PATIENT EVALUATION

Certain hints can predict a higher possibility of cystinuria in a stone patient: prior cystinuria in family members, recurrent disease in patients less than 30 years of age, and characteristic mildly dense "ground glass" calculi. Observation of the characteristic hexagonal crystals in acid or cooled urine also predicts cystinuria. The cyanide nitroprusside screening test for cystinuria can detect concentrations of cystine that exceed 75 mg/g of creatinine. Unfortunately, false positive reactions to this test occur in single allele heterozygotes or because of disulfide-containing medications. Therefore, one must perform a confirmatory quantitative total urinary cystine test for 24 hours if the diagnosis is to be assessed. This measurement of total cystine levels also aids the physician in developing the therapeutic plan.

THERAPY

Cystinurics who excrete 300 to 800 mg/day can usually be controlled by alkalization of the urine to pH more than 7.8, along with substantial water drinking to assure urinary output in excess of 4 L/day. A total of 60 to 80 mL of balanced citrate solution in three or four equally divided doses per day should produce adequate alkalization. As an alternative, patients may ingest 12.6 g or more of sodium bicarbonate, again in divided doses. Patients should initially keep a chart of pH of each voided urine throughout the day. Once they have achieved a stable pH of 8, they need to test the urine only daily on arising.

Water drinking is a habit learned early in childhood. To change this habit requires effort. I usually advise the patients to place a pitcher or other container of 3 to 4 L of water in their office and home. They must drink 250 mL of water every 2 hours while awake (averaging 3,200 mL) and awaken and drink at least 500 mL during sleep. Usually they awaken because they need to urinate. If this does not occur, they must set an alarm clock to awaken them during sleep.

Methionine is the most direct metabolic precursor of cystine. Dietary restriction of methionine results in a very unpalatable diet for most patients. I have used a methionine-restricted diet as a last resort in patients who cannot be controlled by usual methods of treatment.

D-Penicillamine (Cuprimine) offers some hope to cystine stone formers who cannot control their stone formation by the previous methods. It is most often needed in the management of patients who excrete more than 800 to 1,000 mg of cystine daily or to speed attempts at dissolving calculi. It is administered orally at doses up to 1.5 g per day in divided doses. This usually reduces urinary cystine excretion to less than 400 mg/day. This results because urinary cystine in the presence of D-penicillamine forms a soluble cystine–*S*-penicillamine complex. The relative effectiveness of this therapy can be estimated with the nitroprusside test noted earlier or by testing for penicillamine disulfide with a 3% iron chloride solution. Use of penicillamine is limited by a number of allergic reactions; arthralgias, rash, nephrotic syndrome, and fatigue are some of the more common reactions. In addition, drug cost is high.

α-Mercaptopropionylglycine (MPG) now may be used to treat patients with cystinuria. Once again, cystine excretion in a benign form occurs because of formation of thiol disulfide compounds with cystine. Daily dosages range from 300 to 1,500 mg/day in divided doses for prophylaxis. Stone dissolution requires 600 to 1,800 mg of MPG/day. Side effects are minimized by gradual introduction of increasing dosages. It appears that this drug carries less risk of side effects than D-penicillamine.

Complete therapy for cystine stone disease therefore involves substantial urinary dilution, adequate urinary alkalization to pH more than 7.8, occasional medications such as D-penicillamine or MPG, and rarely dietary restriction of methionine.

MANAGEMENT OF THIS PATIENT

Fluid administration and alkalization in this patient seem to be adequate, yet his stone formation continues. Total cystine excretion is about 1,200 mg/day. It is not surprising that fluids and alkali alone are not successful. He is allergic to D-penicillamine, even though gradual adaption therapy was attempted. We must try therapy with MPG. Dosages should be started at 300 mg/day and increased weekly by 300 mg/day until a total daily dose of 1,500 mg has been achieved. This should arrest new stone formation. Urine testing for cystine should indicate reduction of free cystine to less than 300 to 400 mg/day when dosage is adequate.

Therapy may fail, and then procedural or surgical treatment becomes necessary. This is illustrated by a young cystinuria patient who I began treating at age 8 years. She had bilateral complex cystine calculi (Fig 23–1). She was placed on fluid and alkali therapy, and stone growth slowed, but no dissolution occurred. She tolerated D-penicillamine well, and on this therapy the stone on the left dissolved during about 1½ years of treatment (Fig 23–2). The right

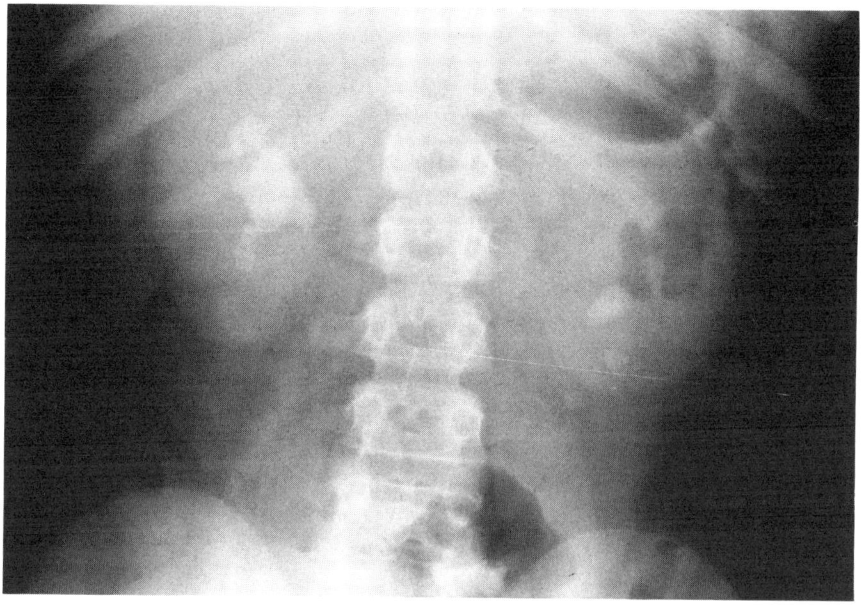

FIG 23–1.
Plain film of abdomen reveals staghorn right kidney stone and three individual lower pole stones of left kidney.

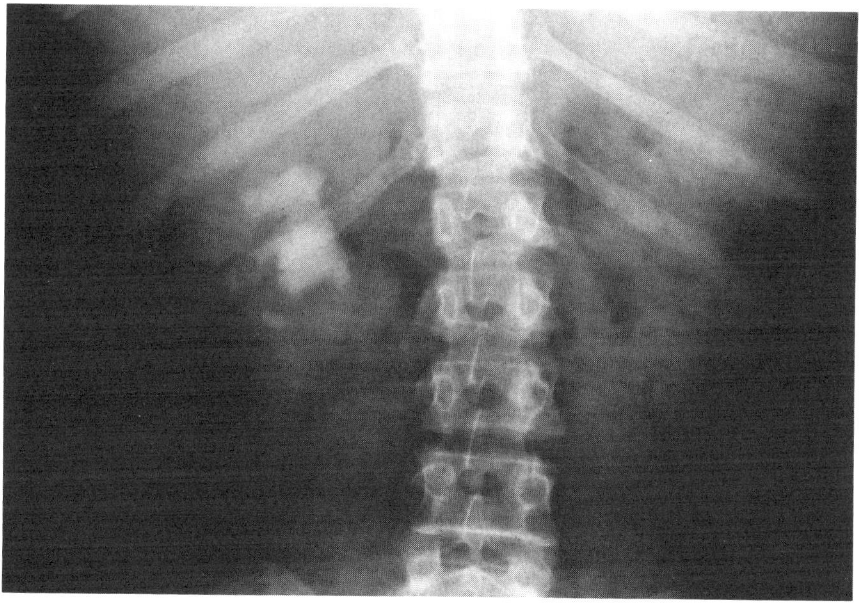

FIG 23–2.
After therapy with D-penicillamine, left renal stones have dissolved, but right renal stone has enlarged.

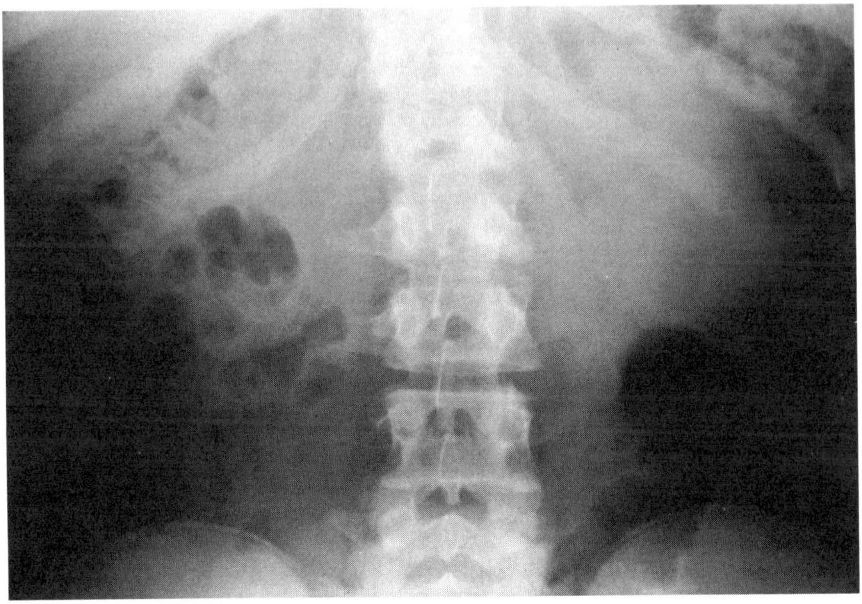

FIG 23–3.
Right staghorn calculus removed surgically. No new stones appear in this film 1½ years after surgery.

renal stone did not dissolve. It was removed by extended pyelolithotomy and proved to be 100% cystine (Fig 23–3). Individual renal function by radionuclide studies is equal, so I have no good explanation for the failure of dissolution of the right stone. This patient remains stone free after another 1½ years, and she illustrates the need for use of all modalities in treatment of cystinuria.

24

Infection-Induced Staghorn Stones

Donald P. Griffith, M.D.

MS, a 42-year-old healthy woman, was seen in 1984 with a 2-year history of recurrent urinary tract infection (UTI). Her symptoms consisted of frequency, urgency, and intermittent low-grade fever (temperature of 38.4°C). She complained of some pain in the left flank. The screening intravenous (IV) urogram is shown in Figure 24–1. Several urine cultures demonstrated *Proteus mirabilis* with a colony count of greater than 10^5 colony-forming units/mL. Her urine pH was 7.8. The patient was considered to be a candidate for percutaneous lithotripsy, surgical nephrolithotomy, and possible extracorporeal shock wave lithotripsy (ESWL). Because of recent publicity, the patient was strongly motivated to undergo ESWL. She did so on Oct. 1, 1984. Twelve hours later she developed severe left flank tenderness with pain and temperature of 39.5°C. Because of the impending urosepsis, she underwent cystoscopy and a ureteral catheter replacement (Fig 24–2). Purulent urine drained. On Oct. 3, 1984, percutaneous nephrostomy was performed on an elective basis. On Oct. 8, 1984, the patient underwent a second ESWL, followed by removal of the ureteral catheter. On Nov. 16, 1984, a third ESWL was performed. On Dec. 18, 1984, only a small quantity of stone debris remained in the kidney, and the nephrostomy tube was removed. The patient remained asymptomatic and underwent routine follow-up studies 6 weeks later (Fig 24–3). The follow-up urogram revealed a small amount of residual stone but no kidney function. Retrograde pyelographic studies demonstrated obstruction to the left ureter. Stone debris was removed ureteroscopically, and a silicone stent was placed (Fig 24–4). This stent was removed several weeks later. The patient remained asymptomatic and received maintenance therapy of 250 mg of amoxicillin three times daily and 250 mg of acetohydroxamic acid (AHA) three times daily for 4 months.

A urogram in June 1985 showed her to be stone free with good kidney function. Urine was sterile when she was receiving antibiotics and AHA. When the drugs were discontinued, the patient did not have follow-up testing for bacteriuria. Eighteen months later symptomatic UTI occurred and was treated appropriately. However, the infection recurred, and in June 1987 a recurrent stone (7 mm) was identified in the left kidney (Fig 24–5).

A fourth ESWL procedure performed in August 1987 left the patient stone free. Antibiotics and AHA were continued for 6 weeks. After discontinuation of medical therapy, urine cultures were made at 3-month intervals for the next year. All were sterile after antibiotics were discontinued.

Radiographic studies in 1989 (see Fig 24–5) were normal, and the patient's urine remained sterile without antibiotic therapy.

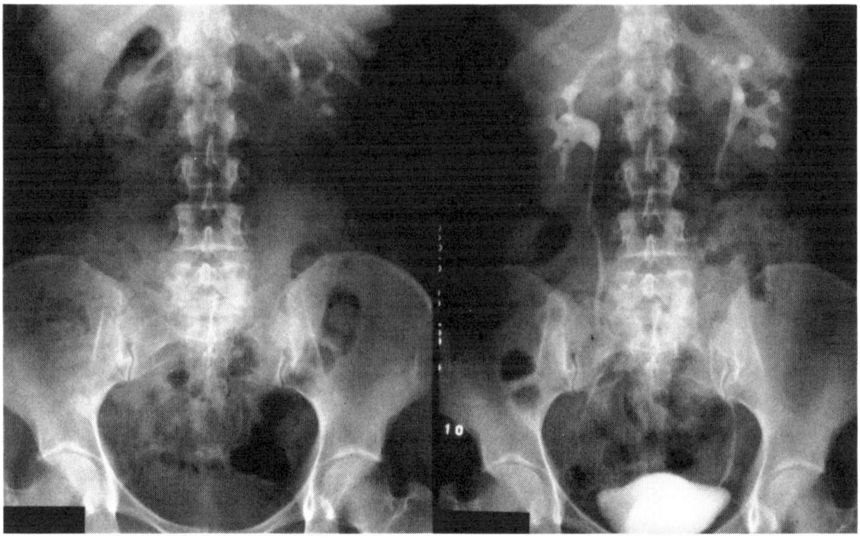

FIG 24–1.
Radiograph of KUB *(left)* and IV pyelogram (IVP) *(right)* before ESWL no. 1.

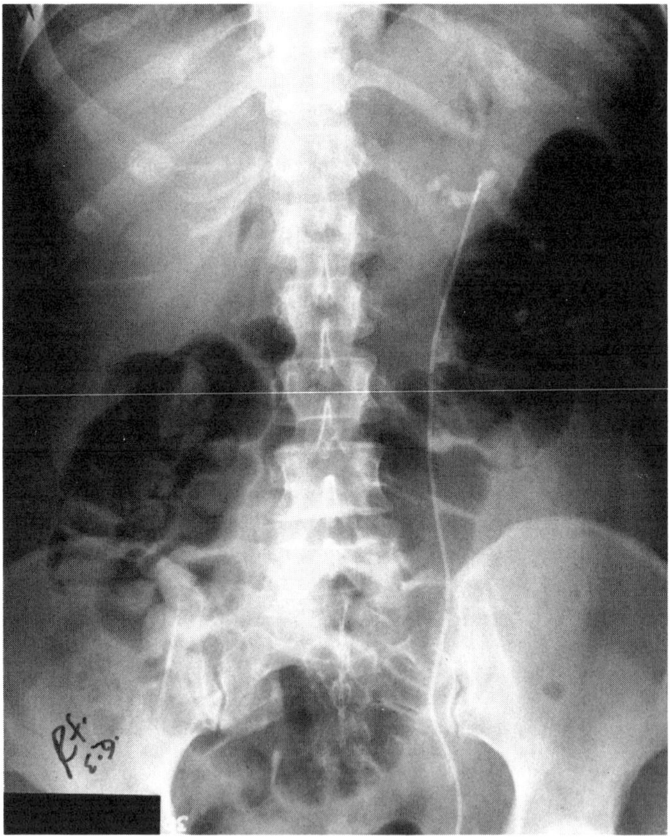

FIG 24–2.
Radiograph of KUB 1 day after ESWL no. 1.

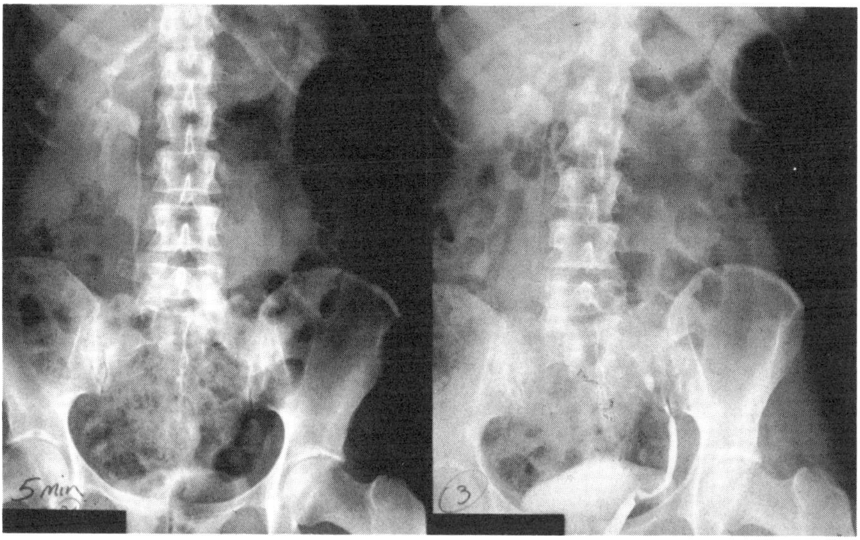

FIG 24–3.
Left, IVP and, *right,* retrograde pyelogram.

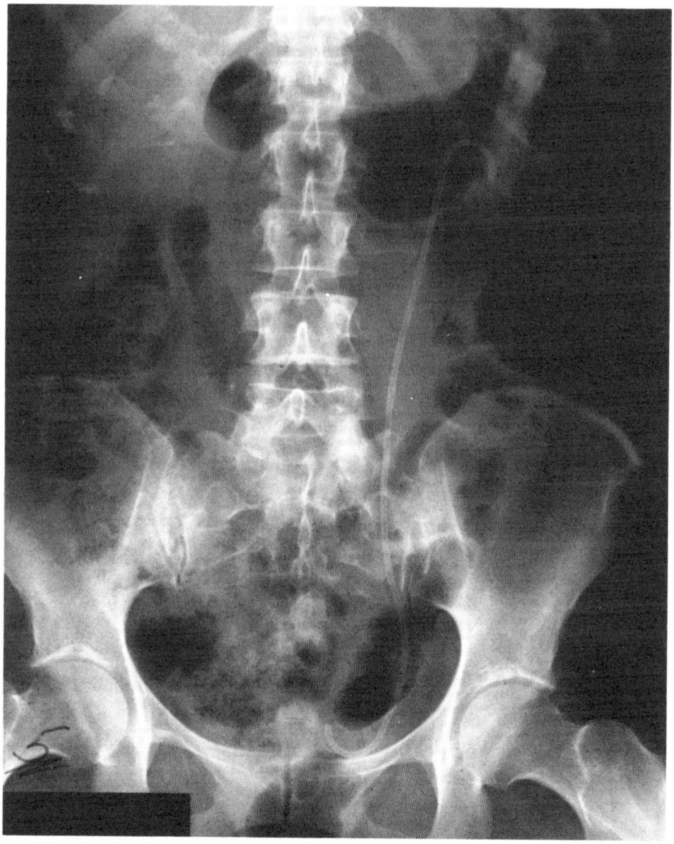

FIG 24–4.
Internal stent with stone debris on KUB radiograph.

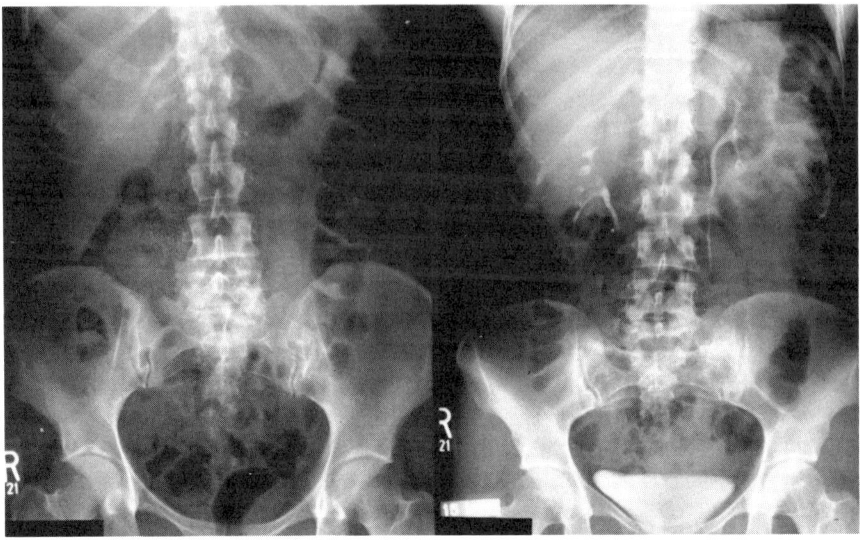

FIG 24–5.
Radiograph of KUB *(left)* and IVP *(right)* after ESWL no. 3 (1989).

DISCUSSION

Considerations of Surgical Management

The initial clinical trials of ESWL in the United States were in progress in October 1984. The patient under discussion was considered to be a marginal candidate. However, she had no interest in nephrolithotomy and insisted on ESWL as her primary treatment. Percutaneous lithotripsy through two puncture sites was the original recommendation. Secondary ESWL was anticipated. However, primary ESWL was undertaken as a consequence of patient insistence.

Complications of ESWL

This case illustrates both a symptomatic and an asymptomatic steinstrasse. This case also illustrates the problems encountered in treating large stones with primary ESWL, namely, problems with particle passage and a need for repeated ESWL procedures. For such cases I currently favor primary percutaneous lithotripsy using multiple access tracts. If patients insist on primary ESWL despite extensive education about the problems involved, I will use it. However, I routinely place one to two ureteral catheters or detachable catheters (KWART, Cook Urological, Spencer, Ind.) preoperatively. I maintain external irrigation for 24 to 48 hours after lithotripsy, during which time much of the struvite debris passes; repetitive catheter irrigation usually is required to prevent catheter obstruction. After passage of most of the stone debris, the external irrigating extension is detached and the internal stent is left in situ for several weeks, during which the need for further treatment is assessed. Elimination of all stone debris is more likely in patients with sharp delicate calyceal systems than in patients with ectatic blunted calyceal systems.[1]

In the absence of routine follow-up, this patient might have experienced permanent loss of most of the function in the left kidney because of the "silent steinstrasse."

Suppression of UTI with penicillin and AHA was successful between February and June of 1985. However, discontinuation of these medications and inadequate follow-up the following year resulted in persistent infection and recurrent stone formation. Bacteriologic follow-up in 1988 was more appropriate.

Medical Management

In patients with infection-induced struvite stones, residual stone debris usually results in persistent infection, thereby setting the stage for stone recurrence. There are, however, scattered reports that UTI has been eradicated with culture-specific antimicrobials after successful stone pulverization with ESWL.[2, 3] Periodic and long-term bacteriologic follow-up of antimicrobials are needed to identify persistent infection. We strive to see patients at monthly intervals for 3 months and at quarterly intervals for 1 year after cessation of antimicrobials. Urine specimens for bacteriologic culture are routinely collected at each follow-up visit.

Antimicrobials

Residual infection is rarely eliminated with "suppressive" medication consisting of sulfas, nitrofurantoins, or methenamine salts. Methenamine salts are to be deplored inasmuch as there are no scientific data to support their use in urea-splitting UTI. There is little rationale for nonspecific antimicrobials.

Culture-specific antimicrobials are the drugs of choice. Standard Kirby-Bauer disk sensitivities, however, may not be helpful in selecting the best agent. In the presence of reasonable kidney function, antibiotics are concentrated 10- to 100-fold over their usual serum concentrations. Inasmuch as Kirby-Bauer disk sensitivities are based on serum concentrations of antibiotic, the achievable urinary concentrations may be bactericidal or bacteriostatic even when the disk sensitivities reflect bacterial resistance. Tube dilution sensitivity techniques may be warranted to assist selection of appropriate antimicrobials, particularly if the agents are to be used for weeks or months.

Penicillin, ampicillin, and tetracycline are good examples of useful agents that may test "resistant" in routine sensitivity testing. Penicillin and ampicillin are effective against more than 90% of *P. mirabilis* strains in urine and are similarly effective against many other *Proteus* strains because of the high concentrations attained in urine.[4] Similarly, tetracyclines are effective against more than 90% of *Pseudomonas* strains in urine.[5]

The norfloxacin group of antimicrobials also are commonly effective against urease-producing organisms.[6]

I favor initiating long-term oral antimicrobial treatment with recommended therapeutic doses. However, after 1 or 2 weeks of treatment, the urine usually is sterile. With demonstrated sterility, I reduce the dosage of antimicrobial and typically continue twice or once daily treatment (usually at bedtime) for up to 3 months. Urine sterility is verified monthly by cultures if breakthrough bacteriuria occurs or if the patient becomes symptomatic; then the therapeutic dose is resumed.

After 3 months of sterile urine, antimicrobials are discontinued; bacteriologic follow-up is maintained for 1 year as described earlier.

Urease Inhibitors

There is good clinical and experimental evidence to support the use of urease-inhibiting drugs.[7, 8] Ureolysis is the primary, and probably the sole, cause for struvite stones in humans. Inhibition of urease retards the growth of existing stones and probably lessens the risk of new stone formation.

The problem with urease inhibitors is their toxicity.[8, 9] Moreover, they are palliative. Acetohydroxamic acid and hydroxyurea are the only two agents available in the United States. Of the two, AHA is the more potent and the least toxic. However, 20% to 30% of patients cannot take AHA at the recommended 250-mg, three times daily dose, because of problematic side effects.

Side effects usually consist of gastrointestinal (GI) upset and neurologic symptoms consisting of headache, tremulousness, anxiety, and, occasionally, hallucinations. Hair loss and a hemolytic anemia have also been reported.

I explain the advantages and disadvantages of AHA to all patients with struvite stones after definitive operative treatment. I strongly recommend long-term antimicrobial treatment (as previously described) and encourage a concomitant therapeutic trial with AHA beginning with 250 mg twice daily. If this initial dose is well tolerated, I increase the dose after 3 to 4 weeks to 250 mg thrice daily.

I do not prescribe AHA for patients with a serum creatinine clearance greater than 2.0 mg/dL inasmuch as therapeutic concentrations in urine are unlikely and the risk of systemic toxicities is increased. I also am hesitant to recommend AHA when the function of the involved kidney is significantly less than that of the normal contralateral one. In this situation the normal kidney excretes high concentrations of AHA, whereas the "sick" kidney may produce dilute urine containing little or no AHA.

Use of AHA is contraindicated in fertile women unless effective contraception is used regularly. Acetohydroxamic acid is clearly teratogenic, but it does not impair fertility, at least in experimental animals.[9] Thus, use of AHA during pregnancy poses a significant risk of fetal anomaly.

Continued use of AHA after cessation of antimicrobials, particularly during the monthly bacteriologic follow-up, is rational inasmuch as the risk of stone recurrence is retarded at a time when emerging bacteriuria is most likely. Acetohydroxamic acid is not antimicrobial, so it does not interfere with bacterial growth or bacteriuric testing.

Acidification

Urinary acidification is desirable. Urine with a persistent pH in the 5.0 to 5.5-range potentiates the antimicrobial effect of penicillins and enhances chemolysis of struvite stones. However, to the best of our knowledge, chronic acidification of urine is pharmacologically impossible with any of the available systemic agents.

Ammonium chloride and other systemic acidifiers acidify urine acutely but not chronically. Compensatory renal mechanisms increase tubular cell production of ammonia, which defuses into urine and binds with the pharmacologically produced hydrogen ion.

The most definitive investigations of systemic acidification of urine were performed in Holland.[10] These investigations found that ammonium sulfate and ammonium nitrate acidified urine better than ammonium chloride. However, ammonium sulfate is a poorly absorbed GI cathartic,[11] and ammonium nitrate is potentially explosive. Neither has become popular in Europe.

Lavage of stone debris with acidic solutions will effect chemolysis of struvite particles and perhaps also of calcium phosphate particles. However, it is unlikely to have a significant impact on calcium oxalate particles. Aggressive lavage, using nephrostomy tubes or ureteral catheters to effect in situ chemolysis will clearly reduce the burden of residual debris and render some patients stone free. However, controlled trials are needed to document the cost effectiveness of this approach compared with that with antimicrobial-urease inhibition.

SUMMARY

Management of infection-induced staghorn calculi must be individualized. No single treatment is uniformly effective. Patient education and clinical judgment are the principles on which management is based. Nephrectomy and no treatment at all are viable options in highly selected patients. However, combinations of operative and pharmacologic treatment are appropriate for most patients. Long-term periodic bacteriologic and radiographic follow-up are needed to identify patients who have chronic problems and who may need additional treatment.

REFERENCES

1. Fuchs G, Rosciszewski A, Royce P: Staghorn stone treatment with ESWL: The fate of residual stones. Paper presented to the Western Section of AUA, San Francisco, Feb 28–March 4, 1988.
2. Michaels EK, Fowler JE Jr, Mariano M: Bacteriuria following extracorporeal shock wave lithotripsy of infection stones. *J Urol* 1988; 140:204–206.
3. Bagley DH: Pharmacologic treatment of infection stones. *Urol Clin North Am* 1987; 14:347–352.
4. Feit RM, Fair WR: The treatment of infection stones with penicillin. *J Urol* 1979; 122:592.
5. Musher DM, Minuth JN, Thorsteinsson SB, et al: Effectiveness of achievable urinary concentrations of tetracyclines against "tetracycline-resistant" pathogenic bacteria. *J Infect Dis* 1975; 131(suppl):S40–S44.
6. Scully BE, Neu HC, Parry MF, et al: Oral ciprofloxacin therapy of infections due to *Pseudomonas aeruginosa*. *Lancet* 1986; 1:819.
7. Takebe S, Numata A, Kobashi K: Stone formation by *Ureaplasma urealyticum* in human urine and its prevention by urease inhibitors. *J Clin Microbiol* 1984; 20:869.
8. Griffith DP, Khonsari F, Skurnick JH, et al: A randomized trial of acetohydroxamic acid for the treatment and prevention of infection-induced urinary stones in spinal cord injury patients. *J Urol* 1988; 140:318.
9. Bailie NC, Osborne CA, Leininger JR, et al: Teratogenic effect of acetohydroxamic acid in clinically normal beagles. *Am J Vet Res* 1986; 47:2604.
10. Froeling, PGAM: Akute zuurbelastingen, in De Zuuruitscheiding bij de Behandeling van Mensen met Nierstenen. Meppel, West Germany, Krips Repro, 1978, pp 93–106.
11. Pizzarelli F, Peacock M: Effect of chronic administration of ammonium sulfate on phosphatic stone recurrence. *Nephron* 1987; 46:247.

25

Complete Metabolic Evaluation of Stone Formers

Charles Y. C. Pak, M.D.

The patient has been forming two or three calcium oxalate stones each year for 7 years. He is only 34 years old now, and he has been unsuccessful at changing his rate of stone formation by increasing fluid intake and following a low-calcium diet. He wishes to have a reasonably thorough evaluation of his problem but does not want to spend time in the hospital for special tests.

DISCUSSION OF CASE

This patient has a metabolically active stone disease, because he has been forming stones at a high rate for some time. Moreover, he is recalcitrant to conservative therapy comprised of high fluid intake and dietary modification. The finding of calcium oxalate on stone analysis does not provide a definitive diagnosis, because calcium oxalate stones are formed by patients suffering from a wide variety of metabolic derangements, such as hypercalciuria, hyperoxaluria, hypocitraturia, hyperuricosuria, and hypomagnesiuria.

The patient therefore deserves a full evaluation directed at a search for underlying metabolic or environmental disturbances responsible for his stone disease. Such an evaluation can now be conducted in an ambulatory setting, perhaps more reliably than is possible in an inpatient setting.

VARIOUS LEVELS OF EVALUATION OF CALCIUM UROLITHIASIS

Several diagnostic protocols are available. They vary in complexity according to the severity of stone disease. The simplest one, designed for patients with single stone episodes, is described in another chapter. A complete evaluation, a model of which is described here, is directed at the assessment of patients with severe recurrent stone disease who are recalcitrant to conservative therapy. Such an assessment is typically practiced at a stone treatment center.

A modified complete evaluation, representing a simplification of a complete evaluation, is designed for use in the setting of a private practitioner for the management of patients with mild-moderate stone disease. Possession of a reliable laboratory is not critical, because the assessment relies on commercial laboratories for the analysis of urinary risk factors. A referral to a stone disease center may be made when this evaluation is inconclusive.

COMPLETE EVALUATION

The objective of a complete evaluation is to identify abnormal environmental and metabolic risk factors that are responsible for stone formation. Diagnostic methods vary among stone treatment centers. Following are the essential features of our protocol,[1] with which we have evaluated nearly 2,000 patients since 1976.

Initial Screen.—The same preliminary evaluation, as described in another chapter, is conducted and includes a careful history of stone disease, diet, and stone-provoking medication, urinalysis, and stone analysis.

Random Urine Collection.—Two 24-hour urine samples are obtained while the subjects continue their customary diet and fluid intake. Drugs that could affect urinary biochemistry are withdrawn temporarily if possible. The samples are analyzed for urinary risk factors, including calcium, oxalate, citrate, uric acid, sodium, phosphorus, sulfate, and magnesium levels, pH, and total volume.

The objective of this analysis is to identify abnormal environmental risk factors, such as inadequate fluid ingestion (low urine volume), exaggerated sodium intake (high urinary sodium), purine gluttony (high urinary uric acid and sulfate), and inadequate magnesium intake (hypomagnesiuria).

Restricted Urine Collection.—Another 24-hour urine sample is obtained after maintenance on an instructed diet restricted in calcium, sodium, and oxalate. The identical analysis for urinary risk factors is performed. In addition, a fasting venous blood sample is obtained to check parathyroid hormone (PTH) and SMA-20 (sequential multiple analysis of 20 chemical constituents).

The purpose of this analysis is to detect the presence of abnormal metabolic risk factors, such as hypercalciuria, hypocitraturia, hyperoxaluria, and undue urinary acidity.

Fast and Oral Calcium Load Test[2].—After collection of a restricted urinary sample, the subjects undergo the study of fast and oral calcium load. A 2-hour urine sample is obtained in the fasting state to determine calcium and creatinine levels. The product of serum creatinine (in mg/dL) and the ratio of urinary calcium/creatinine (in mg/mg) yields fasting urinary calcium concentration in milligrams per deciliter glomerular filtrate. A high fasting urinary calcium level in the setting of normocalcemia suggests renal calcium leak.

A 4-hour urine sample is obtained after an oral ingestion of 1 g of calcium (in a synthetic meal). The calciuric response (expressed in mg/mg creatinine) provides an indirect measure of intestinal calcium absorption.

The fast and calcium load test therefore allows a discrimination of different forms of hypercalciuria.

The diagnostic criteria for some of the major forms of stone disease are shown in Table 25–1. Using this protocol, we can now identify the cause for stone disease in 97% of patients with recurrent nephrolithiasis. The major forms fall into 14 categories: absorptive hypercalciuria type I, absorptive hypercalciuria type II, renal phosphate leak, primary hyperparathyroidism, fasting hypercalciuria with normal parathyroid function, hyperoxaluria (enteric, dietary, primary), hyperuricosuric calcium nephrolithiasis, gouty diathesis, distal renal tubular acidosis, hypocitraturic calcium nephrolithiasis (chronic diarrheal syndrome, thiazide induced hypokalemia and idiopathic), hypomagnesiuric calcium nephrolithiasis, infection stones, cystinuria, and low urine volume.

TABLE 25–1.
Diagnostic Criteria*

	AH-I	AH-II	RH	PHPT	PL	1,25	EH	HUCN	Idiop Hypocit	RTA	GD
Serum Ca	N	N	N	↑	N	N	N	N	N	N	N
P	N	N	N	↓	↓	N	N	N	N	N	N
PTH	N	N	↑	↑	N	↑	↑	N	N	N	N
Urinary Ca											
Fasting	N	N	↑	↑	↑	↑	↓	N	N	↑	N
1 g Ca load	↑	↑	↑	↑	↑	↑	↓	N	N	N	N
24-hr (restricted diet)	↑	N	↑	↑	↑	↑	↓	N	N	↑	N
Oxalate	N	N	N	N	N	N	↑	N	N	N	N
Uric acid	N	N	N	N	N	N	↓	↑	N	N	N/↑
Citrate	N	N	N	N	N	N	↓	N	↓	↓	N
pH	N	N	N	N	N	N	↓	N	N	↑	↓

**AH-I = absorptive hypercalciuria type I; AH-II = absorptive hypercalciuria type II; RH = renal hypercalciuria; PHPT = primary hyperparathyroidism; PL = renal phosphate leak; 1,25 = primary 1,25-$(OH)_2$ vitamin D excess; EH = enteric hyperoxaluria; HUCN = hyperuricosuric calcium nephrolithiasis; idiop hypocit = idiopathic hypocitraturia; RTA = renal tubular acidosis; GD = gouty diathesis.*

MODIFIED COMPLETE EVALUATION

The complete evaluation described earlier is too detailed and expensive to be applicable in the setting of a private practitioner. The recent availability of reliable and economical commercial assays for urinary risk factors has made possible a formulation of a modified protocol, with the following key features.

Stone-Forming Risk Analysis on a Random 24-Hour Urine Sample.—One 24-hour urine sample is collected while the patient continues a customary diet and fluid intake. The sample is then submitted to a commercial laboratory for a full stone risk analysis. The StoneRisk Profile[3] analyzes metabolic risk factors (calcium, oxalate, citrate, uric acid, and pH) and environmental risk factors (total volume, sodium, phosphorus, and magnesium). From these determinations it calculates urinary saturation of stone forming salts and then presents data in a graphic format for easy recognition of abnormal risk factors.

From the StoneRisk Profile report, the physician may recognize an interplay of environmental influences that may have contributed to stone formation. Accordingly, he or she may apply an appropriate dietary modification and fluid adjustment.

StoneTrack Analysis.—After the application of conservative treatment for 1 month, a 24-hour urine sample is collected. The sample is analyzed for seven risk factors considered essential for follow-up response to conservative program: calcium, oxalate, citrate, uric acid, and sodium levels, pH, and total volume. Such an analysis may be obtained commercially as StoneTrack.

This analysis is analogous to the study of the restricted urine sample during a complete evaluation.

Fast and Oral Calcium Load Test.—The fast and oral calcium load test could be done if hypercalciuria is disclosed on StoneRisk Profile and StoneTrack. The objective of this test is to discriminate the cause of hypercalciuria.

REFERENCES

1. Pak CYC, Britton F, Peterson R, et al: Ambulatory evaluation of nephrolithiasis: Classification, clinical presentation and diagnostic criteria. *Am J Med* 1980; 69:19–30.
2. Pak CYC, Kaplan RA, Bone H, et al: A simple test for the diagnosis of absorptive, resorptive and renal hypercalciurias. *N Engl J Med* 1975; 292:497–500.
3. Pak CYC, Skurla C, Harvey J: Graphic display of urinary risk factors for renal stone formation. *J Urol* 1985; 134:867–870.

26

Calcium Urinary Stones: Preliminary Evaluation

Charles Y. C. Pak, M.D.

Your evaluation of this 45-year-old man includes a complete study of his calcium metabolism because he continues to form one or more stones each year, even though he has been taking 50 mg of hydrochlorothiazide daily. You ask him to stop his medication for 5 days and perform your evaluation. His serum calcium, phosphorus, electrolyte, creatinine, and blood urea nitrogen values are normal. On a low-calcium diet (400 mg/day) he excretes 325 mg of calcium/day. After an oral calcium load test, he has a urinary calcium/creatinine ratio of 0.31, whereas his fasting calcium/creatinine ratio was 0.09. He is very distressed by his continued stone formation, even though he has taken his medications faithfully.

DISCUSSION OF CASE

This patient has a metabolically active stone disease, because he is forming stones at a rate of one or more per year. Moreover, he is resistant to thiazide therapy and has a documented metabolic derangement of marked hypercalciuria. Thus, he is a candidate for a complete evaluation,[1] which is described in another chapter.

The initial laboratory work-up suggests that the patient probably had absorptive hypercalciuria type I. Thus, he had normocalcemia and normal fasting urinary calcium levels (absence of renal calcium leak), exaggerated calciuric response to oral calcium load (indicative of high intestinal calcium absorption), and hypercalciuria on a calcium-restricted diet.

Four factors might have contributed to thiazide failure in this patient with absorptive hypercalciuria type I.[2] First, the patient may have developed an attenuation or a loss of hypocalciuric action of thiazide during long-term therapy. Second, thiazide treatment may have caused hypocitraturia, because potassium supplementation was not apparently provided. Third, the dose of thiazide may have been insufficient. Fourth, a concurrent high sodium intake could have blocked thiazide-induced hypocalciuria.

SIMPLE EVALUATION

A simplified protocol may be used for the evaluation of single stone formers[3] without family history of stones or an underlying predisposing disease (e.g., chronic diarrheal state). Such an evaluation could have been applied when the index patient was first admitted with stones. Patients with recurrent stones or single stone formers with a family history of stones or with an underlying predisposing disease are candidates for a more complete evaluation described elsewhere. I recommend the following guidelines for a simple evaluation.

A careful history should be taken for predisposing conditions, medications, dietary aberrations, and insufficient fluid intake. A multichannel blood screen should be performed to identify primary hyperparathyroidism (from high serum calcium levels), renal phosphate leak (from hypophosphatemia), distal renal tubular acidosis (from abnormal serum electrolyte levels), and gouty diathesis (from hyperuricemia). Fresh spot urine sample should be cultured for urea-splitting organisms (suggestive of infection stones) and examined for pH (with a pH electrode) and crystalluria. High pH (>7.5) is compatible with infection lithiasis, and low pH (<5.5) is compatible with uric acid lithiasis. Identification of a particular crystal type in the urinary sediment is compatible with, but not diagnostic of, that type of nephrolithiasis. A qualitative examination of a spot urine sample for cystine (nitroprusside test) provides a clue to the presence of cystinuria. Abdominal roentgenologic examination, with oblique views when necessary, is recommended. Available stones should be analyzed for stone composition. Details of this evaluation are provided later on.

History

A careful history should be taken during the evaluation of the stone-forming patient because it may provide clues to the underlying cause or causes for stone formation. It should include relevant demographic data, medications taken or treatments received, concurrent or other illnesses, and nutritional habit.

Important demographic information that should be taken from every stone-forming patient includes sex, race, and age (current and at onset of stone disease).

Absorptive hypercalciuria and hyperuricosuric calcium nephrolithiasis are more common in men than in women and are rare among blacks. Most commonly afflicted are middle-aged white men. Renal hypercalciuria has less male preponderance than in the previous conditions. Many give a history of urinary tract infection before stone disease. Primary hyperparathyroidism is more common in women than in men, with postmenopausal women being most prone.

Enteric hyperoxaluria and infection lithiasis are more common in women than in men. Cystinuria affects the two sexes equally. Uric acid lithiasis caused by primary gout is much more common in men, but that resulting from gastrointestinal (GI) disease affects women more. Calcium oxalate stone disease in children should suggest idiopathic hypercalciuria of childhood or primary hyperoxaluria. The latter condition should be distinguished by evidence of oxalosis and renal failure.

Medications

Certain medications could cause or exaggerate stone disease; a careful history should be obtained for all medications taken.

Acetazolamide, a carbonic anhydrase inhibitor now used mainly for glaucoma and altitude sickness, induces metabolic acidosis with hypercalciuria, hypocitraturia, and high urinary pH. It may cause development of calcium stones composed of calcium phosphate and calcium oxalate.

Vitamin C supplementation could augment oxalate excretion and in large doses, increase urinary calcium as well. Calcium supplements, vitamin D preparations, and phosphorus-binding antacids (e.g., aluminum hydroxide) could raise urinary calcium levels. The hypercalciuric action of aluminum-binding antacids has been attributed to the reduced GI binding of calcium by phosphate (because of aluminum phosphate precipitation), making more calcium available for absorption, and stimulated synthesis of 1,25-$(OH)_2$vitamin D (from hypophosphatemia). Theophylline and some calcium channel blockers may increase urinary calcium levels by a poorly understood mechanism.

Triamterene therapy may cause deposition of this poorly soluble drug as a sole or a mixed stone. Though rare, allopurinol treatment may cause xanthine crystalluria. Uricosuric agents (e.g., probenecid) may cause transient hyperuricosuria. Because of tissue catabolism, marked hyperuricosuria could result during chemotherapy of malignancy.

Concurrent Illnesses

Renal stones may be a complication of other diseases. A careful history should be taken for them. Patients with gouty arthritis may have uric acid or calcium nephrolithiasis. Chronic diarrheal states may also cause both types of stones. They include gastric resection, pancreatitis, pancreatectomy, malabsorption, regional enteritis, blind loop syndrome, small bowel resection, or ulcerative colitis. The association of primary hyperparathyroidism with nephrolithiasis is well known. Relevant history includes pathologic skeletal fractures, peptic ulcer disease, presence or symptoms of hypercalcemia, and neck surgery indicative of parathyroid surgery. Chronic urinary tract infection may be responsible for infection lithiasis. It may also cause tubular damage and theoretically produce renal tubular acidosis and renal hypercalciuria. Moreover, persistent active urinary tract infection could exaggerate stone disease or cause resistance to certain treatment programs (e.g., potassium citrate and orthophosphate) by destroying urinary citrate and pyrophosphate. Useful history includes the nature of the offending organism (with urea-splitting capacity or not), age at onset, frequency of recurrence, and type of antibiotic used.

Nutritional Habit

A careful nutritional history should be taken, directing particular attention to estimated fluid intake and ingestion of foods rich in calcium, oxalate, purines, sodium, and acid ash. In addition, an inadequacy in the intake of fruits and magnesium should be noted.

Stone Composition

The diagnosis of stone disease is sometimes made on the basis of stone composition. Thus, the disclosure of cystine or struvite and carbonate apatite is diagnostic of cystinuria or infection with urea-splitting organisms, respectively. The presence of 2,8-dihydroxyadenine, triamterene, silica, or xanthine indicates 2,8-dihydroxyadenuria, treatment with triamterene or magnesium trisilicate, or xanthinuria. In these conditions, the crystallographic identification is critical for the diagnosis; laboratory and clinical data provide supporting evidence.

However, for the remaining stones, stone composition is helpful but not conclusive for diagnosis of the underlying disease. The finding of uric acid in stones suggests undue acidity of urine or high urinary urate concentration. However, it cannot distinguish the origin of the stone from gouty diathesis vs. chronic diarrheal syndrome. Stones composed predominantly of hydroxyapatite could arise from distal renal tubular acidosis, primary hyperparathyroidism, or a complication of chronic sodium alkali therapy. Calcium oxalate stones could result from a wide variety of disorders, including hypercalciuria, hyperoxaluria, hyperuricosuria, hypocitraturia, and hypomagnesiuria.

TREATMENT INSTITUTION AND FOLLOW-UP EVALUATION

An appropriate medical prophylactic program should be instituted based on results of diagnostic evaluation rather than before a diagnostic assessment, as was apparently done in the index case. Moreover, once a treatment is instituted, it is critical to obtain a follow-up evaluation to assess the response to treatment and to identify complications of therapy. There is considerable individual variability in treatment response. A follow-up evaluation is necessary so that an appropriate adjustment in dosage may be made. Some patients may develop biochemical abnormalities during treatment, which, if unchecked, may be harmful or affect response to therapy.

I recommend a follow-up evaluation 1 to 4 months after institution of treatment and 4 to 6 months thereafter. A practicing physician may find the commercially available StoneTrack analysis useful. This test provides a measure of calcium, oxalate, citrate, uric acid, and sodium levels, pH, and total volume on a single 24-hour urine sample. The result of the follow-up evaluation is compared with the pretreatment data in a graphic format. A venous blood sample for SMA-20 (sequential multiple analysis of 20 chemical constituents) is also obtained.

MANAGEMENT OF INDEX CASE

This patient with probable absorptive hypercalciuria type I was treated with 50 mg of hydrochlorothiazide daily. The StoneTrack analysis would have been helpful in explaining his resistance to this treatment.

A low urinary citrate level would have suggested thiazide-induced hypocitraturia. Hypercalciuria with high urinary sodium levels would have indicated that the high sodium intake may have attenuated hypocalciuric action of thiazide. High urinary calcium level alone would have suggested that attenuation had developed independent of sodium alone during long-term thiazide use. Hyperuricosuria would have raised the possibility that thiazide therapy may have caused it or contributed to its development. Low urine volume, undue urinary acidity, or hyperoxaluria would have indicated presence of other nondrug-related causes for stone formation.

This index patient apparently was treated with thiazide after only a simple evaluation, and no follow-up assessment was done. This patient deserves a complete evaluation (described elsewhere) after stopping thiazide therapy. If the only identifiable abnormality is absorptive hypercalciuria type I, he might begin treatment with 4 mg of trichlormethiazide/day and 15 mEq of potassium citrate taken twice daily. Trichlormethiazide is better tolerated than hydrochlorothiazide, and is less likely to cause hypokalemia or hypocitraturia. A moderate sodium and calcium restriction should be applied. A follow-up evaluation with a StoneTrack analysis and venous blood SMA-20 should be obtained within the first 4 months.

REFERENCES

1. Pak CYC, Britton F, Peterson R, et al: Ambulatory evaluation of nephrolithiasis: Classification, clinical presentation, and diagnostic criteria. *Am J Med* 1980; 69:19–30.
2. Preminger GM, Pak CYC: Eventual attenuation of hypocalciuric response to hydorchlorothiazide in absorptive hypercalciuria. *J Urol* 1987; 137:1104–1109.
3. Pak CYC: Should patients with single renal stone occurrence undergo diagnostic evaluation? *J Urol* 1982; 127:854–858.
4. Pak CYC: Medical management of nephrolithiasis in Dallas: Update 1987. *J Urol* 1988; 140:461–467.

27

Diet and Fluid Therapy of Urolithiasis

Thomas M. Kinkead, M.D.
Mani Menon, M.D.

The patient is a 24-year-old man who has just passed his first calcium oxalate stone. He has a maternal uncle who has had a stone. Serum calcium and phosphorus levels and creatinine clearance are normal. He excretes 357 mg/day calcium while eating a low-salt, 800-mg calcium diet. He hates taking pills and wonders if there is a simple way to decrease his risk of forming stones in the future.

Urolithiasis continues to be a major health care concern in the United States, both in terms of economics and individual morbidity. Despite the recent development and widespread availability of new surgical therapies for stone disease, such as extracorporeal shock wave lithotripsy (ESWL), percutaneous nephrolithotomy, and newer ureteroscopic techniques, surgical treatment of stone disease is expensive and its aim is solely to eliminate existing stones. Urolithiasis is a disease with a high probability of recurrence, up to or greater than 50% over a 10-year period, and removal of existing stones is unlikely to prevent new stone formation. The yearly expenditure on urinary stone disease in the United States in 1974 was estimated at nearly $50 million, not taking into account time lost from work secondary to pain and complications from these stones. This figure is obviously greatly inflated in current monetary terms. Endourologic stone removal is comparable in price with open stone surgery, approximately $6,000 to $10,000 per case, and the cost of a single ESWL treatment averages $8,000 to $12,000. In contrast, medical treatment and follow-up of a patient with stone disease can be accomplished for less than $1,000 per year. Clearly, our approach to the management of urologic stone disease must incorporate medical treatment aimed at prevention of stone recurrence in addition to surgical treatment, aimed at the removal of existing stones.

As with surgical management, great progress has been made in the area of medical management of stone disease in both the evaluation and characterization of the physiologic derangements responsible for stone formation and in specific therapies, both dietary and pharmacologic, aimed at correcting these abnormalities. We want to implement medical therapies that are practical in terms of patient compliance and cost and that are free of serious side effects. This is why diet and fluid therapy are so appealing as first-line therapy for urologic stone disease. This chapter reviews the rationale for diet and fluid therapy of urolithiasis and identifies which subclasses of stone disease patients and stone types will best benefit from selective diet therapies.

Basically stated, urinary tract stone formation begins when the urine becomes supersaturated with one or more of the chemical constituents of the stone. Crystalluria then ensues, and under appropriate conditions, crystal nucleation, aggregation, and growth follow, with eventual formation of a stone large enough to be retained and cause symptoms. More than 80% of urinary stones are composed of calcium in some form, most commonly as calcium oxalate or a mixture of calcium oxalate and calcium phosphate. Although much of the pathophysiology of calcium stone formation remains unknown, it is well accepted that increased levels of urinary calcium, oxalate, uric acid or combination thereof or a decrease in urinary inhibitors of crystallization such as citrate, phosphate, magnesium, or glycosaminoglycans are important factors for stone formation, as is a low urine volume.

It is also known that the etiology of urinary calculi is multifactorial in the majority of cases, and rarely can one single factor in the patient's history or anatomic or physiologic milieu account for the presence of their stone. For this reason, the initial evaluation of all urinary stone patients should include a thorough general medical assessment, including a complete history and physical examination, to identify any particular "stressors" for stone formation. Specific areas to be addressed include:

1. *Anatomy*. Urinary tract obstruction, either congenital (horseshoe kidney, ureteropelvic junction obstruction, etc.) or acquired (e.g., benign prostatic hypertrophy), leads to urinary stasis and stone formation. Indeed, one group of investigators has found good correlation between caliceal anatomy and stone formation even in patients without urinary obstruction. One percent to 2% of stone disease patients have an associated structural abnormality in the urinary tract. Medullary sponge kidney is the most common renal structural abnormality encountered in patients with calcium-containing stones. Foreign bodies in the urinary tract, usually iatrogenic (sutures, catheters, and stents), may provide the nidus for stone formation. Intestinal disease, usually associated with malabsorption and diarrhea, may lead to increased dietary oxalate absorption in the gut and hyperoxaluria. Such conditions include inflammatory bowel disease, intestinal bypass for obesity, or chronic biliary or pancreatic disease.

2. *Activity level*. Periods of immobilization secondary to illness or injury or even a sedentary occupation may lead to bone demineralization, hypercalemia, and eventually hypercalciuria.

3. *Underlying systemic disease*. Some disease states such as primary hyperparathyroidism, renal tubular acidosis (RTA), gout, and sarcoidosis have a well-known association with calcium stone disease and account for the minority of stones that have a well-defined etiology.

4. *Environmental factors*. Access to and mineral content of drinking water is a possible etiologic factor in stone disease, although there has been conflicting evidence that both soft and hard water contribute to calcium stone formation. People who live and work in hot climates are more prone to sweating, dehydration, and increased urinary concentration, predisposing to stone formation. In most areas, stone occurrence increases during the hot summer months.

5. *Genetics*. A family history of stones may suggest certain etiologies, as in RTA (transmitted as an autosomal dominant trait), cystinuria (autosomal recessive), or absorptive hypercalciuria, seen in one fourth to one third of family members, most commonly males. Blacks seldom form idiopathic calcium-containing stones, and the discovery of such should prompt a search for a secondary cause. The history of a family member having stone disease increases the likelihood of recurrence fourfold.

6. *Infection*. Urinary tract infection, particularly with urea-splitting bacteria such as *Proteus, Klebsiella, Serratia,* and *Enterobacter* species, is well known to predispose to struvite (magnesium ammonium phosphate) stones, the result of precipitation of these substances in an acidic urine. Struvite stones may originate as a metabolic stone that becomes secondarily infected.

7. *Medications*. Corticosteroids, vitamin D, aluminum-containing antacids (which bind phosphate), loop diuretics such as furosemide, and calcium supplements all may cause hypercalciuria. Excessive vitamin C ingestion may lead to hyperoxaluria, and probenecid may cause hyperuricosuria. Antacids and acetazolamide may impair urinary acidification and lead to calcium phosphate stone formation, and, finally, the focus of this chapter,

8. *Diet* and *fluid intake*.

EVIDENCE FOR DIETARY FACTORS IN THE ETIOLOGY OF UROLITHIASIS

That certain dietary habits may predispose to calcium stone formation has long been recognized. Early evidence that dietary factors might be responsible for or contributing to calcium urolithiasis came from international population studies, particularly those implicating increased animal protein consumption as a risk factor.

There has been a tremendous increase in upper urinary tract stones worldwide during the 20th century, most notably in affluent subgroups of economically developed nations, and this has been correlated with increased per capita expenditure on food and animal protein in particular. For example, during World Wars I and II, when economic circumstances necessitated a decrease in animal protein consumption, the incidence of stone disease, as determined by hospital admissions and autopsy findings, decreased in several western European nations, then increased again in the postwar years. People in northern and western regions of India consume approximately 100% more animal protein than in other areas, and the risk of stone formation as measured by hospital admission rates in these regions was approximately four times that in the southern and eastern regions. Other evidence implicating dietary animal protein in the etiology of calcium stone disease comes from studies of British vegetarians who had a stone prevalence of one third of the general population and one eighth of the prevalence in a matched economic class of nonvegetarians.

Subsequently, increases in dietary animal protein were shown to cause increases in the urinary excretion of calcium, oxalate, and uric acid and to decrease urinary pH and citrate excretion in normal individuals, all later shown to be factors favoring calcium stone formation. These alterations persist for as long as protein intake is high and can be reduced by lowering meat intake. These effects are believed to be the result of the high content of sulfur-containing amino acids found in animal but not plant protein. Also, increased acidity of the urine is thought to diminish the inhibitory action of urinary glycosaminoglycans, potent inhibitors of calcium oxalate crystal growth and aggregation. It has been estimated that 50% of the increased levels of urinary calcium, oxalate, and uric acid in stone-forming patients is attributable to a diet rich in animal proteins. More specifically, Burns and Finlayson[1] have shown that the effect of dietary protein on urinary calcium excretion follows the relationship

$$y = 60.8\ B^{0.4}$$

where y equals the increase (in percent) in urinary calcium caused by protein ingestion and B is dietary protein nitrogen (in grams). Using this formula, it can be shown that 10 oz of meat ingested daily will cause a 156% increase in urinary calcium excretion.

It would seem obvious, then, that reduction of animal protein in the diet would be prudent for any patient suffering from urinary stone disease. The difficulty is that no controlled, prospective study has ever demonstrated long-lasting prevention of recurrence of urinary lithiasis as a result of dietary modifications. Similarly, most population studies have shown no significant differences in the diets of recurrent stone formers compared with normal controls. Thus, it has not been unequivocally proved that dietary protein plays an important role in the pathogenesis of urolithiasis in certain patients, but many lines of evidence would indicate that this is so. Some researchers have postulated that patients with recurrent urinary stones are more sensitive to the calciuric action of dietary protein than normal individuals and in some studies have even demonstrated a proportionately greater increase in calciuria in stone patients than in controls for any given increment of dietary protein intake.

Similarly, other dietary components have been implicated as factors in lithogenesis. Ever since Flocks emphasized the importance of hypercalciuria in calcium urolithiasis, dietary calcium restriction in the form of avoidance of milk and dairy products has long been a mainstay of therapy for recurrent calcium stones, based on the theory that decreased calcium absorption in the gut would lead to decreased concentration in the urine. Stone prevalence is high in the so-called dairy belt in the United States, presumably secondary to the increased consumption of dairy products there, which are rich in calcium but also animal protein and vitamin D, the active form of which causes increased calcium absorption from the gut.

Many studies have shown that patients with idiopathic calcium oxalate stone disease have increased intestinal absorption of calcium compared with healthy controls, and hyperabsorption in the gut accounts for the majority of hypercalciuria seen in recurrent calcium oxalate stone formers. It is still unknown whether increased intestinal absorption of calcium is the primary or a secondary event, because a few studies have shown that hypercalciuria persists in some patients despite dietary calcium restriction.

It would seem intuitive that dietary restriction of calcium, the primary component of more than 80% of kidney stones, would be good for a stone former. However, there is plenty of recent evidence to suggest that severe dietary calcium restriction may be unhelpful and even detrimental. Although we know that a low-calcium diet reduces urinary calcium levels to a variable degree, it has been shown that only 6% of an oral calcium load appears in the urine in normal individuals. Dietary calcium usually binds with oxalate in the gut and is excreted in the feces. Restriction of dietary calcium leads to more free intestinal oxalate, which is then absorbed and excreted in the urine, so that the urinary concentration of calcium oxalate may actually rise. Thus, a low-calcium diet must be combined with a low-oxalate diet. This involves avoidance of popular dietary items, including tea, instant and decaffeinated coffee (the processing converts the coffee's glycolate to oxalate), cola beverages, cocoa, nuts, and many vegetables and fruits (e.g., beets, asparagus, spinach, greens, rhubarb, and sweet potatoes, Concord grapes, cranberries, and other berries, plums, citrus fruit, and their juices). Compliance with a diet low in oxalate and calcium is therefore likely to be poor. Furthermore, a diet low in oxalate will also be low in vegetable- and cereal-derived fiber, B vitamins, iron, and zinc.

The role of dietary sodium as a factor in lithogenesis has been emphasized since studies demonstrated that chronic increases in dietary sodium lead to hypercalciuria and that maneuvers (including increased dietary intake) that increase urinary sodium excretion also increase urinary calcium excretion. Calcium and sodium are reabsorbed at many common sites along the renal tubule, and competition for these sites may play a role in this effect, although the exact sites of altered renal transport of these ions have not been precisely identified. Similarly, other studies have shown that dietary sodium restriction leads to notable decreases in urinary calcium excretion. Furthermore, patients with recurrent calcium stones and hypercalciuria are more sensitive to the hypercalciuric effects of dietary sodium, just as with dietary protein. Again, confounding these observations is the lack of any controlled studies demonstrating that recurrent stone formers have a greater mean sodium intake compared with normal controls.

Decreased dietary fiber has been identified in population studies of idiopathic calcium oxalate stone formers. One of the protective effects of a vegetarian diet on stone formation is believed to be its high fiber content, and some studies have revealed that fiber is sacrificed in those eating a high-protein diet. The urinary excretion of calcium has been found to be lower in patients eating a diet rich in fiber. This effect is believed to be mediated by decreased intestinal calcium absorption secondary to accelerated transit of bowel contents and by formation of insoluble calcium-phytin salts. As with other dietary factors in urinary stone disease, no studies have confirmed any beneficial effect of a high-fiber diet on stone recurrence, although several have suggested that this may be the case.

FLUID THERAPY FOR UROLITHIASIS

A low urinary volume has been confirmed as an important risk factor for lithogenesis, and the preventive benefit of a high-fluid intake on stone recurrence has been recognized and practiced as therapy since the days of Hippocrates. Maintenance of a high urine volume through increased oral fluid intake has been claimed to be everything from the most important factor in stone prevention to harmful in that it results in the dilution of urinary inhibitors of stone crystallization. The latter theory has since been disproved.

Evidence implicating low urine volume in stone formation again comes from population studies that consistently demonstrate increased stone incidences in people who live and work in areas of the world with hot climates, even when comparing relatively matched populations. For example, British soldiers stationed in the Middle and Far East had higher stone rates than did their counterparts stationed in England. In Israel, the risk of urolithiasis is much greater in persons living in dry desert regions compared with those living in the more temperate areas. The pronounced seasonal variation in stone incidence in many areas of the world, which peaks during the summer and fall months, provides further evidence. These differences are attributed to increased extrarenal fluid losses (i.e., sweating), which contribute to a lower urine volume in these settings. Similarly, male marathon runners have a threefold to fivefold greater incidence of stones than do age-and sex-matched populations, consistent with the dehydration etiology of stone formation. Nonetheless, it should be noted that many studies do not demonstrate an actual decrease in mean urine volume in recurrent renal stone formers compared with healthy individuals.

A high fluid intake presumably leads to increased urinary volume and decreased supersaturation of calcium, oxalate, calcium phosphate, and monosodium urate and raises the formation product for calcium oxalate and brushite so that crystals are less likely to form and grow. However, the efficacy of a high fluid intake as the sole form of therapy for urolithiasis has never been demonstrated in controlled prospective studies. Part of the problem stems from the difficulty in ensuring reliable controls in a study evaluating fluid intake alone. An exception to this is an Israeli study that found an incidence of stones to be seven times higher at 3 years in a group of recent imigrants who were "uneducated" controls compared with nearby villagers who were educated as to the importance of a high fluid intake in preventing stone formation and who were able to maintain a urine output one third greater than these controls (1,100 vs. 800 mL/day). British naval personnel decreased their stone formation rates by 86% when they were able to increase their average daily urine output from 800 to 1,200 mL/day through increased fluid consumption.

Despite the absence of statistical proof of the efficacy of increased fluid intake, there is little dispute as to its benefits and lack of side effects, and most clinicians recommend increased fluid consumption as the cornerstone and starting point of any regimen aimed at preventing stone recurrence. The benefit of increased fluid intake is used to explain the so-called stone clinic effect described by Hosking. In his study, 100 patients with idiopathic calcium nephrolithiasis were given advice encouraging high fluid intake and avoidance of dietary excesses as the sole therapy in their stone treatment program. Sixty percent of the patients had no evidence of stone growth or new stone formation after a mean follow-up of 5 years. This effect of simply entering someone into a specialized stone program is weak when compared with most studies employing pharmacologic therapies such as thiazide but not insignificant (10%–30% decrease in stone recurrence with most conservative regiments vs. a 90% decrease using thiazides). In this same study, frequency of stone formation was reduced from 0.7 to 0.1 episodes per patient per year, and more important, comparison of initial and follow-up 24-hour urine volumes demonstrated a significant increase (1.6–2.1 L) in those patients whose stones were metabolically inactive at follow-up and no increase in urine volume in patients whose stones were metabolically active. Metabolically active urolithiasis can be defined by one or more of the following criteria: (1) evidence of new stone formation by roentgenograms within the past year, (2) evidence of stone growth by roentgenograms within the past year, and (3) passage of documented gravel or stone within the past year. In contrast, a similar study from Sweden recommending only high fluid intake to those who refused or were not considered to require medical therapy for their stone disease demonstrated a 40% recurrence rate at 3 years and only 15% of patients free from recurrence at 8 years of follow-up.

Although most would agree on the theoretical benefits of increasing fluid consumption for stone disease, there are considerable differences of opinion regarding what constitutes the desirable urine volume to achieve and what fluid recommendations to give to the patient. Recommended urine volumes range from 2 to 4 L/day, which gives an indication of the lack of objective data on which to base these recommendations. To excrete an isotonic urine, the average adult must have a daily urine output of 2 L. In patients undergoing treatment for recurrent calcium stones, a urinary volume of less than 1,400 mL/day is said to convey an increased risk for stone recurrence.

To achieve an increased urine volume, authorities in the treatment of stone disease have recommended ingesting anywhere from 2 and 5 L of fluid daily plus getting up during the night to drink. Those who practice moderation cite the notorious difficulty in getting patients to initiate and sustain their increased fluid intake habits, despite thorough explanations from the clinician as to the benefits of such reforms, because the patients find these increased quantities of fluid intake cumbersome and, in the case of nocturnal drinking, disruptive. The moderates also correctly note the absence of any reliable long-term study showing that massive water drinking prevents calcium oxalate stone recurrence. Clinicians recommending the higher fluid and urine volumes point to a low fluid intake as perhaps the most important and potentially most correctable stress factor for stone formation and that drinking an 8- to 10-oz glass of fluid approximately every hour while awake and again during the night is not unusually cruel or distressing to most patients. In fact, some authors have stated that ingestion of fluids sufficient to maintain such an increased urine output may be a nuisance at first but that the decrease in concentrating ability in the urine induced by diuresis soon stimulates the thirst mechanism so that this new level of fluid intake becomes a habit and a palatable one at that. We believe that patients should adjust their fluid intake to maintain a urine output of a minimum of 2 L and preferably 3 L or more each day.

Most would agree that at least 50% of the ingested fluid should be in the form of water. Maximal intake of fluid should be during certain critical periods when the urine may be expected to be supersaturated with calcium and oxalate, namely, within 3 hours postprandially, during periods of strenuous activity, at bedtime, and during the night, which is the rationale by which many authors recommend deliberate nocturia. The patient should also be informed to avoid drinking large amounts of fluids containing significant amounts of oxalate, including tea, instant coffee, colas, cocoa, and many fruit juices. These may increase urinary oxalate excretion by as much as 60 mg/day when taken in excess.

Whatever the recommendations, fluid therapy should be an integral part of any and all stone prevention programs, for any stone type, including uric acid, cystine, and struvite stones, in addition to calcium stones. Probably the most important factors in assuring patient compliance with fluid therapy include a thorough explanation of the theoretical benefits and goals of the fluid therapy program, a specific prescription or plan dictating the frequency and amount of water and fluid intake, and repeated counselling and reinforcement at follow-up. Compliance will also be better if the family of the patient is involved in these discussions. The patient can provide his or her own feedback by measuring 24-hour urine output at home twice each month. Early on in the program, the patient should bring a 24-hour urine sample to the clinician every month to

3 months for measurement of urinary volume and creatinine clearance. Creatinine clearance is measured to check on the completeness of the collection and to rule out dilution of the urine sample with water by the patient.

It is difficult to predict which patients are most likely to respond to diet and fluid therapy, although increased severity of disease (increased number and frequency of stones) at the time of treatment is associated with a decreased response to therapy. Of course the compliant patient who avoids dietary excesses and who continually maintains his or her urine output at 2 to 3 L/day should fare better than the patient who is sporadically or not at all compliant. Coe and associates have identified three factors that appeared to predict the probability of calcium oxalate stone relapse in a treated population. These include shorter interval of time from last recurrence to initiation of treatment, increased levels of hypercalciuria during treatment, and, most important, failure to increase urinary output during treatment. They developed a discriminant score based on these three factors, as follows:

$$\text{Discriminant score} = 0.2373t - 0.4623C + 1.113\Delta V + 0.9509$$

where t is time in years since last stone, C is urine calcium in mg/kg/24 hours on treatment, ΔV is change in urine volume in liters (treatment − pretreatment). It was calculated that a patient with a positive score has a 90% chance of not relapsing, whereas a negative score portends a 37% chance of relapse.

With this background, let us examine our particular case in more detail. This is a young man without underlying disease who has already passed his first stone, analyzed to be calcium oxalate. His renal function is normal, and primary hyperparathyroidism has been presumptively ruled out by a normal serum calcium level. He has two risk factors for stone recurrence: a family history of stone disease and hypercalciuria.

In general, a healthy white man with his first calcium oxalate stone, if found to have no significant risk factors for stone disease as determined by the careful history taking outlined earlier in this chapter, and who has a normal urinary tract free of stones as demonstrated by intravenous pyelogram, needs no further evaluation and constitutes the ideal candidate for diet and fluid therapy. He should be advised to increase his urine volume to at least 2 L and preferably 3 L/day through increased fluid ingestion and to avoid any dietary excesses of sodium, protein, oxalate, and calcium, if identified. As for further dietary recommendations, moderation is generally in order. Protein intake should not be more than 1g/kg daily, and animal protein should constitute 50% or less of this. Sodium should be restricted to no more than 100 mEq/day, and calcium intake should be around 1,000 mg/day, which is equivalent to about two servings of milk or dairy products per day. Oxalate-rich foods should be avoided whenever possible, and many patients find it helpful when provided lists of the relative sodium, calcium, and oxalate contents of common foods. Dietary fiber should be increased, and a good place to start is by substituting whole grain breads for white bread.

In all other patients besides a healthy young first time stone former, and in all patients with recurrent stones, a more detailed metabolic evaluation is indicated, and this can easily and effectively be performed in an outpatient setting. The purpose of this evaluation is to identify underlying physiologic and metabolic derangements that can contribute to stone formation. These may be detected in more than 95% of patients with stone disease, formerly classified as idiopathic, using an ambulatory protocol as described by Pak. Alone or in combination, hypercalciuria, hyperuricosuria, hyperoxaluria, and hypocitraturia may be identified in up to 50%, 30%, 10%, and 50% of recurrent stone formers, respectively. Uric acid stones and struvite or infection stones each account for 5% to 10% of all renal stones in this country, and cystine stones account for an additional 1% to 2%. Low urine volume can be revealed in up to 50% of stone disease patients.

Briefly, in addition to some baseline blood work, the protocol involves three separate 24-hour urine collections taken over 3 weeks, the first two while the patient is on a regular diet and the third after 1 week on a 400 mg of calcium, 100-mEq of sodium/day diet. A fast and calcium load test is performed on the third visit to differentiate absorptive from renal hypercalciuria. The importance of identifying these various metabolic disturbances is that they carry different therapeutic implications in that some will require pharmacologic therapies and others can be handled more conservatively (i.e., with diet therapy). Medical therapies for stone disease are lifelong, and it should be obvious that we would want to appropriately identify those subgroups of patients who may not require drug therapies with their inherent side effects and costs.

In actuality, our hypothetical patient has already been identified as having a significant metabolic risk factor for nephrolithiasis, that being hypercalciuria. Hypercalciuria is defined as a urine calcium excretion of greater than 300 mg/day for men, greater than 250 mg/day for women, or 4 mg/kg per day for either sex while on their regular diet. Our patient is well above this level, even on a moderately calcium-restricted (800 mg/day) diet. It would be important to know whether the patient's hypercalciuria was absorptive, where the primary defect leading to increased urinary calcium excretion is intestinal hyperabsorption of calcium and which responds to dietary calcium restriction, or renal hypercalciuria secondary to a primary defect in renal reabsorption of calcium, which responds to thiazide therapy rather than dietary modification. Some clinicians believe that differentiating between the various subtypes of hypercalciuria is unnecessary, and any patient identified as having hypercalciuria is instructed to limit calcium intake to 600 mg/day in addition to moderate oxalate restriction and no more than 100 mEq of sodium/day. If this regimen, in addition to fluid therapy, fails to control stone formation over the ensuing 6 months, pharmacologic therapies are probably indicated. In a Japanese study that did not subclassify the stone disease patients with hypercalciuria, 164 patients with "idiopathic" hypercalciuria were given rice bran, 10 g twice daily after meals, and a decrease in urinary calcium excretion was demonstrated in nearly every patient. Fifty two out of 60 patients followed on this treatment for more than 1 year had no recurrence of stones, and stone formation rate decreased impressively from 0.462 to 0.101 per patient year. This effect was even more dramatic in active recurrent stone formers (more than two episodes within the previous 3 years), with stone formation rates dropping from 1.439 to 0.151 episodes per patient year, reemphasizing the importance of dietary fiber in management of the hypercalciuric stone former. Rice bran is also high in magnesium, an inhibitor of calcium oxalate crystallization. Fiber is often prescribed in tandem with thiazide for stone disease associated with diet resistant or renal hypercalciuria.

DIET AND FLUID THERAPY FOR OTHER TYPES OF STONE DISEASE

Uric Acid Stones

In addition to alkalinization of the urine in uric acid lithiasis, increasing urine volume and reduction of urinary uric acid levels are the mainstays of therapy, both of which can be accomplished with diet and fluid therapy. Maintenance of a 2,500 to 3,000-mL urine volume/day is essential to decrease urinary uric acid concentration. Foods high in purines, which are degraded to uric acid, are to be restricted, including animal proteins, such as meat, fish, and poultry, and wine and beer. If diet is ineffective in lowering urinary uric acid, allopurinol therapy (300 mg/day) should be instituted.

Cystine Stones

Cystine stones form in patients with cystinuria when elevated urinary levels of cystine secondary to defective transport of this most insoluble amino acid leads to crystalluria, generally in an acid urine. The solubility of cystine in urine is 200 to 300 mg/L, and therapy is directed at decreasing the concentration of urinary cystine. Recommendations on fluid intake should be even more aggressive than with other stone types. A urine output of 3 to 4 L/day with deliberate nocturia should be the goal of therapy. As far as dietary advice, a low-methionine diet is in order, generally no more than 1 g of methionine/day. Methionine is an amino acid precursor of cystine and is found mainly in animal proteins such as milk, eggs, cheese, and fish, and avoidance of these foods will also help to alkalinize the urine, the other mainstay of therapy in cystine stone disease. Decreased urinary cystine levels may not be apparent for up to 6 weeks after initiation of such dietary therapy. Some investigators have failed to confirm that either dietary restriction or endogenous administration of methionine has any sustained effect on urinary cystine excretion. Furthermore, a low-methionine diet is quite unpalatable to many patients, and assuring compliance with such a diet can be difficult. If fluid and dietary maneuvers fail to decrease cystine concentration in the urine after an appropriate trial period, medical therapies such as penicillamine may be indicated. Also, because cystinuria is a lifelong disorder, this group of stone patients will encompass many children, in whom dietary protein restriction is undesirable. Alternate protein sources such as nuts (peanut butter) and beans should be advised in such situations.

SUMMARY

Diet and fluid therapy have a vital role in the management of this patient with a high risk of stone recurrence. A thorough diet history, preferably in the form of a diet diary kept by the patient, should be included in the initial evaluation of any patient with stone disease. Compliance to treatment should be measured every 3 months with evaluation of urine output, calcium excretion, and discriminant score. The clinician should not hesitate to push for a more thorough evaluation and drug treatment if these measures fail. Institution of such conservative therapies constitutes a reasonable, low-risk, and low-cost approach to first-line therapy of most types of stone disease.

REFERENCE

1. Burns JR, Finlayson B: Strategies for the medical management of patients with urinary stone disease. *Monogr Urol* 1981; 2:106–125.

ADDITIONAL READINGS

Benson EA: Medical management of renal calculi. *AUA Update Series* 1989; 8(21):162–167.

Calculi Update '87 [conference]. AUA Office of Education, Orlando, Fla, 1987.

Coe FL, Parks JH (eds): *Nephrolithiasis: Pathogenesis and Treatment,* ed 2. Chicago, Year Book Medical Publishers, 1988.

Ebisuno S, Morimoto S, Yoshida T, et al: Rice bran treatment for calcium stone formers with idiopathic hypercalciuria. *Br J Urol* 1986; 58:592–595.

Erikson SB: Idiopathic nephrolithiasis, in Rous SN (ed): *Stone Disease: Diagnosis and Management.* Orlando, Fla, Grune & Stratton, 1987, Chapter 7.

Erickson SB: Hypercalciuric nephrolithiasis, in Rous SN (ed): *Stone Disease: Diagnosis and Management*. Orlando, Fla, Grune & Stratton, 1987, Chapter 8.

Flocks RH: Prophylaxis and medical management of urolithiasis: Role of quantity and precipitability of urinary calcium. *J Urol* 1940; 44:183.

Goldfarb S: Dietary factors in the pathogenesis and prophylaxis of calcium nephrolithiasis. *Kidney Int* 1988; 34:544–555.

Hosking DH, Erickson SB, Van den Berg CJ, et al: The stone clinic effect in patients with idiopathic calcium urolithiasis. *J Urol* 1983; 130:1115–1118.

Lindsjo M: Oxalate metabolism in renal stone disease with special reference to calcium metabolism and intestinal absorption. *Scand J Urol* 1989; 119(suppl):1–54.

Menon M, Krishnan CS: Evaluation and medical management of the patient with calcium stone disease. *Urol Clin North Am,* 1983; 10:595–615.

Pak CYC: Medical management of nephrolithiasis in Dallas, update 1987. *J Urol* 1988; 140:461–465.

Smith LH: Stone activity, in Roth RA, Finlayson B (eds): *Stones—Clinical Management of Nephrolithiasis*. Baltimore, Williams & Wilkins Co, 1983, Chapter 6.

Yendt ER: Medical management of calcium stones, in Roth RA, Finlayson B (eds): *Stones—Clinical Management of Nephrolithiasis*. Baltimore, Williams & Wilkins Co, 1983, Chapter 7.

28

Thiazide Treatment of Recurrent Calcium Stones

Bruce Ettinger, M.D.

After his fifth episode of passing a calcium oxalate urinary stone, this patient seeks your help. He has a strong family history of stone disease (father, paternal aunt). Your metabolic evaluation indicates normal serum values. Urine daily uric acid, citrate, and oxalate levels are normal. There is no evidence of hyperexcretion of calcium.

Before initiating prophylactic thiazide therapy for the patient with recurrent calcium oxalate urolithiasis, one must answer a few important questions: What harm would occur from not using any prophylactic therapy? How effective are thiazides? What are the risks of treatment? Finally, some practical decisions need to be made regarding choice of formulation, dosage, monitoring, and duration of treatment.

WHAT IS THE NATURAL HISTORY OF CALCIUM OXALATE LITHIASIS?

Patients suffering from recurrent calcium oxalate lithiasis average one stone event every 3 to 4 years. This rate applies to patients observed prospectively in clinical trials when they are taking a placebo or using no treatment. The rate is artificially elevated to about one stone event every 1.5 years if stone events are examined retrospectively. An even greater distortion may be seen if the stone event rate is calculated from the history obtained from patients referred to stone treatment centers. The higher pretreatment rate reflects selection bias; referral to a special investigative center is usually prompted by a recent cluster of stone events. Any treatment offered is likely to show a 50% or greater reduction if the analysis compares events before and after. This reduction has been coined the "stone clinic effect," but the statistical term is "regression to the mean."

Our hypothetical patient can expect to pass 70% to 80% of his stones without medical attention. Twenty percent will pass spontaneously but will require some medical care, and only 5% to 7% will require urologic intervention, whether manipulation, lithotomy, lithotripsy, or some combination of these procedures. Should our patient simply accept the small risk of serious consequences, or should he begin daily prophylaxis?

If we had a way to predict the likelihood of future stone events, we could encourage or discourage prophylactic therapy. Only two variables have shown predictive power—the previous number and rate of stone events (especially within the past 5 to 10 years) and the presence of calculi in the kidney. The patient with six previous stones has about a 50% higher risk of recurrence than the patient who has had only one previous stone. The presence of residual calcifications doubles the risk of suffering new stone events. About one half of these events are caused by growth or movement of the existing stones, but the remainder come from development of new stones. No other biologic or biochemical markers have predictive value, including the urinary chemistry profile.

HOW EFFECTIVE ARE THIAZIDES IN PREVENTING CALCULI?

Thiazide therapy, although not perfect, significantly reduces the rate of new stone events. Instead of a 50% risk of recurrence in the next 3 to 4 years, the patient using thiazides can expect a 20% risk of recurrence (Table 28–1). Amelioration of stone disease is not limited to patients with hypercalciuria. In fact, thiazides are equally effective in patients with isolated hyperuricosuria, in those with combined hyperuricosuria and hypercalciuria, and in those with no biochemical abnormality of their urine. Therefore, elegant, time-consuming, and expensive tests are not needed to delineate patterns of calcium absorption and excretion. Although it has been suggested that patients with absorptive hypercalciuria will escape from thiazide's control,[10] I have not found a waning of effectiveness with time.

Many theories have been put forth to explain the mechanism or mechanisms responsible for thiazide's protection. The best-supported theory is its hypocalciuric effect, but reductions in urinary oxalate have also been reported, and other nonspecific effects on crystallization and crystal aggregation could account for thiazide's effectiveness regardless of metabolic profile.

Several alternative therapies can be considered; none has been proved effective in rigorously designed clinical trials. Low-calcium diets have never

TABLE 28–1.
Annual Failure Rates During Thiazide Therapy*

Reference	Failure (%)	Patients (n)
Selective use		
Coe[1]	5	212
Pak et al.[2]†	11	27
Pak et al.[2]‡	9	10
Nonselective use		
Ahlstrand et al.[3]	3	85
Backman et al.[4]	4	44
Ettinger et al.[5]	7	42
Laerum and Larsen[6]	7	25
Ljunghall et al.[7]	4	129
Wilson et al.[8]	11	29
Yendt and Cohanim[9]	6	67

**From Ettinger B, Citron JT, Livermore B, et al: J Urol* 1988; 139:679–684. Used by permission.
†Only patients with absorptive hypercalciuria.
‡Only patients with renal hypercalciuria.

been shown to reduce stone recurrences and are no longer recommended. A diet high in fiber and low in sodium, animal protein, and oxalate is often recommended. We have recently completed a randomized study of this diet and found it without value in preventing stone recurrence. Use of cellulose phosphate is fraught with problems. Its long-term effect on the skeleton is unknown, and it is expensive and inconvenient to use, requiring three daily doses, with additional magnesium supplements taken at two other times each day. Potassium citrate is growing in popularity, although no randomized, controlled studies have been published. It requires administration two to three times daily, and it costs more than $1 per day compared with pennies for thiazides. I find 15% to 20% of patients are unwilling to continue potassium citrate because of gastric irritation.

WHAT ARE THIAZIDE'S EXPECTED SIDE EFFECTS AND UNEXPECTED BENEFITS?

Undesirable side effects prompt discontinuation of thiazide treatment in about 20% of stone-forming subjects. Most common complaints are fatigue, weakness, myalgias, and dry mouth. These symptoms are usually observed in the first few weeks of treatment and are not associated with hypokalemia. They are dose related and may sometimes be avoided by restarting at a lower dosage. I find an average decrease in serum potassium concentration of 0.4 ± 0.1 mEq/L (0.4 ± 0.1 mmol/L) in patients taking usual dosages. I have not seen reductions greater than 1.0 mEq/L (1.0 mmol/L), but about 10% to 20% can be expected to have potassium levels less than 3.5 mEq/L (3.5 mmol/L). This effect is dose related but is not progressive after the first few weeks of therapy. It is unclear at present whether a mild degree of hypokalemia has any clinically significant adverse effects on coronary heart disease or glucose tolerance. In most clinical trials, thiazide use is associated with a rise in random blood glucose level of about 10 mg/dL (0.6 mmol/L) and a rise in uric acid level of about 1.0 mg/dL (0.59 μmol/L), yet precipitation of overt diabetes mellitus or gout is unusual.

The cardiovascular risks of thiazide therapy are probably exaggerated.[11] It has been hypothesized that hypokalemia and adverse changes in lipoprotein profile are responsible for some clinical trials showing no benefit or increased risk of coronary heart disease among hypertensive patients given thiazides. The weight of evidence, recently reviewed, suggests that thiazides increase triglycerides and low-density lipoprotein-cholesterol while reducing high-density lipoprotein-cholesterol.[12] These changes are of a small magnitude, appear to be dose dependent, and may not persist after the first year of treatment. Most studies reporting adverse lipoprotein effects used two to four times the dose recommended for preventing calculus recurrence, but others have reported significant increases in cholesterol levels, in the order of 10 to 20 mg/dL (0.26–0.52 mmol/L), with modest doses.[13]

Thiazide's effect on coronary heart disease requires further elucidation, particularly the relations of dosage and duration to lipoprotein changes. Because of the unknown impact, a reasonable approach would be to limit its use in stone prophylaxis to a few years and to monitor possible adverse effects on potassium, glucose, and lipoprotein levels.

In all fairness to thiazide therapy, we should consider its potential benefits aside from stone prevention. Reducing blood pressure would be of benefit to 20% to 25% of stone-forming subjects who also suffer from hypertension. Prevention of bone loss is another possible benefit. Although evidence of metabolic bone disease is not usually found in association with calcium oxalate lithiasis, thiazide therapy of male stone formers was associated with an increase in bone density.[10] Furthermore, in a cross-sectional study of older hypertensive men, those using thiazides had greater bone mass and fewer fractures than those using other antihypertensive therapies.[14] As life expectancy increases, both men and women need to be concerned about osteoporosis; using thiazides might prevent some age-related bone loss.

PRACTICAL CONSIDERATIONS

A number of different thiazides and thiazide-like drugs have been evaluated for their hypocalciuric action, and some have been evaluated in clinical trials of stone prevention. Hydrochlorothiazide, chlorothiazide, bendroflumethiazide, metolazone, and chlorthalidone appear equally effective in preventing stone recurrence. I prefer chlorthalidone because its long half-life (about 60 hours) makes it ideal for long-term therapy, allowing dosing once each day or even every other day. In recent years there has been a tendency to use lower dosages of all thiazides. Because numerous studies have failed to show any relationship between the urinary calcium level and the efficacy of thiazide treatment, I now avoid escalating dosages to achieve some arbitrary degree of hypocalciuria. I have found that 25 mg of chlorthalidone is as effective as 50 mg. In a study still in progress, it appears that 12.5 mg may also be effective; this is not surprising, because 12.5 to 15.0 mg has antihypertensive effects. Although dosing studies have not been performed for other thiazides, I suspect that 25 mg of hydrochlorothiazide, given once or twice each day, will be as effective as larger doses.

Restricting sodium intake may enhance the effects of thiazides. On the other hand, a clinical trial that intentionally avoided prescribing a low-sodium diet found the usual degree of stone protection.[7] Although preliminary studies suggested that addition of amiloride, a potassium-sparing agent, would enhance hydrochlorothiazide's hypocalciuric effect, a double-blind, long-term study found the combination therapy was no better than thiazide alone in terms of both hypocalciuric effect and prevention of stone recurrences.[15] Addition of triamterene to thiazide therapy is contraindicated because deposits of triamterene and its metabolites have been found in calculi. Proponents of combination therapy for stone disease suggest multiple medications to treat all urinary metabolic abnormalities present in each patient. They suggest adding allopurinol if urinary uric acid is in excess and adding potassium citrate if the urinary citrate level is low. No clinical trials have been carried out to test the efficacy of combined regimens. Until such data are available, I prefer monotherapy for its safety, simplicity, convenience, and low cost.

Monitoring drug safety and efficacy enhances patient compliance and improves the benefit/risk ratio as well. Before treating the patient, I obtain, in addition to the chemistry work-up appropriate for urolithiasis, results of fasting glucose, potassium, and uric acid tests and a lipoprotein panel (triglycerides, total cholesterol, and high-density lipoprotein-cholesterol). Follow-up of these chemistry tests after 6 to 8 weeks is reasonable. Thereafter, repeating every 6 to 12 months should demonstrate whether any adverse effects have developed. A yearly evaluation for renal lithiasis is useful, but neither an intravenous (IV) pyelogram nor abdominal flat-plate x-ray studies (kidneys, ureters, and bladder) is recommended for this purpose. The former procedure exposes the patient to unnecessary radiation and the risk of reaction to IV contrast. The latter, by including the pelvis, often excludes the upper poles of the kidneys. By ordering a coned-down view of the kidneys, one can evaluate any change in preexisting stones or evidence of new calcifications. Although ultrasound is free of radiation exposure, it does not allow precise measurement of the size of calcifications. One might consider using this test to follow the patient who begins therapy free of stones, obtaining an x-ray film if a stone is observed.

Finally, some decision must be made regarding the duration of thiazide therapy. I usually recommend that patients discontinue therapy if they are free of renal calcifications and if they have not had a stone event for 3 years. If one or more stones are visible on x-ray films, I recommend continuance of therapy.

Despite the capricious nature of recurrent calculus disease, we have adequate proof of thiazides' efficacy. We have evolved a comparatively safe and simple therapy that can be given to most patients who form calcium oxalate stones, regardless of their urinary biochemical parameters. Thiazides still fail to prevent stone recurrences in some patients. Despite many years of experience with this form of stone prophylaxis, we still do not understand the reasons for its success or failure. Although much has been learned through laboratory investigations, the medical management of the recurrent stone former still remains a clinical art.

REFERENCES

1. Coe FL: Treated and untreated calcium nephrolithiasis in patients with idiopathic hypercalciuria, hyperuricosuria or no metabolic disorder. *Ann Intern Med* 1977; 87:404–410.
2. Pak CYC, Peters P, Hurt G, et al: Is selective therapy of recurrent nephrolithiasis possible? *Am J Med* 1981; 71:615–622.
3. Ahlstrand C, Tiselius H-G, Larsson L et al: Clinical experience with long-term bendroflumethiazide treatment in calcium oxalate stone formers. *Br J Urol* 1984; 56:255–262.
4. Backman U, Danielson BG, Johansson G, et al: Effects of therapy with bendroflumethiazide in patients with recurrent renal calcium stones. *Br J Urol* 1979; 51:175–180.
5. Ettinger B, Citron JT, Livermore B, et al: Chlorthalidone reduces calcium oxalate calculous recurrence but magnesium hydroxide does not. *J Urol* 1988; 139:679–684.
6. Laerum E, Larsen S: Thiazide prophylaxis of urolithiasis: A double-blind study in general practice. *Acta Med Scand* 1984; 215:383–389.
7. Ljunghall S, Backman U, Danielson BG, et al: Prophylactic treatment of renal calcium stones: Experiences with dietary advice, cellulose phosphate and thiazides. *Scand J Urol Nephrol* 1979; 53(suppl):239–252.
8. Wilson DR, Strauss AL, Manuel MA: Comparison of medical treatments for the prevention of recurrent calcium nephrolithiasis [abstract]. *Urol Res* 1984; 12:39–40.
9. Yendt ER, Cohanim M: Prevention of calcium stones with thiazides. *Kidney Int* 1978; 13:397–409.
10. Preminger GM, Pak CYC: Eventual attenuation of hypocalciuric response to hydrochlorothiazide in absorptive hypercalciuria. *J Urol* 1987; 137:1104–1109.
11. Freis ED: Critique of the clinical importance of diuretic-induced hypokalemia and elevated cholesterol level. *Arch Intern Med* 1989; 149:2640–2648.
12. Lardinois CK, Neuman SL: The effect of antihypertensive agents on serum lipids and lipoproteins. *Arch Intern Med* 1988; 148:1280–1288.
13. Oberman A, Wassertheil-Smoller S, Langford HG, et al: Pharmacologic and nutritional treatment of mild hypertension: Changes in cardiovascular risk status. *Ann Intern Med* 1990; 112:89–95.
14. Wasnich RD, Benfante RJ, Yano K, et al: Thiazide effect on the mineral content of bone. *N Engl J Med* 1983; 309:344–347.
15. Ettinger B, Citron JT: Prevention of recurrent calcium-oxalate calculi through use of hydrochlorothiazide combined with amiloride, in Walker VR, Sutton RAL, Cameron ECB, et al (eds): Urolithiasis. New York, Plenum Press, 1989, pp 789–791.

29

Phosphate Therapy In Calcium Oxalate Urolithiasis

Allen D. Seftel, M.D.
Martin I. Resnick, M.D.

After he has passed three kidney stones in the past 2 years, this 27-year-old patient enters your metabolic evaluation program. On a low-calcium (400 mg/day) diet, he excretes 322 mg of calcium/day into his urine. No other metabolic problems exist. In the past he has been given a low-calcium, low-oxalate diet regimen, and he has tried to follow it. It has not helped, in his opinion.

CALCIUM CALCULI

Of all urinary calculi, calcium-containing stones account for more than 70%, with calcium oxalate stones forming the majority of these. In the United States, upper urinary tract calculi (kidney and ureter) occur primarily in patients 20 to 40 years of age. The incidence of calcium stone disease is higher in whites than blacks (4:1) and in men than women (3:1). In the untreated patient the stone recurrence rate has been estimated to be approximately 50% to 70% in 5 to 10 years.

It is generally accepted that initial crystallization associated with urinary calculi formation occurs in the nephron. With growth and agglomeration these concretions pass progressively into the calyces, renal pelvis, and ureter. Once in the ureter, the passing calculi encounter three physiologic narrowings: the first at the ureteropelvic junction, the second at the pelvic brim, and the third at the ureterovesical junction. The patient's symptoms (usually pain) reflect the level at which the stone becomes lodged, which usually results in obstruction and associated hydronephrosis. An obstructing stone usually results in pain that is colicky in nature and usually is localized to the flank. The differential diagnosis of left-sided flank pain should include the possibility of diverticular disease, pain from a leaking or rupturing abdomen aortic aneurysm, and a retroperitoneal inflammatory process. In women, one must also consider pain from a gynecologic source. If the flank pain occurs on the right side of the abdomen, appendicitis and cholecystitis must also be considered. Most stones 5 mL or less will pass spontaneously within 4 to 6 weeks. Larger ones will often require some form of intervention or manipulation.

Physical examination will usually reveal a patient who is in severe pain, and the bowel sounds may or may not be present but are often diminished. Immediate therapy consists of intravenous (IV) hydration and administration of parenteral analgesics. Complete blood cell count, urinalysis, and serum chemistries are performed as dictated by individual protocol. A plain x-ray film of the abdomen (kidneys, ureters, and bladder) is usually obtained and is often helpful in localizing the stone in that most urinary calculi are radioopaque. A serum calcium level should be determined to exclude the presence of hyperparathyroidism in all stone patients. If the stone is recovered, analysis is most helpful in consideration of future therapy toward the prevention of stone recurrence.

PATIENT EVALUATION

After the patient has returned to his or her normal life-style, a metabolic evaluation is performed in an attempt to determine the cause or causes of stone formation. In addition to serum calcium levels, serum uric acid, phosphorus, and creatinine levels are obtained, in addition to urinary parameters.

The most helpful diagnostic study is a 24-hour urine collection, which should be obtained while the patient is maintaining his or her regular diet. The urine is analyzed for the following components: volume; pH; creatinine clearance; sodium, calcium, oxalate, citrate, uric acid, magnesium, phosphorus, and cystine levels. Most authorities rely on two 24-hour urine collections for final diagnosis. This brief survey should identify a metabolic disorder in 80% to 90% of patients. In addition, this metabolic scheme is reasonable in cost to the patient.

A more thorough metabolic evaluation will provide more specific information regarding stone etiology and will also serve as a useful guide to select appropriate therapeutic regimens. After two 24-hour urines are collected while the patient is maintaining a free or ad-lib diet, he or she should be given a 400-mg calcium, 100-mEq sodium diet and maintained on this regimen for 1 week. All patients with absorptive hypercalciuria will have a urine calcium level greater than approximately 300 mg in 24 hours on a random diet, but on a restricted calcium and sodium diet the urine calcium level will fall to less than 200 mg in 24 hours. This is best characterized by absorptive hypercalciuria type II in which calcium excretion levels fall with moderate restriction of calcium intake. This disorder is best treated by a high fluid intake and a low-calcium diet if the patient will follow dietary instruction. If the level of urine calcium excretion remains greater than 200 mg/24 hours on the restricted diet, the patient is further evaluated and fasted overnight, and a 2-hour urine sample is collected. After the 2-hour urine sample is obtained, 1 g of calcium gluconate is administered orally and a 4-hour urine sample collected. These two urine samples are analyzed for calcium and creatinine levels. Urinary pH is also determined on the fasting sample.

The fasting urinary calcium/creatinine (mg/mg) ratio should normally be less than 0.11, and a ratio of greater than 0.11 is diagnostic of renal leak hypercalciuria (i.e., the patient continues to excrete excessive calcium). The calcium load urinary calcium/creatinine ratio will be greater than 0.2 in patients with absorptive hypercalciuria. This disorder can be classified into several subsections. Type II has already been discussed and is characterized by a significant reduction in calcium excretion with moderate dietary calcium restriction. Type I absorptive hypercalcium is characterized by a normal calcium/creatinine ratio and a fasting serum phosphorus level greater than 2.5 mg/dL and with reduction in calcium excretion only with modified limitation in calcium intake. This disorder is best treated with dietary restriction and oral sodium cellulose phosphate. Thiazide diuretics in association with potassium citrate are a reasonable second choice in this disorder. If the serum phosphorus level is less than 2.5 mg/dL the diagnosis is absorptive hypercalciuria type III. This relatively infrequent disorder, also known as hypophosphatemic hypercalciuria or renal phosphate leak, is treated orally with orthophosphates (500 mg three or four times/day). Thiazides can be administered as a secondary measure. As mentioned previously, a high fluid intake and dietary calcium restriction are also integral parts of therapy.

For completeness the other forms of hypercalciuria should also be reviewed. Resorptive hypercalciuria is characterized by an elevated serum calcium level secondary to hyperparathyroidism. Treatment for this disease is surgical removal of the abnormal parathyroid tissue. Renal hypercalciuria represents a renal leak of calcium and is characterized by a normal serum calcium level, hypercalciuria, a fasting urine calcium/creatinine ratio greater than 0.11, and a load calcium/creatinine ratio greater than 0.20. This disorder is best treated with administration of thiazide diuretics.

The metabolic evaluation with this protocol in this patient revealed absorptive hypercalciuria type III. He was treated with orthophosphates and has remained free of recurrent stone disease for 7 years while maintaining his medications.

DISCUSSION

Phosphate Therapy of Calcium Oxalate Urolithiasis

Although the management of patients with calcium urolithiasis often includes some form of intervention (e.g., lithotripsy, ureteroscopy), medical management of such patients is clearly important and is essential in decreasing the rate of stone formation. Management of patients with absorptive hypercalciuria, as well as all patients with urolithiasis, is directed toward maintaining a urine output of 2 or 3 L/day and reducing the excretion of those active products associated with stone formation (e.g., calcium oxalate, uric acid). The importance of this regimen cannot be overemphasized. Individuals with the diagnosis of absorptive hypercalciuria should be placed on a calcium- and sodium-restricted diet. Limiting calcium intake will reduce hypercalciuria, and the low-sodium diet will also aid in reducing calcium excretion. Limitations placed on the ingestion of animal protein and refined carbohydrates will also be helpful in reducing hypercalciuria. Eating foods rich in fiber and bran will also be helpful.

It is clear that orthophosphate therapy is effective in treating specific patients with recurrent calcium oxalate urolithiasis. Phosphates are clearly indicated in patients who are hypercalciuric and are also indicated in patients with idiopathic calcium urolithiasis without a definable metabolic disorder. Phosphate supplements will not effect a change in calcium excretion in patients who are not hypercalciuric but will result in an increased excretion of pyrophosphate, an important inhibitor of calcium oxalate crystal formation.

Two major types of phosphate therapy exist. The first includes oral administration of neutral or alkaline orthophosphates (sodium or potassium salt), which, as indicated previously, are used for treating patients with absorptive hypercalciuria type III. The agent is also used in treating other forms of absorptive hypercalciuria and has been beneficial in patients without identified metabolic disorders. Various commercial preparations of orthophosphates exist. Acid phosphate compounds should be avoided in that they may actually predispose to further stone formation, and phosphate supplements should be limited to the neutral or alkaline form. Many phosphate preparations are available commercially. Experience has shown that a daily dose of 1.25 in women and 1.5 in men are the minimal dosages that will prove effective. Phosphate therapy should be combined with the previously mentioned measures, particularly a calcium-restricted diet.

As an ion exchange resin, phosphate acts in the gastrointestinal tract by exchanging sodium for calcium and thus inhibiting calcium absorption. Phosphate urinary excretion increases twofold to threefold during oral phosphate therapy, and the urinary excretion of oxalate and magnesium usually increases as well. In addition to increasing the urinary concentration of phosphate in the form of pyrophosphate, phosphates also increase urinary levels of citrate. Both pyrophosphate and citrate are known inhibitors of calcium oxalate crystallization. Phosphates should be avoided in patients with urinary tract infections. The increased phosphate load in these patients may predispose to infection (struvite) stones. Obviously antacids that are phosphate binders should be avoided during therapy. For the drug to be effective it must be taken with meals.

Because hypomagnesemia and hyperoxaluria can result from phosphate therapy, oral magnesium supplementation should be given and dietary oxalate should be restricted. As may be expected, phosphates usually induce a mild dose-related change in serum concentration of calcium and phosphorous. The sodium-containing mixtures may cause an exacerbation of high blood pressure in hypertensive patients. These patients may be best treated with the sodium-free neutral mixture of potassium phosphates.

Phosphate therapy is also indicated in those patients who have medullary sponge kidney, as well as those with idiopathic hypercalciuria. Although helpful in the treatment of patients with hyperparathyroidism, surgery remains the first line of therapy. Phosphate should not be administered to patients who are azotemic who may tend to become hyperphosphatemic. Phosphates are also not indicated for patients with distal renal tubular acidosis and, as mentioned previously, are contraindicated in patients with struvite calculi. Diarrhea and abdominal bloating are the most common side effects of phosphate therapy, but the diarrhea is mild and often subsides with continued therapy. Other reported side effects include soft tissue calcification and parathyroid stimulation, but the consequences of these occurrences are unknown. The second important type of phosphate compound is sodium cellulose phosphate. This compound is a cellulose resin in the sodium form that contains approximately 0.1 of phosphorus/g of resin. Cellulose phosphate binds divalent cations and has been advocated as a means of controlling absorptive hypercalciuria type I. It is apparently not absorbed and is hydrolyzed in the intestinal tract. It is usually administered in doses of 5 g two to three times daily with meals and has been reported to regularly reduce urinary calcium and magnesium excretion. Urinary phosphorus excretion is only minimally increased. It has the same undesirable consequences as other forms of phosphate therapy, namely, it also increases urinary oxalate and magnesium levels; therefore, patients should be placed on magnesium supplements (10 mEq of magnesium citrate twice daily) and be instructed to reduce oxalate intake. Its sole indication appears to be in patients with absorptive hypercalciuria type I. Because the agent stimulates parathyroid activity, it is contraindicated in other forms of hypercalciuria. It should be used with caution in pregnant women and children because of its potential effect on stimulating bone loss and impairing skeletal growth. It is somewhat more expensive than the other phosphate compound previously mentioned.

SUMMARY

Urolithiasis is a diverse disorder, with calcium oxalate stones playing a prominent role. Oral orthophosphate and sodium cellulose phosphate therapy has had a major impact on the formation of recurrent calcium calculi, and phosphate therapy should be used in conjunction with dietary manipulation and increased fluid intake. Phosphate therapy in the properly selected patient has clearly been shown to be effective in the reduction of recurrent calcium calculi.

BIBLIOGRAPHY

Menon M, Krishnan CS: Evaluation and medical management of the patient with calcium stone disease. *Urol Clin North Am* 1983; 10:595–615.

Pak CYC: Medical management of nephrolithiasis. *J Urol* 1982; 128:1157–1164.

Pak CYC, Peters P, Hurt G, et al: Selective therapy of recurrent nephrolithiasis possible. *Am J Med* 1981; 71:615–622.

Thomas WC Jr: Use of phosphates in patients with calcareous renal calculi. *Kidney Int* 1978; 13:390–396.

30

Magnesium Therapy of Urolithiasis

George W. Drach, M.D.

A 53-year-old man requests your assistance in the metabolic management of his urolithiasis. He has had more than 20 stones. Most passed spontaneously. Nevertheless, he has required surgical upper ureterolithotomy for removal of right ureteral stone and has had two nephrolithotomies for removal of multiple calculi on the left. One of these resulted in a lower pole nephrectomy. His stones have been mixed calcium oxalate and phosphate. Metabolic evaluation revealed marginal absorptive hypercalciuria (calcium/creatinine index after load 0.23; normal <0.21) and markedly low fasting magnesium/calcium ratio (26; normal >33). Other portions of the study were normal.

Magnesium therapy of calcium urinary lithiasis reduces incidence of new stone formation and decreases rate of growth of previously formed stones. Its effect is presumed to be its action as an inhibitor of calcium precipitation in urine. I suspect that the explanation is more complex than just inhibition of precipitation. For example, in an extensive study of effects of magnesium therapy on stone formers, no difference could be found in the magnesium metabolic processes or urinary composition of stone formers vs. normals. Yet patients treated with magnesium demonstrated a much lower rate of stone formation than did patients who were treated with a placebo drug. In other words, it works but we do not know why it works.

This patient demonstrates the findings of most of our small group of patients who have clear-cut magnesium deficiency in relation to calcium. Because magnesium is absorbed by the intestine across the same pathway as calcium, you would expect that it would keep pace with the calcium and there would be no magnesium deficiency. (There is a second pathway for absorption of magnesium, I must admit, so a patient should easily be able to absorb adequate amounts.) In magnesium-deficient patients, there seems to be a preferential absorption of calcium rather than magnesium. They become magnesium deficient on a chronic basis. Our own studies illustrate this deficiency. In a group of stone formers that we have reported previously, fasting serum magnesium/calcium ratio was abnormally low, along with the abnormal urinary ratio (Table 30–1). Hence, for practical purposes, one need measure only the fasting urinary magnesium/calcium ratio.

Some investigators criticize the magnesium/calcium ratio because they say it reflects only preferential postprandial absorption of calcium over magnesium, as might be illustrated by this patient. Hence, patients with absorptive hypercalciuria could have low magnesium/calcium ratio because of the large increase in calcium. I agree that this might be true. Our group of patients had abnormal postprandial ratios also (see Table 30–1). But again, for clinical purposes I prefer to measure and consider the fasting ratio only.

Another group of patients who demonstrate magnesium deficiency (without an abnormally low magnesium/calcium ratio) is found among those who have

TABLE 30–1.
Magnesium/Calcium Ratios of Significance

	Normals		Stone Formers		
	$\bar{X}$	S.D.	$\bar{X}$	S.D.	Significance *(p)*
Fasting serum	0.25	0.02	0.23	0.03	0.017
Fasting urine	0.69	0.15	0.4	0.27	0.001
Postload urine	0.62	0.15	0.4	0.2	0.002

enteric diseases associated with hyperoxaluria. Most of these patients require potassium citrate therapy to counteract their metabolic acidosis and magnesium gluconate therapy (500 mg two or three times daily) to restore urinary magnesium levels.

Why do the nonenteric disease patients become magnesium deficient? I suspect it is related to their abnormal absorption of magnesium. Others present an alternate hypothesis, however. Much of the produce of the United States is grown in the West, especially California. Lands used in such agriculture lose magnesium rapidly, and it is not always replaced in the fertilizer. Vegetables grown under these conditions become magnesium deficient. Patients eating the vegetables could become magnesium deficient. But because most of our patients eat considerable animal protein and animal cells are high in magnesium, they should acquire enough magnesium in their diets. I doubt this dietary deficiency hypothesis, therefore.

In the past, a magnesium/calcium ratio (calculated from milligrams) of less than 40 was considered abnormal. More recently, a level less than 33 indicates an abnormally low ratio. Most patients with hypomagnesiumuria have ratios of 26 to 33, so this patient falls at the lower end of the patient group. I find that about 10% of my patients fit this category of hypomagnesiumuria. In the past, therapy consisted of 120 mg of magnesium oxide three times daily with meals. One commercial product combined 500 mg of magnesium oxide with 50 mg of vitamin B_6. Some patients preferred this once daily dosage if they could tolerate it. Some magnesium oxide is converted to magnesium hydroxide in the gut, so intolerance to magnesium oxide usually manifests itself as diarrhea and flatulence. The majority of patients (80%) demonstrate this only temporarily and then adjust to the medication. If they do not, another class of medication must be prescribed. Patients should be cautioned to buy tablets with the United States Pharmacopeia (USP) designation. This means that the tablets will dissolve properly. I have seen non-USP magnesium tablets that entered and left the gastrointestinal (GI) tract looking just the same.

Another magnesium compound, magnesium gluconate, has become available in the United States. I have used this lately because it seems to cause less GI distress. Dosage averages 500 mg twice daily with meals.

Some cautions are necessary. Magnesium therapy should not be used in patients with renal failure (serum creatinine levels >3 mg/dL). If patients take antacids containing magnesium and take magnesium to treat stone disease, they may develop diarrhea that will worsen stone disease. Indeed, that happened in this patient. He suddenly began to form stones again after a period of total freedom from stones of more than 4 years. I learned that his internist had prescribed an antacid containing magnesium. Our mutual patient was having three to four loose stools each day. His medication was changed to an alternate antacid that did not contain magnesium, and the stone formation ceased.

Magnesium cannot be used as shotgun therapy of stone disease. It is best applied only when the patient has had a metabolic evaluation that demonstrates fasting hypomagnesiumuria. On the other hand, it is relatively nontoxic and inexpensive, so it represents a simple means of therapy that will stop stone formation in the proper patient.

BIBLIOGRAPHY

Drach GW, Gaines J, Donovan J: Is magnesium metabolism related to calcium urolithiasis? in *Urolithiasis and Related Clinical Research.* Schwille PO, Smith LH, Robertson WG, et al (eds): New York, Plenum Press, 1985, p 241.

Johansson G, Backman U, Danielson BG, et al: Magnesium metabolism in renal stone formers. Effects of therapy with magnesium hydroxide. *Scand J Urol Nephrol* 1980; 53(suppl):125.

31

Citrate Therapy of Urinary Stones

Glenn M. Preminger, M.D.

The patient forms and passes two or three calcium oxalate and calcium phosphate renal stones per year. She is 34 years old and had her first stone at age 19 years. She did require shock wave lithotripsy for a 1.5-cm renal stone 3 years ago. At this time, she has two 3-mm stones in the left kidney. Several metabolic evaluations implied that she had no specific metabolic defect, except that she seldom had a urinary pH less than 6. She did acidify the urine after an acid load test. She had been given oral neutral phosphates, then thiazides, and finally both medications with no prolonged decrease in her stone disease. She appeared to follow her low-calcium, low-oxalate diet well, and she drank more than 2,000 mL of fluids/day. Repeat metabolic evaluation after cessation of medications for 5 days indicates that her calcium metabolism is normal, but her urine citrate level is 135 mg/24 hours.

Numerous inhibitors of urinary calcium–containing calculi have been identified, including mucopolysacchrides, polypeptides, and RNA. However, although these various inhibitors may play a role in stone formation, most of these substances are often difficult to identify and quantitate. Moreover, even if reliable and easy to manage assays were available for their identification, it would be difficult to administer specific medications to increase the production of these substances.

It is the ease and reliability of identifying urinary citrate, combined with its wide clinical applicability and proved efficacy, that makes this inhibitor a clinically proved treatment for a wide variety of metabolic stone problems.

METABOLIC EVALUATION AND DETERMINATION OF URINARY CITRATE

The goal of any diagnostic evaluation of a patient with recurrent nephrolithiasis should be to identify as efficiently and economically as possible the particular physiologic defect present in a given patient with nephrolithiasis to enable selective, rational therapy of his or her stone disease. Such a metabolic evaluation should be able to identify specific medical disorders responsible for recurrent stone disease. These problems include some of the causes of hypocitraturia, such as renal tubular acidosis (RTA) and chronic diarrheal syndromes. In these conditions it is generally agreed that selective medical therapy is indicated not only to prevent further stone formation but also to correct the underlying physiologic disturbances that may lead to other metabolic or physiologic problems.

The magnitude of the metabolic evaluation in a stone-forming patient should be gauged on the "severity" of the patient's disease. For example, in a first-time stone former who has no specific risk factors for recurrent stone formation such as a strong family history for stones or a metabolic abnormality that may predispose toward recurrent stone formation, one may perform a simplified metabolic evaluation that includes looking at the serum electrolytes levels, performing a urinalysis and urine culture, and analyzing the stone composition. However, the patient in this case is truly a metabolically active stone former and has additional risk factors for recurrent stones, such as early age of onset and persistent stone production while on medical therapy; therefore, an extensive metabolic evaluation is indicated.

After all medications are discontinued, two 24-hour urine collections are obtained with the patient on a random diet reflective of her usual dietary intake. A third 24-hour urine sample is collected after 1 week of a calcium- and sodium-restricted diet. This dietary restriction is imposed to standardize the diagnostic tests, to better assess the etiology of hypercalciuria, and to prepare for the fast and calcium load test, which is performed on the second visit. Blood samples are obtained during both visits.

The collection of a 24-hour urine sample should not be a complex endeavor. For the accurate determination of stone-forming risk factors, all that is needed is a refrigerated 24-hour urine sample. The main purpose of refrigeration is that the cold will inhibit bacterial growth within the urine, which can often degrade some of the stone-forming risk factors, especially the urinary citrate. At the completion of the 24-hour urine collection, the urine should again be kept refrigerated or on ice until it is brought to the hospital laboratory for processing.

INTERPRETATION OF TESTS

Results of the urine samples obtained during a random diet, especially when compared with the urine samples collected during the restricted diet, will permit an assessment of environmental risk factors. The patient in question has already undergone several metabolic evaluations that have implied that she had no specific metabolic defect. The only factor of note was the finding that her urinary pH was rarely less than 6.0. The finding of a persistently alkaline urine should alert one to the suggestion of distal RTA or chronic urinary tract infection (UTI). Moreover, the patient was also noted to have profound hypocitraturia, a finding that is also consistent with either distal RTA or infection lithiasis. Let us explore both of these possibilities in further detail.

Distal Renal Tubular Acidosis

The metabolic defect in patients with distal RTA entails the patient's inability to adequately acidify the urine. This accounts for the finding of a persistently alkaline urinary sample. It is unusual for a normal person to routinely produce urine samples with a pH greater than 6.0.

The definitive test to identify a patient with distal RTA is the ammonium chloride load test. The finding of inadequate urinary acidification after ammonium chloride load will confirm the presence of an acidification defect in the distal tubule.

It has been noted that our patient was able to adequately acidify her urine after an acid-loading test, which by definition will exclude the diagnosis of definitive distal RTA. However, one must still be concerned that an incomplete form of distal RTA may be present, as suggested by the persistently alkaline urine and the significant hypocitraturia.

The cause of hypocitraturia in patients with distal RTA has been attributed to hypokalemia and chronic metabolic acidosis, both persistent findings in patients with distal RTA. Both of these conditions will enhance renal tubular reabsorption and reduce tubular synthesis of urinary citrate, factors contributing toward low urinary citrate levels.

Infection Lithiasis

Patients with persistent UTIs often form recurrent urinary calculi if the offending organisms produce urease, a urea-splitting enzyme. These organisms cause ammonia to be dissociated to form ammonium and hydroxyl ions. The resulting alkalinity of urine augments the dissociation of phosphate to form triphosphate ions and reduces the solubility of struvite, calcium carbonate, and calcium phosphate. Moreover, persistent infection will also produce citrate-lyase, an enzyme that will degrade urinary citrate. Hence, patients with persistent UTIs often demonstrate profound hypocitraturia. Although our patient has persistent hypocitraturia, neither her history nor stone analysis suggest infection lithiasis as the cause of her recurrent stone disease.

Other Potential Causes of Hypocitraturia

As mentioned earlier, any condition that shifts the patient's acid-base status toward chronic metabolic acidosis will cause persistent hypocitraturia. In patients with chronic diarrheal syndromes such as Crohn's disease, intestinal malabsorption, or short-bowel syndromes, chronic diarrhea causes significant bicarbonate loss with resultant metabolic acidosis.

Thiazide therapy for either hypertension or recurrent stone disease may induce hypokalemia, which contributes to intracellular acidosis and hence hypocitraturia. Moreover, studies have demonstrated that a high–animal-protein diet with an elevated acid-ash content can also contribute to an overall acidotic milieu and can contribute to hypocitraturia. Finally, approximately 5% to 10% of patients may have idiopathic hypocitraturia where their only metabolic finding is that of low urinary citrate excretion without other identifiable metabolic abnormalities.

Our patient had been on thiazide therapy in the past, which may have contributed to her hypocitraturia. Another possibility might be that the patient has idiopathic hypocitraturia. Whatever the cause, correction of the hypocitraturia must be accomplished to prevent this patient's recurrent stone disease.

SPECIFIC MEDICAL THERAPY OF HYPOCITRATURIA

In patients with hypocitraturic calcium oxalate nephrolithiasis, potassium citrate therapy is capable of restoring normal urinary citrate levels, lowering the urinary saturation of calcium oxalate and calcium phosphate, and inhibiting the crystallization of calcium salts. The major metabolic finding in our patient is that of hypocitraturia. Because the mean normal urinary citrate excretion is 640 mg/day, this patient would definitely benefit from alkali therapy.

Historically, sodium alkali has been the treatment of choice for chronic therapy in patients who require alkali administration, such as those with distal RTA. This therapy has been given either in the form of sodium bicarbonate or a combination of sodium citrate and citric acid. Although sodium alkali therapy is efficacious in correcting the metabolic acidosis and hypocitraturia in patients with distal RTA, the excess sodium load may have potential unfavorable affects on recurrent calcium nephrolithiasis. Indeed, sodium alkali has been shown to increase the risk of calcium stone formation. In contrast, potassium citrate therapy has been demonstrated to provide an adequate alkali load while effectively reducing the formation of calcium oxalate and calcium phosphate stones in patients with incomplete distal RTA, chronic diarrheal syndromes, thiazide-induced hypocitraturia, and idiopathic hypocitraturia. Potassium citrate therapy is able to restore urinary citrate excretion in all of these conditions, with doses varying from 40 to 120 mEq/day, depending on the severity of metabolic acidosis.

I usually begin citrate therapy at 60 to 80 mEq/day in divided doses. Patients are instructed to take their potassium citrate tablets within ½ hour of meals to prevent gastrointestinal (GI) upset (because of the potassium). Because urinary pH is generally high in the aforementioned conditions, the overall rise in urinary pH is small. In patients who have difficulty tolerating potassium citrate tablets or have problems with citrate absorption (e.g., in chronic diarrheal states), a liquid preparation of potassium citrate rather than the slow-release tablet preparation may be prescribed. In addition, a frequent dosage schedule (three to four times per day) for the liquid preparation is necessary because this form of the medication has a relatively short duration of biologic action. A less frequent dosage schedule (two to three times per day) is acceptable if the solid preparation is adequately absorbed because of its slow-release characteristics.

Although thiazide diuretics have been widely used for the medical management of hypercalciuric calcium nephrolithiasis, some patients may continue to form stones while on thiazide therapy. This poor clinical response may be the result of thiazide-induced hypocitraturia. Thiazides have been shown to reduce urinary citrate excretion because of hypokalemia, with resultant intracellular acidosis. The reduced citrate excretion caused by thiazide administration may therefore increase the risk for calcium stone formation and attenuate the beneficial effects of thiazide therapy, such as a decline in urinary calcium excretion. It should therefore be common practice to administer potassium supplementation, preferably in the form of potassium citrate, to patients receiving thiazide diuretics for the treatment of hypercalciuria. The addition of potassium citrate to thiazide therapy has been shown to prevent the development of hypokalemia and cause a sustained increase in urinary pH and citrate levels. Most patients will require only 60 mEq/day in divided doses.

In patients with idiopathic hypocitraturia, potassium citrate therapy has been shown to produce a sustained increase in the urinary citrate excretion from initially low values to within normal limits. This treatment results in a significant decline in the urinary saturation of calcium oxalate and has been demonstrated to significantly reduce the stone formation of calcium oxalate and calcium phosphate calculi in these patients.

GENERAL COMMENTS ON CITRATE THERAPY

It is apparent that potassium citrate therapy can be used successfully in a variety of conditions. Combined data from recent long-term clinical trials utilizing potassium citrate show no significant change in serum potassium levels, hematocrit values, bone density, or creatinine clearance during treatment. Although the slow-release tablet preparation of potassium citrate is associated with occasional GI complaints in a number of patients, the liquid preparation of potassium citrate is well tolerated. After potassium citrate therapy is instituted, serum potassium and urinary potassium and citrate levels are determined to assess the effect of citrate therapy. Observing whether the urinary potassium excretion remains increased will allow an easy way to monitor patients' compliance in taking their medication.

Various forms of potassium citrate are currently available for the treatment of hypocitraturia. Plain potassium citrate preparations include a slow-release tablet form, as well as potassium citrate liquid and crystals. In addition, potassium citrate can be formulated with citric acid or sodium citrate. However, as previously noted, my preference is to limit the amount of sodium intake in the calcium stone formers, and I would therefore recommend staying with potassium citrate alone or potassium citrate or citric acid preparations.

Although citrate is readily available from citrus juices and urinary citrate levels may be increased by a modified diet of reduced acid-ash content, potassium citrate preparations will offer the easiest (and probably most economical) method of obtaining a significant increase in urinary citrate excretion.

BIBLIOGRAPHY

Nicar MJ, Peterson R, Pak CYC: Use of potassium citrate as potassium supplement during thiazide therapy of calcium nephrolithiasis. *J Urol* 1984; 131:430.

Nicar MJ, Skurla C, Sakhaee K, et al: Low urinary citrate excretion in nephrolithiasis. *Urology* 1983; 21:8–14.

Pak CYC, Britton F, Peterson R, et al: Ambulatory evaluation of nephrolithiasis: Classification, clinical presentation and diagnostic criteria. *Am J Med* 1980; 69:19–30.

Pak CYC, Fuller C, Sakhaee K, et al: Long-term treatment of calcium nephrolithiasis with potassium citrate. *J Urol* 1985; 134:11–19.

Preminger GM, Sakhaee K, Pak CYC: Alkali action on the urinary crystallization of calcium salts: Contrasting responses to sodium citrate and potassium citrate. *J Urol* 1988; 139:240.

Preminger GM, Sakhaee K, Skurla C, et al: Prevention of recurrent calcium stone formation with potassium citrate therapy in patient with distal renal tubular acidosis. *J Urol* 1985; 134:20.

32

Hyperoxaluric Urolithiasis

John G. Gregory, M.D.

A 46-year-old male pilot who had an ileal bypass procedure because of obesity 7 years ago is now found to have two 3-mm calculi in the area of the left kidney. The patient has formed at least nine calcium oxalate monohydrate calculi since his bypass procedure. The patient strongly refuses reversal of his surgery because he has maintained his weight within the limits for his aviation physical examination. On the other hand, he is now threatened with losing his flying license because of stone disease. The patient is 6 ft tall and weighs 233 lb. His physical examination is unremarkable except for a well-healed midabdominal scar. Serum electrolyte analysis shows a low potassium level, elevated chloride levels, and low carbon dioxide level. Serum creatinine clearance is 1 mg/dL. His urinary excretion of calcium is 52 mg/day and oxalate is 134 mg/day.

During the 1970s small bowel bypass procedures began to be frequently performed, and it was soon recognized that stone formation was an early complication of this procedure. It was initially assumed that the stones produced by these patients were the same as those produced by patients suffering and undergoing treatment for regional enteritis. In the first reports dealing with bypass stone disease, it was suggested that the calculi were uric acid induced by conditions of dehydration, protein catabolism, and acidosis. It soon became evident, on examination of the calculi, that the stones formed after small bowel bypass procedure were constructed entirely of calcium oxalate. Although the mechanism of stone formation that occurs after intestinal resection is only partially understood, it does appear that if considerable segments of ileum and jejunum are removed and the colon is left intact, hyperoxaluria will occur. This hyperoxaluria will produce a propensity in those patients for stone formation of calcium oxalate calculi. That this hyperoxaluria is dependent on the intact colon is demonstrated in those few patients having both small bowel resections and ileostomies who do not become hyperoxaluric.

The source of the oxaluria is predominantly exogenous. Dietary oxalate is absorbed from the colon of bypass patients up to 300 times more efficiently than it is absorbed from the intact gut in the same patients. It is believed that after the bypass procedure, unabsorbed fat combines with calcium in the gut lumen, reducing the amount of ionized calcium present in the bowel content. With insufficient calcium available to combine with oxalic acid, thus making it relatively insoluble, the highly water-soluble oxalate passively diffuses through the gut lumen. The absorbed oxalate, which is a metabolic end product, is excreted by the kidney, and in the kidney it combines with urinary calcium to create calculi. After the small bowel bypass procedure, the patients are relatively oliguric because the short-bowel syndrome results in a watery diarrhea and because the patient attempts to decrease this diarrhea by restricting fluid intake. A fluid-restricted patient with urinary oxalates often in excess of 150 mg/24 hours is at a high risk of stone formation. In fact, up to 16% of the small bowel bypass patients did form calculi. Of interest is the fact that not a higher percentage formed calculi. All patients who had ever had a calculus before having the small bowel bypass procedure did form postbypass calculi, suggesting once again that there is an as yet not understood propensity for stone formation. In individuals with this propensity, once the conditions of stone formation are reached, crystallization will occur.

Of some benefit for the small bowel bypass patients is the fact that after bypass, patients are generally hypocalciuric. Urinary calcium levels less than 50 mg/24 hours are not uncommon. Thus, although the oxalate level is increased, the calcium level is decreased, and the calcium oxalate ion product may remain unchanged.

The endogenous nature of the oxaluria is also illustrated by the fact that it is possible by totally avoiding dietary oxalate to prevent the resultant hyperoxaluria. Small bowel bypass patients given synthetic diets devoid of oxalate can drop their urinary oxalate values to normal levels. Unfortunately, such diets are unpalatable for long periods. Because oxalate is an ubiquitous substance present in many food products, it has been difficult to design an effective low-oxalate diet.

STONE FORMATION

The incidence of stone formation after intestinal resection varies with the extent of the resection. In our series of 660 patients followed for more than 6 years, the incidence of stone formation was 17.1%. Fifty-two percent of these patients formed only one calculus, and only 1.3% had such frequent calculogenesis to warrant consideration of bypass reversal. Sixty-five percent of the calculi formed were noted within 1 year of bypass—a period of time when the patient is maximumly oxaluric and also a period of time when the urinary calcium level is in the process of falling but has not yet reached its low postoperative level.

TREATMENT OF ENTERIC CALCULI

The treatment of enteric calculi is based on methodology designed to:

1. Reduce the level of endogenous oxalate production.
2. Prevent the absorption of exogenous oxalate.
3. Prevent the urinary saturation of calcium oxalate.

PREVENTION OF ENDOGENOUS OXALATE PRODUCTION

The prevention of endogenous oxalate is difficult to achieve and of limited significance insofar as less than one fifth of the oxalate excreted by the postbypass patient is of endogenous origin. Increasing the levels of pyridoxin and folic acid in the diet can lead the oxalate metabolic pathway to products other than oxalate. Likewise, the avoidance of entry compounds capable of being converted to oxalate (e.g., vitamin C) will reduce endogenous production. Reliance on these measures alone is not sufficient.

PREVENTION OF EXOGENOUS OXALATE ABSORPTION

As stated earlier, oxalate absorption can be eliminated by a diet that contains no oxalate. Obese patients are obese because of an inability to diet, and an impractical diet has no chance of success. Of some practicality is the avoidance of foods known to be high in oxalate; spinach, okra, rhubarb, and loose tea have the highest levels of oxalate, and the avoidance of these materials is sensible.

Chelating agents such as cholestyramine bind oxalate and prevent absorption but not with enough efficiency to make this a practical therapy.

The most effective agent to reduce exogenous oxalate absorption is calcium. Although it might seem initially counterproductive to give oral forms of calcium to patients suffering calcium oxalate stone disease, the intent is to decrease the gut absorption of oxalate by increasing the possibility of the formation of insoluble calcium oxalate gut complexes. Calcium does, if given in high enough quantities, reduce the level of oxaluria in small bowel bypass patients. Other divalent ions such as magnesium and lanthanum have been used as alternatives for calcium as a gut-binding agent. Although these agents seem theoretically preferable to calcium, their efficiency at reducing stone formation has not been borne out in clinical trials.

PREVENTION OF CRYSTALLIZATION

Hydration

As in all instances of stone formation, modalities that decrease the urinary concentration of solute are most advantageous. With sufficient hydration it is possible to prevent crystal components from demonstrating spontaneous nucleation. Immediately after the bypass procedure, hydration is difficult because of the associated diarrhea. But by 1 year after bypass, hydration to a greater or lesser extent is possible for most patients using diphenoxylate hydrochloride (Lomotil) or (less desirable) codeine as a means to prevent gastric motility and the associated diarrhea.

Allopurinol

The aciduria seen after bypass is associated with urate precipitation. This crystal precipitation removes from the urine those proposed but incompletely identified inhibitors of calcification. The use of allopurinol, at least in theory, prevents the urate crystallization and thus increases the inhibitor activity of the urine. I recommend that bypass patients take 300 mg of allopurinal daily.

Alkalinization

It has been shown that at an alkaline urinary pH the level of calcium oxalate saturation is increased, as is the urinary crystal formation point. Experimentally and clinically it has been possible to reduce calcium oxalate crystallization after small bowel bypass by adequate systemic alkalinization. Unfortunately, in these patients alkalinization is difficult to achieve. Doses of bicarbonate up to 1 g four times daily can be successful but is associated with extreme flatulence. Citrate combinations such as Polycitra and Citrolith are more palatable.

For patients with existing stones, alkalinization can be problematic. In fact, in two patients whose urine was alkalized after discovery of renal calcium oxalate stones, a considerable mass of calcium phosphate was laid down on the existing calcium oxalate nuclei.

SUMMARY

The measures taken for this pilot should include hydration to decrease the relative concentration of calcium oxalate, liberalization of his calcium intake to increase the intestinal precipitation of oxalate and thus decrease oxalate absorption. Allopurinol should be added to both decrease heterotropic nucleation and aid in increasing those factors inhibitory of nucleation. Alkalinization by bicarbonate or preferably citrate may help to decrease the likelihood of calcium oxalate nucleation. The pilot should be informed that the majority of post–small bowel bypass stones are formed within the first year of the bypass procedure. With subsequent diminution in the formation rate, hydration improves and diarrhea decreases. Unfortunately, to date, a group of patients without identifiable characteristics continue to form stones at a fairly steady rate years after bypass. If the pilot in question finds himself in this latter group, he must choose between an alternative form of weight reduction and stone formation. Alternatively, if the stone formation rate can be reduced to a relatively reasonable frequency, it should be possible to diagnose by renal ultrasonography and to treat by extracorporeal shock wave lithotripsy any resultant calculi. Although such diagnosis and therapy are relatively noninvasive, the cost would not be inconsequential, and the possibility that the patient could develop painful obstructive stone disease at a particularly inopportune moment would always remain. It would seem reasonable to advise the patient to consider alternative employment if careful attention to this regimen does not dramatically decrease his stone formation to less than the currently described rate of 1.3 per year.

33

Nephrolithotomy

William H. Boyce, M.D.

You examine a 48-year-old slightly obese woman who has been referred to you because of a staghorn calculus of the left kidney that extends to all calyces. She has moderate tenderness to palpation of the left flank and a well-healed right flank scar. Right nephrectomy was performed 12 years previously because of pyonephrosis. She continues to have *Proteus mirabilis* urinary tract infections (UTIs). Serum creatinine level is 1.3 mg/dL, and her creatinine clearance is 64 mL/minute, corrected. Intravenous (IV) urogram reveals that at least two of the middle posterior calyces have narrowing of the infundibula.

Three well-defined techniques for removal of staghorn renal calculi are extracorporeal shock wave lithotripsy (ESWL), percutaneous nephrostolithotripsy (PNL), and anatrophic nephrolithotomy (AN). Fully 90% of all renal calculi seen in the past 5 years were treated by ESWL, PNL, or both. The remaining 5% to 10% required open surgical procedures (AN) because of anatomic or infectious considerations or a wide range of systemic or urinary diseases. Virtually all stones treated by AN should be in this category of complicated calculous disease. The problems arise in guidelines for physicians' choice and patient acceptance of the decision. When we have had time to fully evaluate the results, we may find that all true staghorn calculi are most effectively treated in combination with AN.

Noninvasive techniques of PNL and ESWL were introduced to America in 1982 and 1983. The distribution of equipment, the "learning curve," and Food and Drug Administration approval required 2 to 3 years. The emphasis in the past 5 years has been to test the technical capability for removal of urinary calculi and hence to push these techniques to their limits. The two current and most comprehensive symposia on treatment of urinary calculi clearly attest to this fact, because neither of them includes a section on open surgery or medical management of calculi, which must be an integral part of treatment.[1, 2] Renal calculi are, in fact, a symptom of one of many well-recognized disease syndromes. Because stones are a solid symptom, they may create additional disease. Calculous disease therefore frequently presents itself in a baffling array of etiologic, anatomic, physiologic, and even sociologic combinations. Effective therapy includes correction of the etiologic factors, preservation of renal function, and comfort without disability at reasonable cost. To concentrate all our attention on removal of the calculus is a reversal of medical advance in the field in this century.

IS THERE GREATER DANGER WHEN OPERATING (AN) ON A SOLITARY KIDNEY THAN WHEN EMPLOYING EITHER ESWL OR PNL?

"Danger" is interpreted as a major life-threatening complication, such as renal damage requiring nephrectomy, dialysis, or pulmonary embolus, or cardiovascular accident, such as stroke. The incidence of such complications in 1,065 operations resulted in a mortality rate of 0.38% within 3 months of surgery; no nephrectomies were done.[3] The incidence of complications was no greater in patients with solitary kidneys than in those with two kidneys. Assimos et al.[4] have recently completed a retrospective comparison of 36 patients with staghorn calculi in which one third were treated by AN and two thirds were treated by PNL with or without ESWL. The assignment to AN or PNL was made on the basis of anatomic considerations. There were equivalent numbers of solitary kidneys in each group. The complications of those with solitary kidneys were no different from those with two kidneys and regardless of the disease state of the opposite kidney. No case of major complications or mandatory nephrectomy occurred in either group. Therefore, the tentative conclusion is that a solitary kidney per se is not a contraindication to any of the three techniques. We must bear in mind that injury to a solitary kidney by any means is far more threatening (dangerous) than when a functional contralateral kidney is present.

NEPHRECTOMY IN THE TREATMENT OF STAGHORN CALCULI

In the decade immediately following World War II, nephrectomy was not uncommon treatment for staghorn calculi in patients who had a normal contralateral kidney. It was only when surgeons began to operate on solitary kidneys that they discovered the frequency of acute tubular necrosis (ATN) in kidneys subjected to the surgical techniques of the day. The results of surgical treatment were so adverse that many internists and surgeons alike preferred to delay or postpone forever surgery of some staghorn calculi. In 1983 a review of 1,065 intrarenal nephrotomies, of which 315 required extensive reconstruction of the collecting system, reported no obligatory nephrectomies at the time of or following surgery.[3] This is not to say that nephrectomy should not be done in some patients. At least six individuals in this series had no appreciable function preoperatively and never developed function in the operated kidney. This does emphasize the fact that all methods for evaluating renal function must reflect actual function of the aggregate of nephrons at the time and condition of the test. There is no test with reliable predictive value as to recovery after treatment of disease. The clinical assessment of potential recovery is colored by the observation that few nephrons recover from chronic disease compared with the recovery rate from ATN.

None of the previous reviews[1, 2] has addressed the incidence of obligatory nephrectomy after PNL or ESWL treatment of infected staghorn stones. Conditions that may be expected to set the stage for hemorrhage or sepsis requiring nephrectomy include poor renal function with poor concentration of antibiotics in the kidney, release of bacteria from fragmentation of stones, hemorrhage from vascular injury, and obstruction to poorly functioning urinary conduits.

One of the first rules of AN is never to operate on a staghorn kidney without maximal preoperative antibiotic suppression of the infection. To do so is to risk operating on an acutely inflamed, hyperemic, friable, and easily injured kidney. It is not always possible to predict general or localized acute or subacute infections in staghorn calculi from the systemic signs and symptoms. Open surgery would seem to be a much safer and more reliable way to prevent sepsis or to avoid nephrectomy in this situation than either PNL or ESWL.

WHAT ARE THE IMPLICATIONS OF STRUCTURAL (CICATRICIAL OR CONGENITAL) INCOMPETENCE OF THE URINARY CONDUITS?

When one compares the incidence of calculi in matched patients with and without congenital ureteropelvic obstruction, there is no convincing evidence that such obstruction per se contributes significantly to the diathesis for stone formation. However, once the stone diathesis has been activated, especially in the presence of infection, stasis is a major determinant in the severity of the disease. It also has influence on the effectiveness of therapy as judged by persistence, recurrence, or progression of the infectious process. Clinical observation strongly supports the analogy that cicatricial obstruction of the ureteropelvic junction and intrarenal conduits secondary to stones and infection has similar effects. However, to suggest that percutaneous incision without repair relieves such stasis and is, in fact, comparable with reconstructive intrarenal surgery belies all the principles of plastic surgery and all of our past experience with intubated ureterotomy and pyeloureteroplasty.

It is never possible to resurrect or regenerate back to normal structure and function the irreversibly dilated calyces with papillary and parenchymal atrophy. However, it is possible to significantly improve treatment of infection by reconstructive renal surgery, which removes all stone fragments and improves drainage.[4] It should be emphasized that identification of mechanical obstruction by purely pyelographic observation without pressure gradients, calibration, or volume flow is always inconclusive. An example is the differentiation of true ureteropelvic stricture from spasm in the presence of pelvic stone or pyelitis. Stasis may reflect either obstructive resistance to flow (high pressure) or reduced volume per time (low pressure). The decision to repair or remove a dilated calyx or group of calyces depends on the weight accorded an impressive number of factors. The final analysis should be made at the time of open surgical inspection, but much of the data should be collected before the choice of procedure for stone removal. Examples of necessary data are:

1. Of prime consideration is the amount of functional parenchyma supplied by the dilated calyces relative to the total functional reserve of the patient.

2. The position of the calyx is important because with all other factors being equal, success is more often achieved with preservation of the superior calyces.
3. The technical feasibility of successful calycoplasty is influenced by the opportunity for combination with adjacent infundibulum or pelvis.
4. The presence of abnormal peripelvic or parenchymal lipomatosis is a very poor prognosis for recovery or even stabilization of renal function. The process of lipid replacement of the obstructed kidney is rare but once in progress appears to be irreversible.
5. Selective parenchymal biopsy of the kidney at the time of surgery is virtually a routine part of AN. A frozen section can provide invaluable assessment of functional capability of the parenchyma.
6. Determination of basal renal arterial blood flow and especially the response to measured ischemia are proven indicators of renal functional capability.[5] Whether velocimetry by Doppler ultrasound with other forms of renovascular stimulation in vivo may accomplish the same result is yet to be investigated.

Whatever one's convictions of the necessity of these considerations, there can be little argument that their assessment and disposition are best accomplished by open surgery. Thus, the signal indication for anatrophic reconstructive surgery is anatomic abnormalities of the kidney.

BODY HABITUS

Body size and thickness of the subcutaneous and perirenal fat pads have an important bearing on choice of therapy for staghorn calculi. Shock waves are difficult to focus precisely at the greater distance, the change in energy level at point of impact is unpredictably altered, and repeat treatments are more frequent in excessively large people. Although the problems of too short instruments for PNL have been solved by the manufacturers and by precise computerized measurements of distance from skin to renal capsule and calculus, this has not completely removed the difficulties of precise placement and manipulation of percutaneous instruments. It is my experience that obesity adds time and some frustration to preoperative and postoperative care but has never impaired one's ability to accomplish any of the surgical objectives of AN. The patient population of 951 individuals undergoing nephrolithotomy over a 20-year period included some truly giant individuals, many with bilateral stones.[3] There was no unsatisfactory result in any, and no patient was refused operation because of body size or habitus.

RENAL DISEASE

The patient under consideration has excellent preservation of renal reserve. The question is: When does renal function become a factor in the choice of procedure equation? It is beyond the scope of this review to discuss all of the forms of renal disease that may sway the choice. Certain ones are already flagged for caution in ESWL therapy. These include hypertensive disease, peripheral vascular disease (especially those with increased capillary fragility), and diabetes mellitus. The ubiquitous distribution of nephrotoxins and their potentiations by interaction with other agents or physiologic changes such as renal perfusion or tubular injury are well known (e.g., aminoglycosides). It has long been a rule of hypothermic surgery not to operate with a detectable plasma level of aminoglycosides.

In 951 patients undergoing nephrolithotomy with hypothermia, the adjusted creatinine clearance (two or more specimens) was less than 20 mL/minute in 86 (9%) and between 40 and 20 mL/minute in 255 patients (27%). Thirty-six percent were thus classified as in marginal or established renal failure. Many (estimated 36) of the patients with less than 20 mL/minute clearance were subjected to preoperative or postoperative dialysis (usually peritoneal). Only one continued dialysis 3 months after surgery, and this patient had been using shunt dialysis before surgery. In these azotemic patients recovery of depressed function was infrequent, but stabilization of attrition and general improvement as a result of recovery from infection were usual results.

SUMMARY

The positive contributions of ESWL, PNL, and PCN to urologic patients with uncomplicated stones less than 2 cm in diameter fully justifies the enthusiastic acceptance these techniques have been accorded. The case is not so acceptable for true staghorn calculi, perhaps because the follow-up period and the documentation of results are so much more demanding than for smaller uncomplicated calculi. To suggest that ESWL or PNL may have some limitation in effectiveness or may on occasion create disease more serious than that which they were treating detracts in no way from the accomplishments of these instruments or from those individuals who have created and developed them. We, as a scientific discipline, should not continue to extend their usage by good faith analogies rather than by scientific monitoring of the subject.

Reliable answers can evolve only from a scientifically crafted, prospective, randomly assigned comparison of equally competent applications of the three methods with proper collection and analysis of the data under rigorous scrutiny. This is feasible and possible if the scientific community wills it to be so.

REFERENCES

1. Assimos DG, et al: The role of open stone surgery since extracorporeal shock wave lithotripsy. *J Urol* 1989; 142:263–267.
2. Resnick MI (ed): Update on urinary stone disease. *Urol Clin North Am* 1990; 17:157.
3. Boyce WH: Surgery of urinary calculi in perspective. *Urol Clin North Am* 1983; 10:585–594.
4. Assimos DG, et al: A comparison of anatrophic nephrolithotomy and percutaneous nephrolithotomy with and without ESWL for management of patients with staghorn calculi. *J Urol* 1991; 145:710–714.
5. Metzner PJ, Boyce WH: Engineering in urology, in Ray CD(ed): *Medical Engineering*. Chicago, Year Book Medical Publishers, 1974, pp 558–566.

34

Posterior Lumbotomy for Removal of Ureteral Calculi

Dean G. Assimos, M.D.

Extracorporeal shock wave lithotripsy failed to fragment this 44-year-old man's 2-cm right proximal ureteral stone. Plain abdominal films 3 weeks after that treatment showed no change at all. His father developed severe hemorrhage during a percutaneous removal of his renal stones, and the patient does not want that procedure. In addition, he is an active volleyball player and does not want his "muscles cut." He consults you because he has heard that you can do a simple operation that does not need to cut the muscles.

INDICATIONS FOR PROCEDURE

Since the development of percutaneous nephrolithotomy, ureteroscopic lithotripsy, and extracorporeal shock wave lithotripsy (ESWL), very few patients, probably less than 1% to 2%, needing stone removal require an open surgical approach. This small subset of individuals usually have associated complex anatomic and physiologic abnormalities such as infundibular stenosis, large patulous multicalyceal collecting systems, and extreme morbid obesity that preclude less invasive forms of therapy. Patients with impacted ureteral calculi that are refractory to ESWL, ureteroscopic lithotripsy, and percutaneous nephrolithotomy are also candidates for open surgery.

Posterior lumbotomy remains an excellent approach for open stone removal in selected cases. Because the renal pelvis and ureter are positioned dorsally, it can provide excellent exposure for proximal ureterolithotomy and pyelolithotomy. This incision may also be used for pyeloplasty, renal biopsy, and the removal of small kidneys. This approach should be avoided in extremely obese patients or in those harboring complex branched calculi where anatrophic nephrolithotomy is contemplated. Because muscles are not transected with this incision, patients usually have less pain than experienced with standard flank incisions and therefore typically have a brief convalescence.

ANATOMIC CONSIDERATIONS

The gateway of the posterior lumbotomy is the lumbodorsal fascia, which is composed of three layers, or lamellae. This fascia extends from the sacrum and iliac crest to the thoracic area interdigitating with the fibers of the latissimus dorsi and serratus posterior inferior muscles. The posterior lamella spans from the spinous processes of the vertebra extending to the angles of the ribs and covers the sacrospinalis muscle. The middle lamella courses posterior to the quadratus lumborum, whereas the anterior lamella is situated just anterior to this muscle. All three lamellae fuse into a single layer from which the transverse abdominis muscle originates (Fig 34–1). The iliohypogastric and subcostal nerves travel obliquely over the anterior lamella. The paranephric fat and Gerota's fascia are located just anterior to this layer.

TECHNICAL ASPECTS OF PROCEDURE

In most cases, this approach is done with the patient receiving general anesthesia, but in selected situations it can be accomplished with regional or local anesthesia. The patient is placed in a modified lateral position with the affected

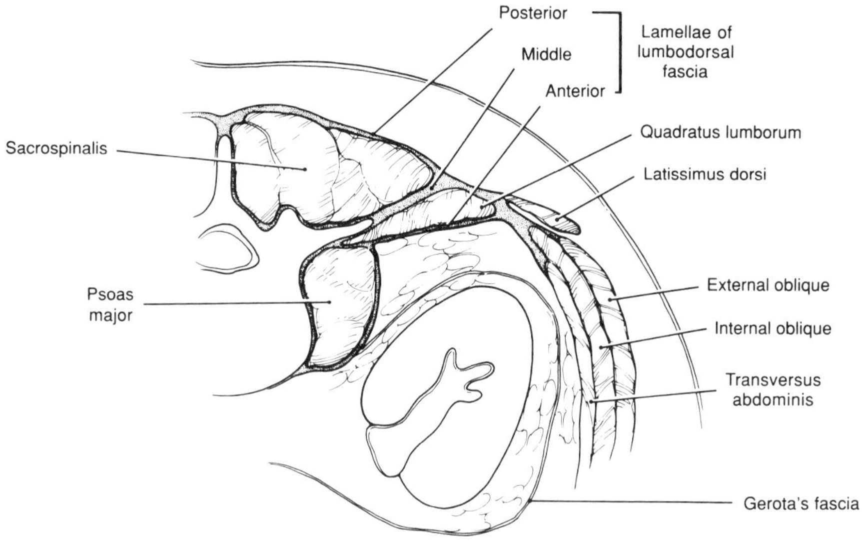

FIG 34–1.
Anatomic relationships of the lumbodorsal fascia.

side up and rotated forward 15 to 45 degrees. The table is slightly flexed, or a sandbag can be placed underneath the opposite loin to increase the space between the lower ribs and iliac crest. The bottom leg is partially flexed, and the top remains straight. Wide tape is placed across the hips and attached to the table to further stabilize the patient's position. The extremities are carefully positioned and padded to prevent nerve palsy (Fig 34–2).

The skin incision is made starting at the lateral border of the sacrospinalis muscle at the level of the costovertebral angle and is extended slightly obliquely down to the middle portion of the iliac crest. The posterior lamella of the lumbodorsal fascia is incised vertically, exposing the sacrospinalis muscle, which is retracted medially (Fig 34–3). This maneuver exposes the middle lamella, which is divided in a similar fashion. The quadratus lumborum muscle is retracted toward the vertebral column, and the underlying anterior lamella is incised between the subcostal and iliohypogastric nerves (Fig 34–4). A self-retaining retractor is placed and opened to expose the paranephric fat and underlying Gerota's fascia. If further superior exposure is needed, the costovertebral ligament can be divided, segments of the 11th and 12th ribs can be resected subperiosteally, or the incision can be extended anteriorly at a right angle to the superior aspect of the wound. When any of the aforementioned maneuvers are undertaken, the pleura is carefully mobilized superiorly.

When proximal ureterolithotomy is performed through this incision, the lower pole of the kidney is lifted superiorly and the ureter is located in the ret-

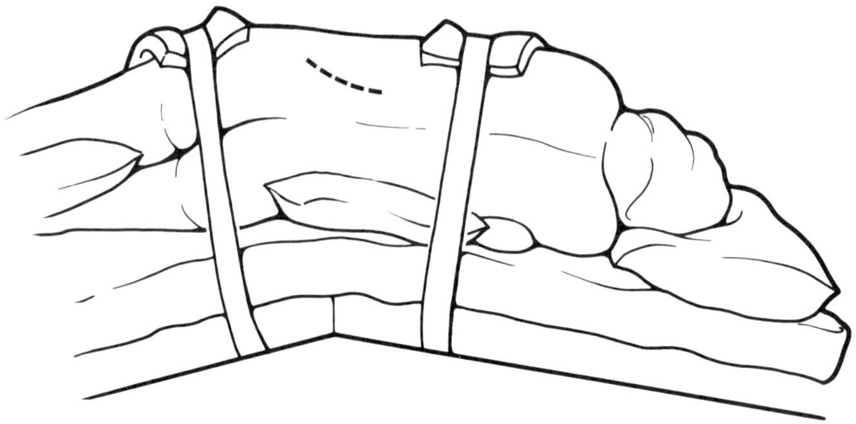

FIG 34–2.
Proper patient positioning for posterior lumbotomy.

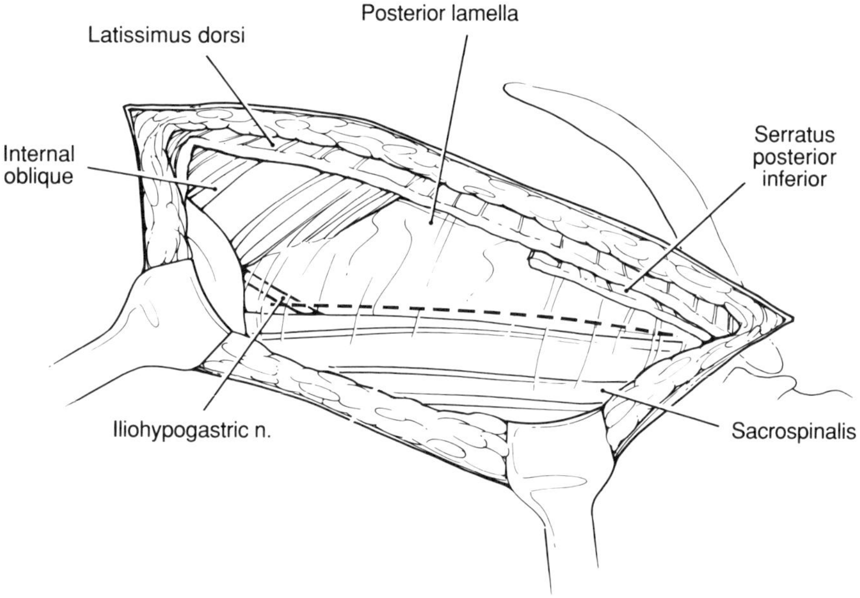

FIG 34–3.
A vertical incision through the posterior lamella of the lumbodorsal fascia exposes the underlying sacrospinalis muscle.

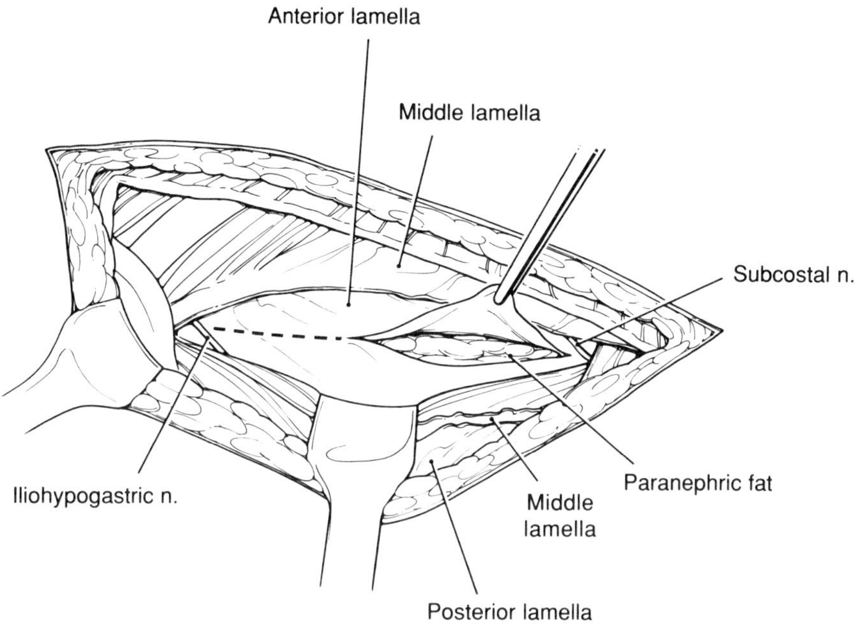

FIG 34–4.
Medial retraction of the sacrospinalis and quadratus lumborum muscle exposes the anterior lamella of the lumbodorsal fascia, which is incised between the subcostal and iliohypogastric nerves.

roperitoneal space. Vessel loops are placed around the ureter above and below the calculus to prevent stone migration. A curved scalpel blade is used to longitudinally incise the ureter over the stone. After the stone is extracted, a silicone stent is placed down the ureter into the bladder and up into the renal pelvis. The ureterotomy is closed with an extramucosal running 5-0 or 6-0 absorbable suture (Fig 34–5).

During pyelolithotomy, Gerota's fascia is incised longitudinally and the renal hilar area exposed. The space between the renal pelvis and parenchyma is gently dissected to expose the renal sinus. Two Gil-Vernet retractors are placed to enhance exposure. If multiple renal calculi are present, a coagulum pyelolithotomy can be performed. A wide U-shaped incision is made in the renal pelvis, avoiding the area of the ureteropelvic junction. A stone forceps is used to carefully extract calculi. If necessary, flexible nephroscopy is employed to extract hard to reach calculi. An intraoperative radiograph should be obtained to confirm total stone removal. A stent is passed antegradely into the bladder and carefully positioned in the renal pelvis. The pelvic incision is closed with a running 5-0 or 6-0 absorbable suture.

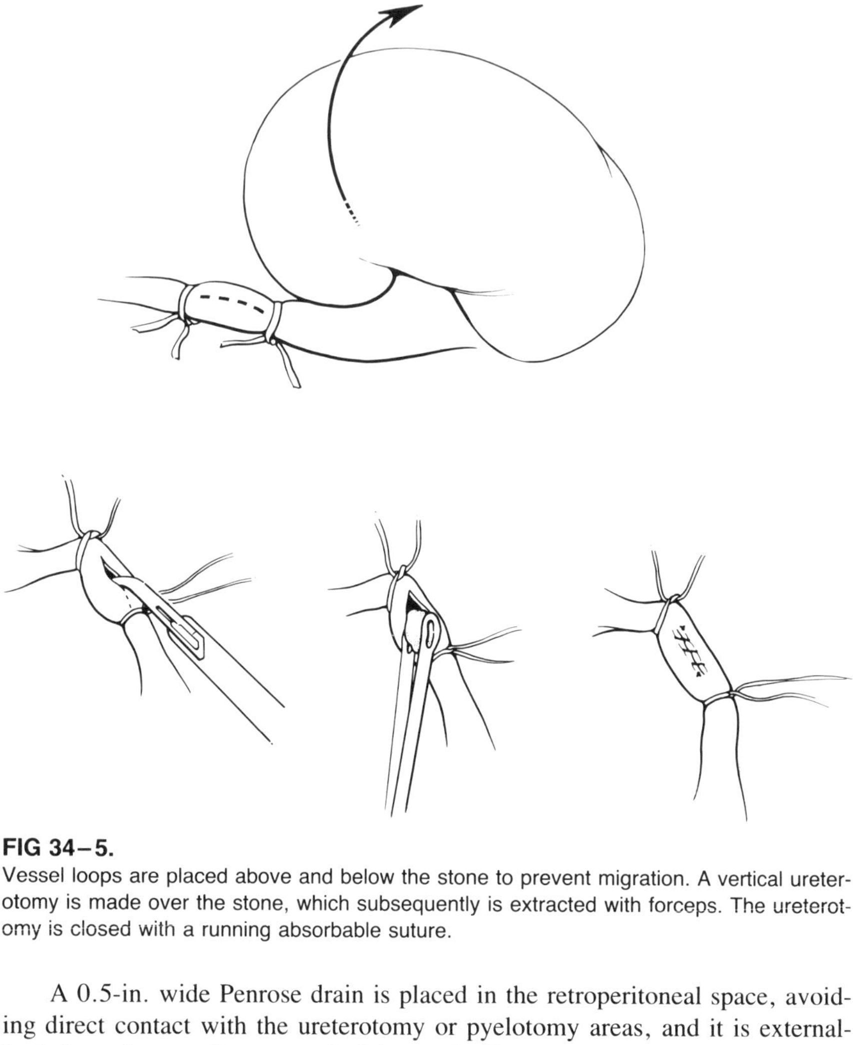

FIG 34–5.
Vessel loops are placed above and below the stone to prevent migration. A vertical ureterotomy is made over the stone, which subsequently is extracted with forceps. The ureterotomy is closed with a running absorbable suture.

A 0.5-in. wide Penrose drain is placed in the retroperitoneal space, avoiding direct contact with the ureterotomy or pyelotomy areas, and it is externalized through a small separate incision and affixed to the skin. The middle and posterior lamella of the lumbodorsal fascia are closed separately with a running 2-0 or 0 absorbable suture. The subcutaneous tissue is approximated with a running 3-0 or 4-0 absorbable suture, and the skin is closed with a running subcuticular suture. The Penrose drain is removed when drainage ceases. The stent is usually removed endoscopically on the first postoperative visit, usually 2 weeks after discharge.

35

Percutaneous Nephrolithotripsy

Joseph W. Segura, M.D.

You have shock wave lithotripsy and percutaneous lithotripsy facilities at your hospital. This 38-year-old patient asks you to perform shock wave lithotripsy on her cystine stones of the left kidney. One is a 3.5-cm renal pelvic stone that extends branches into two lower calyces, and the second 1.5-cm stone sits beside it in a posterior calyx.

This woman has doubtlessly has had experience with many other cystine stones in the past and typically would have undergone previous surgical procedures for her stones. Also, because she has these symptomatic, surgical stones, she has failed medical therapy. Although we do not know the reason for this, it is an important consideration in selecting therapy and in determining whether a given procedure is successful.

Patients in this situation have three choices for management of the stone: (1) open surgery, (2) percutaneous lithotripsy (PL), and (3) shock wave lithotripsy.

SURGERY

Open stone removal should be avoided because these patients usually have had previous surgery, resulting in a procedure of increased difficulty. Also, because they represent failures of medical therapy, they are likely to reform surgical stones.

SHOCK WAVE LITHOTRIPSY

The usual question is whether the situation is appropriate for treatment with the shock wave machine. The response of cystine stones to extracorpeal shock wave lithotripsy (ESWL) is variable and not predictable. Further, because this stone is a high-volume stone, even should fragmentation occur, multiple treatments will probably be required to generate fragments small enough for spontaneous passage. Further, it is very likely that stent insertion will be necessary to prevent ureteral colic; also, ureteroscopy may well be required if large fragments end up in the ureter. The size of this stone precludes the use of ESWL, although this technique is occasionally more reliable with smaller cystine stones.

PERCUTANEOUS LITHOTRIPSY

This patient is a good candidate for a percutaneous procedure for stone removal because of the size of the larger stone. Direct access should enable the operator to remove this stone in one procedure. The approach should be into one of the two lower calyces, probably the more superior calyx, to maximize the possibility that the calyceal extentions can be accessed by manipulating the nephroscope in the tract.

I prefer to use the ultrasonic probe on a stone such as this because the pieces will be removed as they are created. How long this will take depends on how hard the stone is, as well as its size. Bhatta and Dretler[1] have recently demonstrated that there are two types of cystine stones, a rough and a smooth variety, which vary in their hardness. This may explain why some cystine stones respond quickly to ultrasound and others do not. If the procedure is becoming tedious because of stone hardness, the electrohydraulic probe should be used to break off pieces of stone, which can then be treated with ultrasound.

It should be possible to remove the entire pelvic portion of this stone together with its calyceal extentions in one procedure. The question is whether the posterior calyceal stone can be accessed through this tract or whether some other maneuver will be necessary. Hopefully the nephroscope can be oriented so that the infundibulum can be seen and the ultrasonic probe placed through it, directly on the stone. If this is not possible, the flexible nephroscope may be maneuvered to visualize the infundibulum, after which the electrohydraulic probe can be used on the stone. In situations where the infundibulum is about the size of the stone, a 22-gauge needle can sometimes be employed to push the stone into the pelvis, where it is then easily reduced with ultrasound. Extracorporeal shock wave lithotripsy could be used in the hope that this stone may respond, but this will ensure another percutaneous procedure to remove the pieces. The simplest and surest thing to do is to create a second tract through the posterior calyx and remove the stone directly. If things are going well and bleeding is minimal, this should be done as part of the original procedure. Otherwise it can be done as a second procedure.

It is essential that all the stone be removed. One might suspect that after debulking, medical therapy might be expected to dissolve the remaining stone, but this has not proved to be the case. Review of our cystine stone formers treated by percutaneous methods revealed that if they were not stone free after the procedure, they would not be stone free at follow-up (mean follow-up, 22 months). The corollary of this is that if postprocedure films reveal residual stones, a second look through the tract should be done to remove this stone. We have alkalinized the urine in these patients and have the impression that this has made the residual stones easier to remove than they were during the first treatment.

The nephrostomy tube and percutaneous stent inserted in all PL patients is removed when the patient is stone free. If success was achieved at the initial procedure, removal is after 48 hours. I also like to perform a nephrostogram to be certain that there is no unrecognized obstruction. A leak not recognized at the original procedure is very uncommon. If a second procedure is not required, the patient is in the hospital 4 days (procedure day 1). They may return to average physical activity 7 to 10 days after the procedure. Statistically, cystine stone patients have about a 40% chance of needing a second procedure, and this will add 2 days to their hospital stay. Percutaneous lithotripsy can be repeated in these patients, if necessary.

SUMMARY

In this patient with cystine stones, PL is the single procedure most likely to clear her of stone with the least invasion and probably least cost. If she is to be stone free, previous experience dictates that she must be made so at the time of PL.

REFERENCE

1. Bhatta KM, Prien EL Jr, Dretler SP: Cystine calculi—rough and smooth: A new clinical distinction. *J Urol* 1989; 142(4):937.

36

Percutaneous Treatment of Calyceal Stone, Narrow Infundibulum

Robert M. Moldwin, M.D.
Arthur D. Smith, M.D.

Two stones, 5 mm each, lie in a single dilated calyx of the midportion of the left kidney. On an intravenous (IV) urogram, the infundibular outlet appears to be narrow. The patient describes intermittent bouts of left flank pain, which is accompanied by microscopic hematuria.

Calyceal stones in the face of infundibular narrowing frequently come to the urologist's attention because of the patient's complaints of intermittent flank pain or infection. In many instances these stones behave in a manner similar to that seen with ureteropelvic junction obstruction. The etiology of the associated obstruction may be one or a combination of the following:

1. Congenital. On rare occasions, extrinsic infundibular compression is caused by a crossing interlobar artery.[1]
2. Acquired scarring or edema secondary to chronic mucosal irritation.
3. Functional. The stone in these instances may elicit an "outlet spasm."
4. Factitous. A narrowed infundibulum seen on an IV pyelogram (IVP) may be artifactual if the patient is dehydrated during the study.

We have found conservative management using oral chemolytic agents has little value in the treatment of these stones. The exception are small uric acid or possibly cystine calculi, which we treated with a trial of urine alkalinization. Endourologic methods and occasionally extracorporeal shock wave lithotripsy (ESWL) have been our mainstay treatments for these calculi. Infundibular narrowing unfortunately often presents a frustrating technical problem for both of these lines of management. In the case of ESWL, although many patients seem to be relieved of their painful symptoms, passage of stone fragments has been disappointing. Percutaneous removal of these calculi can be difficult when one attempts to dilate the narrowed infundibulum, particularly when one is dealing with an anterior calyx. Careful patient selection and preoperative strategy are, therefore, essential to achieve a successful result.

PREOPERATIVE EVALUATION

A complete history and physical examination are mandatory. With specific reference to those patients whose sole complaint is flank pain, neurologic and gastrointestinal (GI) etiologies should be excluded. A complete blood cell count, analysis of serum electrolytes, blood urea nitrogen, serum creatinine, coagulation studies are routinely done. A urinalysis and urine culture are obtained. If bacteriuria is present, the urine should be sterilized with an appropriate antibiotic before treatment. All patients receive IV antibiotic prophylaxis before surgery and in the immediatc postoperative period.

A high-dose IVP is the single most important preoperative test. The IVP should be performed with oblique and lateral views to precisely evaluate whether the stone lies in an anterior or posterior calyx. Stone position is particularly important when one is contemplating a percutaneous approach (discussed later on). The addition of a furosemide bolus to the IVP will often reveal an otherwise nonvisualized infundibulum. Retrograde pyelography is useful for patients in whom an IVP does not give acceptable results.

OPERATIVE MANAGEMENT

Before deciding on therapy, we discuss the benefits and complications of the various treatment modalities.

Extracorporeal Shock Wave Lithotripsy

We will generally offer ESWL therapy to patients with calyceal stones associated with a narrowed infundibulum. Patients excluded from this form of therapy are those with associated urinary tract infections, cystine stones, or large (>2 cm), hard (calcium monohydrate) stones. Although fair results have been achieved for relief of patient's symptoms, subsequent passage of the fragmented stone burden has been disappointing. Psihramis and Dretler[2] recently reviewed ten patients who underwent ESWL therapy for calculi located within a calyceal diverticulum (a similar clinical situation to the narrowed infundibulum). With a mean of 5.9 months' follow-up, they reported seven patients having relief of their flank pain but only two patients having complete passage of their stones. In addition, three patients required two ESWL treatments for complete stone fragmentation probably because of the small confines within the diverticulum. Van Cangh et al.[3] identified only a 50% stone-free rate in patients who had undergone ESWL vs. 95% in patients treated by percutaneous techniques. Extracorporeal shock wave lithotripsy was associated with a 45% retreatment rate, no change in the diverticula postoperatively, and 62% of patients remaining symptomatic.

Patients undergoing ESWL must be well aware of these mediocre results before choosing this form of therapy.

Percutaneous Approach to the Calyceal Stone

Percutaneous approaches to calyceal stones may be broadly divided into two categories: antegrade and retrograde. The goals of therapy are twofold: to remove the stone and to create a widely patent infundibulum. An outline of our operative strategies follows.

Direct Puncture

This is the most common approach that we use. The direct approach is most useful with stones located in a posterior calyx.

A no. 6 French open-ended ureteral catheter is placed preoperatively. The patient is then rotated onto the operating table into the prone position with appropriate bolsters in place. Contrast medium is then infused through the ureteral catheter to opacify the collecting system and to visualize the narrowed infundibulum. An 18-gauge trocar-cannula needle is introduced into the chosen calyx directly in the standard fashion. Every effort is made to create a nephrostomy tract that lies below the 12th rib to avoid entry into the pleural space. The needle is directed onto the stone burden. The guidewire is advanced onto the calyx, and an attempt is made to direct it into the renal pelvis during nephrostomy tract dilation. With access achieved, a small J-tipped 0.038-in. or Bentson (Cook Urological) guidewire is gently introduced into the dilated calyx. Advancement of the wire is performed under fluoroscopic guidance in an attempt to manipulate it across the narrowed infundibulum (Fig 36–1,A). If access to the renal pelvis is accomplished, sequential dilatation of the tract into the chosen calyx is performed to no. 34 French size using an Amplatz system. An additional "safety" guidewire is introduced during tract dilation. The calculi are then extracted using grasping forceps or ultrasonic lithotripsy. The infundibulum can then be dilated with the Amplatz system to size no. 34 French. Alternatively, the narrowed infundibulum may be balloon dilated.

The most common problem encountered when one is dealing with infundibular stenosis is the inability to pass a wire into the renal pelvis. In these instances, we will gently coil the guidewire in the involved calyx (Fig 36–1,B). Occasionally a Cobra catheter can be introduced into the calyx over the guidewire. This catheter may then be used to manipulate the guidewire through the infundibular outlet under fluoroscopic control. If access to the infundibulum is not achieved, the nephrostomy tract is carefully dilated, taking care to avoid guidewire displacement. When the no. 34 French Amplatz sheath is introduced, the stone fragments are removed (Fig 36–1,C). Nephroscopy then continues with the hopes of identifying the infundibular outlet. When the outlet has been identified, a Bentson guidewire is passed into the renal pelvis. The infundibulum is then dilated in the usual fashion. Again, a reentry tube is left in place across the infundibulum.

If the infundibulum cannot be identified, one may infuse a mixture of contrast media and methylene blue in a retrograde fashion through the previously placed ureteral catheter. The infundibulum can then be identified through the nephroscope and under fluoroscopic guidance.

Infundibulotomy is an alternative to dilation and may be helpful with difficult guidewire passage. One must be acutely aware of the segmental arteries that lie beside each infundibulum.[4] A straight cold knife is used to create incisions that are no greater than 1 to 2 mm in depth and 120 degrees apart from one another (Fig 36–2,B). Alternatively, infundibulotomy may be performed

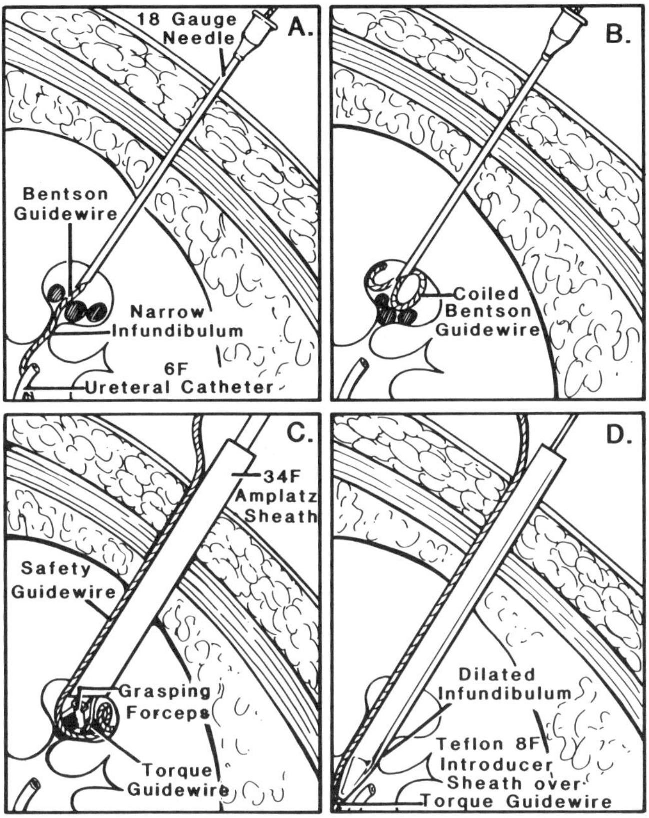

FIG. 36–1.
A, a no. 6 French open-ended ureteral catheter is placed into the renal pelvis in a retrograde fashion. Contrast media is infused into the collecting system, and an 18-gauge trocar-cannula needle is used to puncture into the dilated calyx. **B,** in the event that the guidewire cannot be passed through the infundibulum, it is coiled into the calyx. **C,** dilation of the established tract is carefully performed into the calyx. Note that a second torque guidewire was added for the larger-diameter dilators. **D,** the calyceal stones have been removed. A guidewire has been advanced into the renal pelvis, and the infundibulum has been dilated.

using an Nd:YAG (neodymium–yttrium–aluminum-garnet) laser or coagulation electrode.

Nephroscopy continues into the renal pelvis, where the previously introduced ureteral catheter is grasped and brought through the nephrostomy site. The catheter is then exchanged for a 0.038-in. torque guidewire. A no. 24 French reentry nephrostomy tube is placed over the guidewire. With correct po-

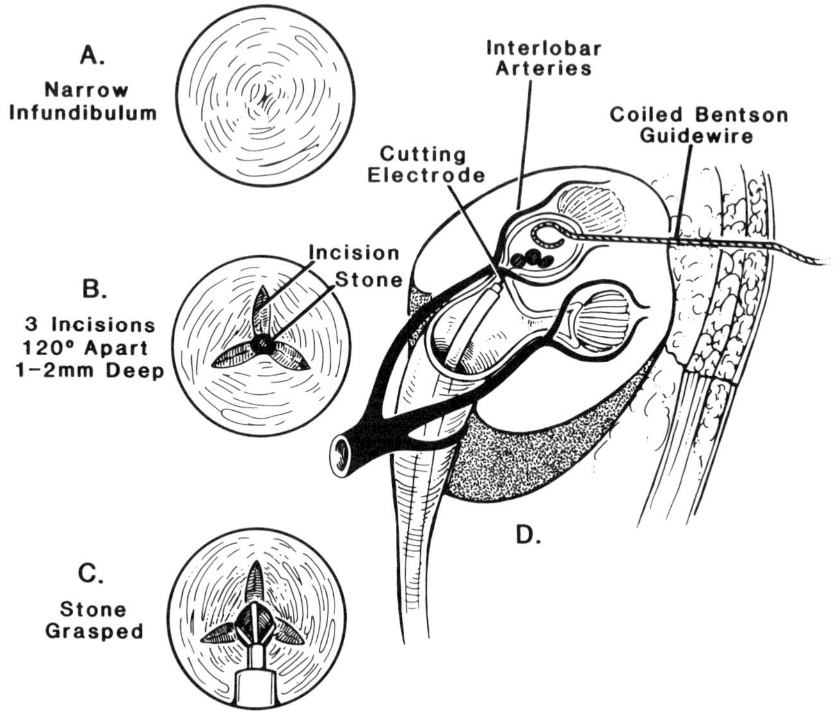

FIG 36–2.
A, an antegrade or retrograde view of a narrowed infundibulum. **B,** superficial incisions are created to widen the infundibulum while avoiding the segmental and interlobar arterial blood supply. **C,** the stone can then be removed with grasping forceps. **D,** an approach to the anterior calyx. If a direct puncture into the calyx is performed, access to the renal pelvis is difficult because of the orientation of the infundibulum (see text).

sitioning of the nephrostomy tube confirmed, the tube is secured in place and the guidewire removed. We remove the nephrostomy tube after a nephrostogram (performed 48 hours postoperatively) assures the absence of stones or significant extravasation.

Problems With Difficult Access

Upper pole and anterior calyces present the most difficult technical challenges for stone extraction and infundibular dilatation. Upper pole calyces are generally approached indirectly through a lower pole puncture. The infundibulum is, therefore, approached in a retrograde fashion. As with direct caliceal puncture, the infundibulum may be incised or a guidewire placed for subsequent dilation (Fig 36–2,D).

Access to the upper calyx may also be obtained by downward renal displacement.[5] This is performed by establishing a nephrostomy tract through a middle pole calyx. The tract is dilated, and a no. 30 French Amplatz sheath is left in place. The tip of the sheath is then angulated inferiorly, thereby displacing the upper calyx into a position that can be accessed below the 12th rib.

Anterior calyces present a technical problem because of difficulties in gaining access to the infundibulum. If a rigid nephroscope is admitted directly into the anterior calyx, the endoscopist would need to then direct the scope backward to visualize the infundibulum. To circumvent this problem, we keep a flexible nephroscope available to locate the infundibulum and pass a guidewire. If access cannot be achieved, we will leave the guidewire coiled in place, then gain retrograde access through another calyx as discussed earlier. If the calyx can be entered in this fashion, the previously placed coiled guidewire can be grasped and pulled through the second nephrostomy tract. Dilatation of the infundibulum is performed, and a circle nephrostomy tube is placed.

Ureteroscopy is yet another approach for managing these calculi. The ureteroscope must be flexible with active and passive control of its distal limb. As with the nephroscope, one must be certain that instruments of sufficient size will be able to advance through the working channel, even when the distal limb of the instrument is angulated. The pulse-dye laser is particularly helpful in these situations because the fibers are very flexible and accomodate most working channels. Electrohydraulic lithotripsy has also had reported success when flexible instruments are used.[6]

The ureteroscope may be advanced over a previously introduced guidewire. The guidewire is then removed, leaving the working channel free. If repeated access is necessary, we will advance a no. 12/14 French "peel-away" sheath (Cook Urological) upward to the ureteropelvic junction during these manipulations.[7] Infundibulotomy is advised in these cases because stenting of a dilated infundibulum postoperatively is not possible.

CONCLUSION

Calculi residing in obstructed calyces frequently present challenging management problems. Oral chemolysis and ESWL therapy have limited roles in treatment because of their poor success rates for ridding patients of their stone burden. Moreover, these methods do not address the remaining infundibular stenosis, which predisposes the patient to recurrent stone disease. Our mainstay of therapy has been a percutaneous approach to the involved calyx, with subsequent dilatation of the narrowed infundibulum. Although this technique is usually successful, difficulties at gaining control of the involved infundibulum frequently arise. One should therefore be familiar with multiple approaches to this problem to achieve optimal results.

REFERENCES

1. Fraley EE: Dismembered infundibuloplasty, in Whitehead ED, Leiter E (eds): *Operative Urology,* ed 2. New York; Harper & Row, 1984.
2. Psihramis KE, Dretler SP: Extracorporeal shock wave lithotripsy of caliceal diverticula calculi. *J Urol* 1987; 138:707.
3. Van Cangh PJ, AaD AA, Lorge FJ, et al: Management of symptomatic calculi located in caliceal diverticula: A review of 38 patients. Paper presented at the 84th Annual Meeting of the American Urological Association, Dallas, May 1989.
4. Kaye KW, Goldberg ME: Applied anatomy of the kidney and ureter. *Urol Clin North Am* 1982; 9:3.
5. Karlin G, Smith AD: Approaches to the superior calyx: Renal displacement technique and review of options. *J Urol* 1989; 142:774.
6. Bagley DH: Removal of ureteral and renal calculi with the flexible ureteropyeloscope [abstract]. *J Urol* 1988; 139:188A.
7. Saltzman B, Smith AD: Percutaneous renal surgery. *Semin Urol* 1986; 4:153.

37

Selection of Patients for Extracorporeal Shock Wave Lithotripsy

Christian Chaussy, M.D.
Gerhard J. Fuchs, M.D.

You receive a telephone call from your urologic colleague in another country. He inquires about your thoughts on the treatment of a 57-year-old woman who has a 1.3-cm stone impacted in the right ureter at the level of the transverse process of L4. The stone sits in the notch created by the spine and the iliac crest. Should he treat it in situ or push it back into the kidney? Is it advisable to pass a stent first? He is concerned by all of the literature that seems to contradict itself.

EXTRACORPOREAL SHOCK WAVE LITHOTRIPSY OF URETERAL STONES

Approximately 80% of all urinary stones pass spontaneously; only 10% to 15% need interventional therapy, such as extracorporeal shock wave lithotripsy (ESWL) or ureteroscopy (URS). The basic indications for surgical treatment of ureteral stones are (1) unresolving pain; (2) stone size too large for spontaneous passage; (3) persistent obstruction regardless of stone size; (4) anatomic alterations, such as stricture distal to the stone; and (5) emergent treatment to avoid severe complications.

Indications for emergency treatment of ureteral stones are (1) obstructive pyelonephritis because of the impending risk of sepsis and (2) anuria in the case of either bilateral ureteral obstruction or obstruction of a solitary kidney.

Unremitting pain unresponsive to oral analgesics and antispasmodics may become an indication for a more urgent treatment strategy, especially in the elderly and debilitated patient because of the risk of severe pain triggering a myocardial infarction or a stroke via hypertension secondary to the pain.

The treatment strategy for patients with obstructive pyelonephritis is geared toward immediate renal decompression via ureteral drainage or percutaneous nephrostomy tube placement and initiation of broad-spectrum intravenous (IV) antibiotic coverage. After resolution of the acute symptoms, further treatment follows the established guidelines for elective treatment of ureteral stones (Tables 37–1 and 37–2).

Elective treatment of ureteral stones is determined by the stone location, stone size, degree of stone impaction, the anatomy of the upper urinary tract, and the availability of modern technology such as ESWL and URS. Assuming that all of the new technologies are available to the operator, the strategy for elective treatment of ureteral stones is directed primarily by the stone location and the technical features of the lithotriptor available (anesthesia vs. anesthesia-free, fluoroscopy vs. ultrasound localization). Endourologic skills, such as ure-

TABLE 37–1.
Treatment Algorithm for Ureteral Stones

Symptom	Action
Pain	
Intermittent	Elective treatment
Incidental finding	Elective treatment
Unremitting	Drainage via double-J or direct ureteroscopic stone removal
Fever (obstructive pyelonephritis)	Drainage (percutaneous or ureteral stent) IV antibiotics and fluids

TABLE 37–2.
Selection Criteria for ESWL of Ureteral Stones

Variables determining treatment approach
Approach individualized according to expansion space and stone location
No standard treatment protocol for all ureteral stones
Depending on lithotriptor used (x-ray or ultrasound stone localization)
Depending on endourologic experience

teroscopy and percutaneous antegrade access to the ureter, are important for the management of complicated stone disease and ESWL failures. Open surgical procedures are reserved for the concomitant repair of severe anatomic anomalities of the upper urinary tract and for the management of complications.

Selection Criteria

Stone Location

Three different areas in the ureter, namely, the proximal ureter above the iliac crest, the midureter between the iliac crest and pelvic brim, and the lower or pelvic ureter below the pelvic brim, are distinguished, and different protocols for the management of ureteral stones in each of these locations have to be implemented.

Proximal Ureter.—The factors determining the selection of the best treatment strategy for the management of proximal ureteral stones are the existence of a sufficient expansion space, the availability of "anesthesia-free" lithotriptors, and the availability of ureteroscopic lithotripsy.

For a patient with a 1.3-cm stone at the level of L4, the preferred treatment in the United States since 1990 is retrograde stone manipulation with the intent to reposition the stone into the renal collecting system, followed by ESWL fragmentation under the same anesthesia. This treatment philosophy is based on the use of a first-generation fluoroscopy localizing lithotriptor, which in a one-stage procedure yields the highest success rates, but at the expense of the need for regional anesthesia and an auxiliary endoscopic procedure with limited invasiveness. A success rate greater than 85% can be achieved for retrograde stone manipulation, and a greater than 90% stone-free rate is seen after ESWL of the repositioned stone. Whenever retrograde repositioning of the stone into the kidney is not feasible, creation of an artificial expansion chamber using ureteral stents yields stone-free rates of up to 92%. If the stone can not be successfully manipulated using the previous approach, the success with in situ ESWL is approximately 50%, and these patients therefore are not good candidates for ESWL; instead, they are best treated by direct contact lithotripsy with electrohydraulic, laser, or ultrasonic fragmentation for a success rate of close to 100% in experienced hands. Operators of the newer anesthesia-free lithotriptors mostly favor direct in situ treatment of stones in the proximal ureter to capitalize on the anesthesia-free feature. This is especially true when fluoroscopy localizing lithotriptors are used, which allow successful localization of the stone in most of the cases. In situ treatment without attempted retrograde manipulation can result in a stone-free rate of up to 75%; however, a significant number of patients need multiple treatments and subsequent auxiliary endoscopic procedures that require regional or general anesthesia. Technical difficulties in ultrasonic identification of proximal ureteral stones below the lower margin of the kidney preclude in situ ESWL treatment of such patients with the newer lithotriptors featuring ultrasound stone localization. To overcome this impasse, manufacturers have equipped a number of recently introduced lithotriptors with dual imaging capabilities of ultrasound and fluoroscopy. No larger clinical series using these machines have been published, so that assessment of this approach is not possible at the present time.

Midureter.—Originally called the "stone cracker's no man's land," stones located in the midureter (i.e., between the iliac crest and the pelvic brim) can now be treated with the newer, fluoroscopy localizing lithotriptors. The patient can be positioned prone, so that no bone is interposed between the shock wave source and the targeted stone. Stone-free rates of up to 60% can be achieved using this approach. Although the anesthesia-free feature makes this approach appealing, the treatment outcome is less than certain because of imaging problems (stone overlying bony pelvis). This approach requires the use of an x-ray table version second-generation lithotriptors, which are not yet widely available. Most urologists still prefer the classic approach of retrograde stone manipulation, followed by ESWL, which for stones in this area allows successful repositioning into the kidney in approximately 75% and ESWL stone-free rates of approximately 90%. Direct contact ureteroscopic lithotripsy is yet another approach that, in experienced hands, results in success rates of almost 100% at the expense of slightly increased invasiveness.

Distal Ureter.—Stones in the distal and prevesical ureter were the first ureteral stones approached using the in situ ESWL treatment technique with the first-generation lithotriptors. Despite the difficulty of patient positioning for stone visualization with the fluoroscopy imaging systems, stone-free rates of up to 90% have been reported. Alternatively, direct ureteroscopic stone retrieval or ureteroscopic lithotripsy can be employed, which has yielded success rates close to 100% with minimal complications in almost all larger series published. Localization of the stone with ultrasound localizing lithotriptors is feasible but technically difficult and time consuming. Using these lithotripters, one can image the distal ureter through a full bladder with the patient in the prone position. In these instances, the stone-free rates are similar to those with fluoroscopy localizing ESWL.

Stone Size

Stone size greater than 8 mm precludes spontaneous stone passage in more than 90% of cases; therefore, in our experience conservative management using the strategy of watchful waiting is limited to smaller stones. Patients with stones larger than 8 mm who have preserved kidney function are scheduled for elective treatment. When the kidney is nonfunctioning on IV pyelogram (IVP) studies, renal function tests are performed and the obstruction is relieved before the definite stone treatment.

Stone Impaction

The degree of impaction of ureteral stones has been shown clinically and experimentally to be an important predictor of the outcome of ESWL when ESWL is employed to treat these stones in situ. The more a stone is wedged in the reactive edema surrounding it, the lesser the chances for spontaneous stone passage after ESWL. Unfortunately, there are no accurate imaging studies to correctly assess the degree of stone impaction, and therefore no prediction of the outcome of in situ ESWL is possible. Even a most recent IVP demonstrating contrast passing by the stone does not ensure a successful treatment outcome. Overall, in situ ESWL of ureteral stones yields stone-free rates between 50% and 70% in one treatment session. In our health care environment in the United States this is not acceptable. We therefore rely on retrograde ureteral stone manipulation as a minimally invasive and time-efficient adjunct to ESWL. Retrograde stone manipulation is successful in approximately 80% of all upper and midureteral stones. Stones resisting attempts at retrograde manipulation at best have a 50% clearance rate after in situ ESWL and therefore should be treated directly with ureteroscopic lithotripsy. The major advantages of ureteroscopy are consistently high success rates, with stone-free rates greater than 90% and more than 95% of patients having only one treatment session. This is achieved at the low expense of an anesthetic with an overall complication rate of less than 5%. For these reasons this approach has become the treatment of choice for ureteral stones in the United States. The use of anesthesia-free ESWL appears to offer no advantages in our health system as far as the treatment of ureteral stones is concerned.

Upper Urinary Tract Anatomy

Anatomic alterations of the ureter precluding retrograde ureteral stone manipulation or spontaneous passage of fragmented stone material may require corrective endourologic or open surgical procedures, with ESWL being utilized as an auxiliary procedure at best.

URETEROSCOPIC REMOVAL OF URETERAL STONES

Ureteroscopic removal of ureteral stones with or without direct contact fragmentation is the treatment of choice when ESWL (1) is not available, (2) is not the most appropriate choice, or (3) has failed. Review of several larger series reveal average success rates with ureteroscopic ureteral stone removal of 70%, 85%, and 95% in the upper, middle, and lower ureter, respectively. However, the higher invasiveness compared with ESWL and the rate of complications of 10%, 5%, and 3%, respectively, have to be considered.

Ureteroscopy, especially for more complex stones that cannot be repositioned or have failed ESWL, requires special endoscopic skills and should be reserved for the more experienced endourologists. Antegrade URS using a percutaneous approach is indicated when retrograde access to the stone cannot be gained (stricture, urinary diversion) and open surgery is not necessary for correction of an anatomic problem.

EXTRACORPOREAL SHOCK WAVE LITHOTRIPSY OF RENAL STONES

As described earlier, the traditional approach for treating ureteral stones with ESWL has involved retrograde stone repositioning into the renal collecting system, based on the fact that small- to medium-size stones located in the kidney can achieve stone clearance rates greater than 90% with ESWL. As of 1990, approximately 70% of patients with renal stones can be treated with ESWL-monotherapy, and 20% of patients with more complex renal stones can receive ESWL treatment in conjunction with endoscopic surgery. The remaining 10% of patients require either percutaneous endoscopic surgery alone or open surgery. Ten years of clinical experience with ESWL have led to the identification of the stone- and patient-related parameters governing the treatment outcome of ESWL technology. The determinants for the selection of the appropriate treatment for renal stones are (1) stone burden, (2) intrarenal and upper urinary tract anatomy, (3) concomitant disease, and (4) patient compliance. In addition, a small number of exclusion criteria still have to be observed, such as uncorrected bleeding disorder, uncorrected hypertension, and aortic or renal artery

TABLE 37–3.
Selection Criteria for ESWL of Renal Stones

Variables determining treatment approach
Stone burden (period of stone passage and rate of auxiliary procedures increase proportionally with stone size)
Intrarenal stone distribution (pelvis vs. calyces)
Presence of intrarenal stenosis
Isolated dilatation of calyces (diverticulum, history of surgery)
Stone composition (calcium oxalate monohydrate and cystine stones respond poorly to ESWL)
Patient compliance (prolonged period of time before treatment is completed)

aneurysms (Table 37–3). Exclusion from ESWL treatment for technical reasons is rare and depends on the type of lithotriptor used. However, patient habitus may present problems because of the stone location relative to the energy source and the patient positioning system (determinants: patient size, patient obesity, skeletal anomalies, and ectopic kidneys) Urologic contraindications are severe anatomic or functional alterations precluding proper elimination of debris (stenosis distal to the stone, e.g., at the calyceal neck, the ureteropelvic junction and in the ureter), hypertrophy of the prostate requiring surgical correction, urethral stricture, a grossly distended stone-bearing calyx (especially dependent calyces), and severe functional impairment of ureteral mobility (neurogenic, immobile patient). In these situations percutaneous surgery or open surgery may be preferable (Table 37–4).

Selection Criteria

Stone Burden

Solitary stones or multiple stones of an added diameter up to 2.5 cm are considered ideal conditions for ESWL treatment, provided there is no hindranced to the spontaneous elimination of gravel. Stone clearance rates between 90% for stones 1 cm and 70% for stones up to 2.5 cm can be expected. For such stones the clinical experience does not identify significant differences in terms of success and complication rates comparing first- and later-generation lithotriptors. Fluoroscopy localizing lithotriptors offer the advantage of a better assessment of stone fragmentation, whereas ultrasound localizing lithotriptors allow treatment of radiolucent and semiopaque stones without auxiliary administration of contrast dye. Most newer, so-called second-generation machines en-

TABLE 37–4.
Exclusion Criteria for ESWL

Medical	
	Uncorrected bleeding disorder
	Uncorrected hypertension
	Patients unfit for anesthesia (for ESWL or auxiliary procedure, if needed)
	Pregnancy (stone treatment rarely necessary, placement of internal stent or percutaneous nephrostomy)
	Aortic or renal artery aneurysm (calcifications of aorta and renal artery are relative contraindications)
	Pacemakers (standby, cardiologist recommended)
Technical	
	Depending on type of lithotriptor
	General problems: stone location relative to energy source and patient positioning system (determinants: patient size, patient obesity, skeletal anomalies and ectopic kidneys, radio-opacity of stone)
Urological	
	Severe anatomic or functional alterations precluding proper elimination of debris
	Stenosis distal to the stone (calyceal neck, ureteropelvic junction, ureter, hypertrophy of prostate requiring surgical correction, urethral stricture)
	Stone-bearing calyx grossly distended (especially dependent calyces)
	Functional impairment of ureteral mobility (neurogenic, immobile patient)
	Gross anatomic anomaly (horseshoe kidney, ectopic kidney, duplicated kidney and/or ureter)
	Attempted manipulation of ureteral stone not successful (relative, has lower ESWL success rate)
	Large stone burden (combination with percutaneous stone removal)

able anesthesia-free ESWL; however, this is done at the expense of a higher retreatment rate than the first-generation lithotriptors (30% vs. 10%). Although it has been proved that even staghorn stones can be treated with ESWL monotherapy, increasing stone burden resulting in lesser stone-free rates and higher complication rates (ureteral obstruction, obstructive pyelonephritis, prolonged period of stone passage, unpredictability of outcome) have significantly dampened the initial enthusiasm with ESWL of staghorn stones. Major stone referral centers with experience in endourology prefer percutaneous debulking for these patients, using ESWL as an auxiliary procedure for stone parts that cannot be reached from the percutaneous access. Average stone-free rates of approximately 50% for ESWL vs. approximately 85% for percutaneous surgery combined with ESWL, as well as annual recurrence rates of 25% and 10%, respectively, speak in favor of the combined or primary percutaneous approach.

Nephrolithiasis is a relatively rare incident in the pediatric age group. In this patient population ESWL has become particularly advantageous because clinical experience has shown no deleterious effects, even when multiple sessions are required. Concerns have been raised with regard to the effect of high-energy shock waves on immature bony tissue, growing renal tissue, long-term renal function, or the induction of hypertension. The available clinical results indicate that ESWL does not lead to deterioration of renal function or altered renal development, and no juvenile hypertension has been noted after ESWL. Recently conducted research on the effects of high-energy shock waves on immature bony tissue and renal growth confirms the safety of this treatment modality. Cautious use of the energy with adherence to certain limits, however, is advocated, and treatment should be performed at major referral centers where all treatment options are readily available.

Upper Urinary Tract Anatomy

Anatomic alterations of the renal collecting system or ureter precluding spontaneous passage of fragmented stone material may require endourologic or open surgical procedures, only to be followed by ESWL as an auxiliary procedure.

Patient Compliance

Extracorporeal shock wave lithotripsy therapy consists of two parts: fragmentation of the stone and spontaneous elimination of the stone debris. Depending on the size of the original stone, a large amount of stone debris may have to clear the ureter, resulting in a prolonged period of stone passage. During this period of time, the patient is at theoretical risk of ureteral obstruction and obstructive pyelonephritis, which may result in loss of renal function or a life-threatening septic complication if not treated appropriately. Patients need to be made aware of this possibility, and the need for compliance with a timely follow-up protocol has to be stressed. Patients who appear unfit to comply with the follow-up protocol should not receive ESWL treatment of complex stones but should undergo percutaneous or open surgery instead.

In 10 years of clinical use, ESWL has proved itself as an efficient and safe treatment of urinary stones with minimal invasiveness. It has become a most valuable asset to the urologist and greatly benefits urologic stone patients. During the short period of time since the advent of ESWL, the management of urinary stone disease has completely changed. Extracorporeal shock wave lithotripsy has almost completely supplanted open surgical, and to a lesser extent, endourologic approaches. Approximately 70% of patients can benefit from ESWL as monotherapy; however, more complex stones require auxiliary procedures, namely, endourological procedures or open surgery. Those 25% to 30% of cases, which require combined endourologic or open surgical techniques, are technically demanding and at times should be reserved for the stone treatment centers where extensive experience with all alternative techniques of urinary stone treatment exists.

BIBLIOGRAPHY

Chaussy C, Fuchs G: Extracorporeal shock wave lithotripsy (ESWL) for the treatment of urinary stones, in Gillenwater J (ed): *Textbook on Adult and Pediatric Urology,* Chicago, Year Book Medical Publishers, 1986.

Chaussy C, Schmiedt E, Jocham D, et al: First clinical experience with extracorporeally induced destruction of kidney stones by shock waves. *J Urol* 1982; 127:417–420.

Chaussy C, Schmiedt E, Jocham D, et al: *Extracorporeal Shock Wave Lithotripsy,* ed 2. Basel, Karger S, 1986.

Drach G, Dretler S, Fair W, et al: Report of the United States cooperative study of extracorporeal shock wave lithotripsy. *J Urol* 1986; 135:1127.

Eisenberger F, Fuchs G, Miller K, et al: Extracorporeal shock wave lithotripsy and endourology—an ideal combination for the treatment of kidney stones. *World J Urol* 1985; 3:41–47.

Miller K, Fuchs G, Rassweiler J, et al: Treatment of ureteral stone disease: The role of ESWL and endourology. *World J Urol* 1985; 3:445.

38

Treatment of Renal Stones by Piezoelectric Lithotriptor

Richard G. Middleton, M.D.

You have just examined a 37-year-old man who has intermittent left flank pain related to a 1.3-cm renal pelvic calculus. This is his first stone, and he is otherwise healthy.

This patient is a suitable candidate for treatment on the Wolf piezoelectric lithotriptor (Richard Wolf Medical Instruments Corp., Rosemont, Ill.), a device with which we have had 2 years of experience at the University of Utah.[1, 2] The procedure is virtually painless. No preparation of the patient is necessary, and there is no interruption of meals or regular activities. No premedication is given at all, and no anesthesia is used. All treatments are carried out on an outpatient basis.

The patient lies on the lithotriptor table. Underlying the patient is the shock wave–generating dish, a 50-cm concave spherical structure containing about 3,000 piezoelectric elements arranged in a mosaic-like fashion. Between the generating dish and the patient's flank is a cylindrical tub containing water that is heated and degassed. The water fills this space to come in contact with the patient's skin. At the same instant, an electric discharge causes each of these individual piezoelectric units to produce a single shock wave. The shock waves all converge at the same point, an area of about 4 by 8 mm. The focal point, or the convergence of the shock waves, is the point for positioning the patient's stone.

Visualization of the kidney and the stone is achieved by two real-time B mode ultrasonic scanners mounted obliquely in the dish. The scanners can be rotated 90 degrees. The scanners can also extend like a telescope for zooming in on a particular area. The urologist sits at the console alongside the patient, who is lying on the lithotriptor table. Bringing the patient's stone into the focal point can be accomplished by moving the generating dish in three planes, extending or retracting the ultrasound scanner, and adjusting the patient's position. Most often the patient is treated in a supine position, but occasionally an oblique or lateral position is preferred.

A standard treatment session lasts about 45 minutes and consists of up to 4,000 shocks. Four levels of pressure intensity are available, ranging from 400 to 1,000 bar at the focal point. Usually the highest energy level is used, except in children or extremely thin patients. Patients experience little or no pain. Usually they detect only a mild vibratory sensation. After the lithotripsy session, patients return to work or other normal activities. They are advised that their urine will likely be mildly bloody for a few hours. They are also given a prescription for an oral narcotic agent, should they have colic with the passage of the stone fragments. Of course, they are asked to strain the urine for the collection of stone material. The following morning an x-ray film of the kidneys, ureters, and bladder (KUB) is obtained. If any significant stone fragments remain, repeat lithotripsy is carried out. When only tiny fragments are seen on the x-ray film, no repeat treatment is needed; but when any doubt exists about the adequacy of stone fragmentation, retreatment is always performed. Retreatment at daily, or at least frequent, intervals has been our approach until we are convinced that only small fragments remain. We have seen no disadvantage or adverse effect from aggressive and prompt retreatment when necessary. The retreatments are painless; patients' normal routine is minimally interrupted, and the expense to patients is the same in our institution whether they have one or several treatments.

For the patient in this case, with a 1.3-cm stone in the renal pelvis, no preliminary double J stent would be employed. We have not used stents before lithotripsy except in selected patients with very large or infected stones or when stones have been manipulated or pushed from the upper ureter into the collecting system before renal lithotripsy.

RESULTS OF PIEZOELECTRIC LITHOTRIPSY

A 2-year experience with the Wolf piezoelectric lithotriptor at the University of Utah is available for review (Table 38–1). This experience occurred from January 1988 through December 1989, with a follow-up of at least 3 months in all cases except for 18 renal units (kidney and upper ureter) that were lost to follow-up. There were 884 treatments to stones in 388 renal units in 220 patients. Actually the stones were located in the renal pelvis, infundibula, or calyces in 375 kidneys. Treatment of upper ureteral stones occurred in only 13 instances. (The Food and Drug Administration–approved protocol for this device excluded treatment of ureteral stones, but occasional exceptions were made when clinically appropriate.) Bilateral renal calculi were common in our series; 168 of 220 patients underwent bilateral lithotripsy.

There were 370 renal units treated for stones and followed for 3 months. At 3 months after treatment, 279 of 370 renal units (75%) were free of stone by KUB x-ray examination, and another 75 (20%) had residual stone fragments less than 3 mm and judged capable of spontaneous passage. Thus, thorough pulverization or stone fragmentation was achieved in 90% of cases. Twelve

TABLE 38–1.
Results With the Wolf Piezoelectric Lithotriptor

	Renal Units	
Results	*n*	%
Stone free	279	75
Fragments <3 mm	75	20
Fragments >3 mm	12	3
Failures	4	1
TOTAL	370	100

kidneys (3%) still contain fragments larger than 3 mm, which will require retreatment. In four patients (1%) sizable ureteral fragments after lithotripsy led to referral to another facility for lithotripsy with a different type of device.

One hundred eighty three renal units (49%) received only one treatment for adequate stone fragmentation, whereas 187 (51%) required two or more lithotripsy sessions to achieve thorough fragmentation (Table 38–2). Small stones, 1 cm or less in diameter, required a mean of 1.5 treatments. Medium-sized stones, 1 to 2 cm in diameter, received a mean of 2.1 treatments. For large stones, those greater than 2 cm in diameter, the mean number of treatments for total fragmentation was 4.9

After lithotripsy with this machine, there has been no case of significant blood loss; no blood transfusion has been given. No perinephric or intrarenal hemorrhage has been detected. Ninety percent of patients passed fragments after treatment with relative ease; either they had no colic or the pain was controlled by oral narcotic agents. Severe colic after lithotripsy requiring parenteral narcotic administration occurred in 38 patients (10%). After treatment nine patients (2%) required a ureteral stent or percutaneous nephrostomy for pain and ureteral obstruction by stone fragments. One patient required ureteroscopic extraction of an obstructive fragment, and two patients underwent ureterolithotomy after ureteroscopic efforts to deal with ureteral stone fragments were unsuccessful. One patient required pyelolithotomy and pyeloplasty for a large fragment collection that could not pass through an obstructive ureteropelvic junction. One patient required admission and treatment for pyelonephritis shortly after lithotripsy. No patient had significant deterioration of renal func-

TABLE 38–2.
Number of Treatments With Piezoelectric Lithotripsy*

	Stone size							
	Small		Medium		Large		All Stones	
No. of Treatments	RU	%	RU	%	RU	%	RU	%
1	138	68	42	38	3	6	183	49
2	42	21	44	39	13	24	99	27
3	15	7	9	8	6	11	30	8
4	4	2	10	9	9	17	23	6
5	2	1	4	4	3	6	9	2
6	3	1	2	2	4	7	9	2
7–10	0		1	1	14	25	15	4
11–13	0		0		2	4	2	0.5
TOTAL	204		112		54		370	
MEAN	1.5		2.1		4.9		2.2	

RU = renal unit.

tion, but five patients (1%) had moderate hypertension after treatment. This hypertension resolved in all but one patient who ultimately required an antihypertensive medication to restore his blood pressure to normal.

ADVANTAGES AND DISADVANTAGES OF THE PIEZOELECTRIC LITHOTRIPTOR

The original Dornier HM-3 (Dornier Medical Systems, Inc., Marietta, Ga.) has proved to be an effective lithotriptor, but it requires an anesthetic and the installation of the water tank and associated equipment. Modifications have reduced the pain and thus the need for anesthesia. Still, premedication with narcotic drugs and sedatives is used with many lithotriptors to help the patient tolerate the pain of the shock wave treatment. As mentioned earlier, a remarkable characteristic of the Wolf piezoelectric lithotriptor is that the patient feels no pain or, at most, a mild vibratory sensation. The patient is treated easily in an ambulatory setting and requires no premedication of any kind. He or she returns to normal activity after the completion of the treatment, which usually lasts about 45 minutes. Two children, ages 6 and 7 years, were given a pretreatment "cardiac cocktail" to ensure that they would hold still. Two children who were 11 and 12 years of age have been treated without premedication and without fear after they were allowed to observe another patient undergoing lithotripsy with this device.

The need for retreatment is commoner with the Wolf piezoelectric lithotriptor than is seen with some other devices. However, retreatment is easy for the patient and apparently harmless, and the cost to the patient is not increased by retreatment. Our philosophy, therefore, has been to use retreatment promptly and aggressively until the stone appears totally fragmented. When doubt exists about the adequacy of treatment, retreatment is the preferred approach. Retreatment with some other lithotriptors exposes the patient to repeat anesthesia, premedicating drugs, disruption of normal daily activities, and extra cost. The ease of retreatment with the piezoelectric lithotriptor means that retreatment is no longer a disadvantage. Retreatment can be carried out freely to hasten the eradication of the stone.

The use of ultrasound guidance is an advantage in that all ionizing radiation is eliminated, and uric acid stones, as well as calcium stones, can be localized. The position of the stone can be monitored constantly, and alterations of the stone or changes in stone location during treatment can be visualized. Renal anatomy can be inspected; masses can be discovered, and hydronephrosis is readily identified and monitored. On the other hand, a KUB film is needed to assess the adequacy of stone fragmentation. Ultrasonic characteristics can suggest to the operator that effective stone breakup is occurring, but the x-ray film reveals the ultimate result of the treatment. Also, the operator needs training in renal ultrasound and in the localization of stones ultrasonically. Several weeks may be needed for the operator to become proficient. More retreatments may be required during the operator's learning phase. The average urologist can learn the techniques in 1 or 2 weeks and will become expert in several additional weeks of experience with this lithotriptor.

The ultrasonic identification of stones in the upper ureter presents difficulty. The urologist who develops confidence and proficiency with renal stone identification may take longer to learn to recognize ureteral stones, which can be subtle. Our treatment protocol has generally excluded lithotripsy for stones lying in the ureter, so we have usually manipulated the stones upward into the collecting system for renal lithotripsy. We have, however, gained some experience with ureteral stone identification and treatment. When there is some degree of hydronephrosis and hydroureter above the stone, and with the patient positioned in an oblique or lateral position, stone localization and treatment of an upper ureteral stone is possible. Our experience at this point is simply limited.

CONCLUSION

The Wolf piezoelectric lithotriptor is safe and effective for the eradication of renal calculi. The success rate is high; treatment is remarkably benign and essentially painless to the patient, but the retreatment rate is higher than that with many other lithotriptors. Retreatment is so simple and convenient with this device that it ceases to be a significant disadvantage. Experience with the treatment of upper ureteral calculi is limited.

BIBLIOGRAPHY

Bowsher WG, Carter S, Philp T, et al: A clinical experience using the Wolf Piezolith device at two British stone centers. *J Urol* 1989; 142:679.

Marberger M, Turk C, Steinkogler I: Painless piezoelectric extracorporeal lithotripsy. *J Urol* 1988; 139:695.

39

Outpatient Extracorporeal Shock Wave Lithotripsy

John R. Burns, M.D.

You review radiographs that indicate a single 1.2-cm stone in the right renal pelvis in this otherwise healthy 24-year-old woman. Her internist has asked you for your opinion on the advisability of extracorporeal shock wave lithotripsy (ESWL). She has passed a prior stone of calcium oxalate. She is self-employed and does not want to miss work days if possible.

Extracorporeal shock wave lithotripsy (ESWL) has become the preferred treatment for removing most urinary calculi. It is generally accepted that the patient described is an ideal candidate for ESWL. The chances that ESWL will fragment a calculus into pieces small enough to pass are 98%. The residual stone rate in this patient would be approximately 10 to 15%, and probably no second treatment or other ancillary procedure would be necessary. Although it is not stated whether the calculus is symptomatic, treatment is indicated, because most renal pelvic calculi eventually become symptomatic. Urologists have been reluctant to recommend surgical treatment for asymptomatic calyceal calculi, but ESWL of a calyceal calculus might be indicated if it is judged to be too large to pass spontaneously. Marberger[1] recently reviewed 63 patients with primary asymptomatic calyceal calculi followed for a mean of 7.4 years. The calculi migrated to the renal pelvis and ureter in about one half of the patients, and about 80% of those eventually required surgical intervention to remove the calculi. Those results should be interpreted in the context of a patient's clinical situation. For example, an asymptomatic calyceal calculus in a 75-year-old patient in poor health might be followed conservatively, whereas the same calculus in a younger patient in good health would be treated promptly.

CRITERIA FOR OUTPATIENT ESWL

When ESWL was introduced into the United States, the Food and Drug Administration (FDA) required that all patients be hospitalized for several days after lithotripsy. After general FDA approval was granted, lithotriptors became widely available, and patients could be treated as outpatients. The practice of outpatient lithotripsy, initially discouraged because of fear of unrecognized serious complications, has become more popular during the last few years.

Extracorporeal shock wave lithotripsy is associated with minimal complications. Lingeman et al.[2] reported on 982 patients treated with ESWL. Nonoperative complications, such as temperature of more than 39°C, pulmonary or cardiovascular problems, or excessive bleeding requiring transfusions, occurred in only four patients. Because the complication rate is extremely low, outpatient ESWL should be safe for most patients. In 1987, we[3] reviewed the records of the first 246 patients treated at our institution. Fifty percent of our ESWL treatments were performed on outpatients. The remaining patients were hospitalized for a number of reasons, often not related to medical necessity. For example, several insurance carriers required admission as a condition for reimbursement, and some referring physicians were uncomfortable with the idea of outpatient lithotripsy and requested hospital admission. Of the first 123 patients treated as outpatients, only 8 required hospital admission within 3 days after ESWL. All patients were treated with a Dornier HM-3 lithotriptor (Dornier Medical Systems, Inc., Marietta, Ga.). I now perform almost all ESWL treatments on outpatients. I have also found that patients who require ureteroscopy in conjunction with ESWL can usually be treated as outpatients. The introduction of second-generation lithotriptors has made outpatient ESWL even more practical. I currently treat many of my patients with a Wolf Piezolith 2300 (Richard Wolf Medical Instruments Corp., Rosemont, Ill.), which requires no anesthesia or sedation and is ideally suited for outpatient use.

A patient's general medical condition might warrant hospital admission for ESWL. Patients thought to be at high risk of post-ESWL bleeding should be observed after the procedure. A patient on chronic anticoagulant therapy is generally instructed to stop warfarin sodium (Coumadin) 2 days before hospital admission, and is then started on intravenous (IV) heparin therapy. When the prothrombin time has returned to normal, the patient is scheduled for ESWL the next day. Heparin is stopped 6 hours before ESWL and reinstituted the following morning if the patient's urine is clear. Warfarin sodium therapy is then restarted, and the patient is discharged when prothrombin time reaches a therapeutic level. Patients with uncontrolled hypertension are at increased risk of a perirenal hematoma after ESWL and should probably be admitted for observation. Any patient with a serious arrhythmia or serious cardiovascular disease should be observed for at least 24 hours after ESWL and should have a follow-up electrocardiogram (ECG) before discharge. Outpatient treatment of a patient with one kidney is controversial. Early in our experience, two such patients treated as outpatients developed steinstrasse. Both became anuric and required emergency cystoscopy and ureteral stenting. I still perform outpatient ESWL in patients with one kidney, but I routinely place a double J ureteral stent, which is removed at a follow-up visit.

PATIENT EVALUATION BEFORE ESWL

Pretreatment evaluation begins with a detailed history and physical examination. In the case presented, we are told that the patient has a prior history of calcium oxalate calculi. If a patient is young and has no prior history of urolithiasis, an initial cystine screen is warranted. A prior history of surgical procedures on a kidney or ureter might make percutaneous stone removal a better treatment option. A patient with a ureteropelvic junction obstruction, a ureteral stricture, or a ureteral reimplantation is not a good candidate for ESWL because any of these conditions can prevent passage of stone fragments. Endoscopic treatment of a steinstrasse is likely to be impossible in a patient with a previous ureteral reimplantation.

The size of the calculus should be considered in determining proper treatment. If a calculus is 2 cm in diameter, residual fragments will probably be present 3 months after ESWL in about one half of the cases. A patient with a calculus of 2 to 3 cm in a lower pole calyx has only about a 1 in 3 chance of becoming stone free after ESWL; many of the retained fragments will eventually grow to clinically important size, so percutaneous stone removal might be a better initial treatment. Patients should be informed of such probabilities to permit more informed decisions.

The extent of pretreatment laboratory evaluation varies according to patient age and medical history. All patients are initially admitted to a holding area, where they are prepared for ESWL. A hematocrit and urinalysis are performed for each patient. If the patient is more than 40 years old or has a history of cardiovascular disease, an ECG is done. Clotting studies are not done unless indicated by patient history (e.g., in cases of bleeding disorders or recent aspirin ingestion). Levels of serum electrolytes, glucose, and creatinine are measured if a patient is taking antihypertensive medication or has a chronic illness. When a patient is scheduled for ESWL, the referring physician is asked to perform a urine culture if the urinalysis is abnormal. A patient with a positive urine culture should be treated for 48 hours before ESWL. As an added safeguard, each patient is given a single dose of gentamicin immediately before ESWL.

ANESTHESIA FOR ESWL

The type of anesthesia administered for ESWL often depends on the physical arrangement of the lithotripsy suite. At our facility, almost all patients are treated with epidural anesthesia. Because the cystoscopy room is not adjacent to the lithotripsy suite, patients must be moved through the hallways of the operating room. That is easier when they are under regional anesthesia. It also reduces turnover time between cases, because anesthesia can be administered in a holding area, thereby reducing the time spent in the lithotripsy suite. It is true that high-frequency jet ventilation anesthesia will reduce diaphragmatic excursions and allow shock waves to be delivered to a calculus more precisely, but this is seldom important in a clinical situation.

USE OF STENTS

The use of double-J ureteral stents after lithotripsy is controversial. Libby et al.[4] demonstrated that the use of double-J stents reduced post-ESWL complications in patients with renal calculi more than 2.5 cm in diameter. For calculi less than 1.5 cm in diameter, the use of stents did not appear to be indicated.

For calculi 1.5 to 2.5 cm in diameter, the use of stents decreased the need for ancillary procedures, although the difference was not statistically significant.

Most of my ESWL procedures are performed on outpatients, and I use double-J stents liberally. When a calculus is larger than 1.5 cm, I routinely use a double-J stent. An exception would be a patient with a calyceal diverticulum in which stone fragments would be expected to pass slowly, if at all. Another exception would be a patient with a lower-pole calculus and a narrow infundibulum. If a calculus is impacted at the ureteropelvic junction, I attempt to push it back into the renal pelvis with a spiral-tip ureteral catheter. If that is successful, I decide whether to use a double-J stent accordingly to stone size, as described earlier. If, however, the calculus cannot be dislodged, I pass a Glide Wire (Microvasive, Watertown, Mass.) beyond the calculus and then pass a double-J stent over the wire and position it in the collecting system; I do that regardless of stone size, because impacted ureteropelvic junction calculi are difficult to fragment adequately in the absence of a stent and obstruction after ESWL is common.

In the case of ureteral calculi, many of our patients have a double-J stent already in place. If the calculus is small (<7 mm in diameter) and not extremely radiodense, I treat it in situ. The patient is given a maximum of 1,800 shocks at 22 kV, and a radiograph is obtained. If partial breakup is evident, I give as many as 600 additional shocks. If no fragmentation is evident on the radiograph, I take the patient to the cystoscopy suite and attempt to push the calculus back into the kidney. To do that, I remove the double-J stent, pass a spiral tip ureteral catheter up the ureter to the calculus, and then either physically push the calculus up the ureter or flush the catheter with normal saline solution, advancing the calculus into the collecting system. If those maneuvers are unsuccessful, I pass a Glide Wire beyond the calculus and dilate the intramural ureter with a 5-mm Olbert balloon catheter (Surgimed Inc., Summerville, S.C.). I then pass a no. 10 French rigid ureteroscope up the ureter as far as possible. If the ureteroscope can be passed to the level of the calculus, I can use the scope to push the calculus into the collecting system. If the calculus is densely impacted, it can be fragmented with either an electrohydraulic electrode or an ultrasonic probe and the pieces flushed into the kidney. If the ureteroscope cannot be advanced to the calculus, forceful injection of saline solution through the ureteroscope will often flush the calculus back into the collecting system. If none of those maneuvers is successful, the double-J stent is replaced over the Glide Wire, and the patient is given a total of 2,400 shocks.

If a ureteral calculus is large (>7 mm) or very radiodense, I reposition it into the kidney before ESWL with the measures just described. If a patient with a ureteral calculus does not have a ureteral stent, I use those measures to reposition the calculus into the kidney; if that is not possible, I pass a double-J stent over a Glide Wire and treat the calculus in situ. In the rare case when even a guidewire cannot be advanced beyond the calculus, a ureteral catheter is left in place just below the calculus and in situ treatment is performed.

POST-ESWL TREATMENT

All patients are given 20 mg of furosemide intravenously at the completion of lithotripsy. That allows the inevitable gross hematuria to clear rapidly and avoids clot retention. Patients are taken to the recovery room, stay there for about 1 hour, and are then returned to the holding area. They are observed until they have recovered full movement, are able to eat, and can urinate. Discharge medications usually include a broad-spectrum antibiotic (commonly trimethoprim-sulfamethoxazole) for 3 days and an oxycodone-based analgesic for pain. Any patient who has a temperature of more than 38°C after lithotripsy is given either a second dose of gentamicin or a long-acting cephalosporin. A patient who remains febrile either is admitted into the hospital or remains overnight in the hospital motel, where skilled nursing care is available. Patients are instructed to resume full activities as soon as possible. The exception is the patient with persistent gross hematuria, who is instructed to refrain from any vigorous physical activity until the urine looks clear. Many of our patients return to work the day after ESWL. If a patient has a large number of fragments in a lower pole calyx after ESWL, postural drainage with flank percussion is taught to a family member. It is my impression that that is helpful in promoting passage of fragments, although I cannot document it. At the time of discharge from the holding area, patients are instructed to contact their local urologist if problems such as pain or fever develop.

FOLLOW-UP AFTER ESWL

Follow-up after ESWL is outlined in Figure 39–1. The first follow-up appointment is scheduled for 7 to 10 days after lithotripsy. If the patient did not have a double-J stent placed for lithotripsy, an excretory urogram (EXU) is ordered. Blood work is not routinely ordered. Blood pressure is recorded at each follow-up visit. If the EXU shows normal function of the treated kidney and stone breakup appears complete, a plain abdominal radiograph of the kidneys, ureters, and bladder (KUB) is taken in 3 months. It is extremely unusual to develop a delayed (>1 week after ESWL) clinically significant steinstrasse, so repeated EXUs are not indicated unless symptoms develop. If the treated kidney is unobstructed but takes up contrast medium slowly, I order an abdominal

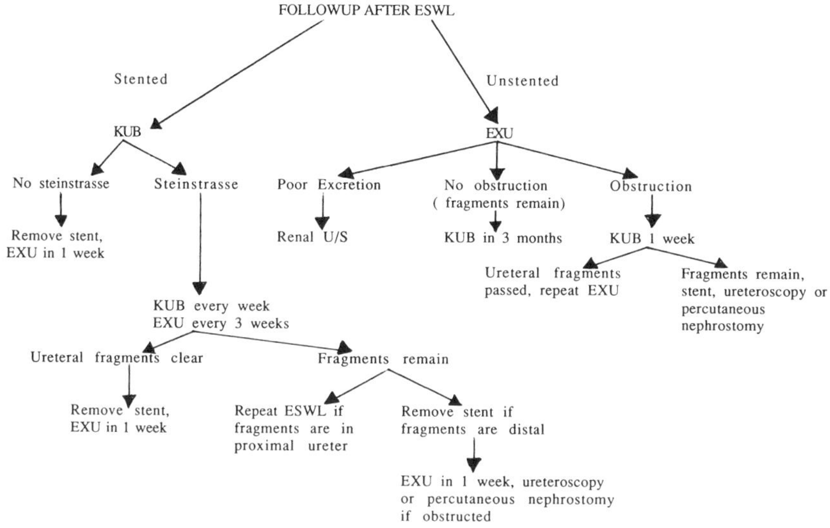

FIG 39–1.
Follow-up after ESWL.

ultrasonograph to look for a subcapsular or extracapsular hematoma. If the initial EXU shows any degree of obstruction from fragments in the ureter, I take weekly KUB radiographs until the fragments have cleared. These fragments should clear in 1 to 2 weeks. A follow-up EXU is then taken to document a lack of obstruction. If residual fragments of larger than 4 mm remain in the kidney, I counsel the patient about repeat ESWL or observation. Because residual fragments often grow, repeat ESWL seems a reasonable approach.

If a double-J stent was placed at the time of ESWL, a KUB radiograph is ordered at the first follow-up visit. If some of the fragments have passed and a steinstrasse is not present, the stent is removed and an EXU is performed the following week. If a ureteral steinstrasse is found, the stent is left in place and the KUB radiograph is repeated every week until the ureteral fragments have passed. If the patient becomes symptomatic, an EXU is obtained to ensure that the stent is functioning properly. Even if a patient with a steinstrasse has no symptoms (i.e., pain, fever, or nausea), I will order an EXU every 3 weeks while waiting for fragments to pass. I have seen several patients with steinstrasse and a nonfunctioning double-J ureteral stent who have lost a kidney in the absence of any symptoms. It is a mistake to remove a functioning double-J stent prematurely in the belief that the stent is preventing the passage of stone fragments. Many patients who have been treated for partial staghorn calculi with ESWL have passed their entire stone burden around double-J stents.

If a steinstrasse has not diminished in size after 6 weeks, further improvement is unlikely. In such a case, a large leading fragment is usually preventing passage of the more proximal fragments. The patient is then treated with repeat ESWL (if the steinstrasse is above the iliac crest), or the stent is removed (in the case of a distal steinstrasse). In the latter situation, obstruction might occur; if so, ureteroscopy can be performed to evacuate the steinstrasse. Alternatively, a percutaneous nephrostomy tube can be placed. Fragments can then pass during the next few weeks even without the flow of urine down the ureter. When the ureter is free of fragments, a follow-up EXU is obtained.

In some institutions, the follow-up EXU is replaced with a KUB radiograph and renal ultrasonograph. At our institution, those two are more expensive than an EXU. The incidence of contrast medium–induced reactions is quite small; almost all the patients have already had EXUs to establish the presence of a calculus. Although ultrasonography is superior in diagnosing subcapsular hematoma, clinically significant hematoma is extremely uncommon and will cause enough abnormalities on an EXU to suggest fluid collection; an ultrasonograph can be obtained for confirmation.

SUMMARY

Outpatient lithotripsy is suitable for most patients with urinary calculi. I have confined this discussion to treatment with the Dornier HM-3 lithotriptor because it is the most widely available unit. Outpatient lithotripsy will become even more practical with the introduction of second-generation lithotriptors. Many of the newer machines require no anesthesia and little or no sedation. Despite improvements in technology, however, it is important to remember that obstruction by retained fragments will continue to be the most important complication of ESWL. No matter what type of lithotriptor is used, close follow-up of patients is mandatory.

References

1. Marberger M: Renal calyceal calculi, in Resnick MI, Kursh E (eds): *Current Therapy in Genitourinary Surgery*. Toronto, BC Decker, 1987, p 387.
2. Lingeman JE, Coury TA, Newman DM, et al: Comparison of results and morbidity of percutaneous nephrostolithotomy and extracorporeal shock wave lithotripsy. *J Urol* 1987; 138:485.
3. Breaux E, Burns JR: Outpatient extracorporeal lithotripsy. *Urology* 1987; 29:131.
4. Libby JM, Meacham RB, Griffith DP: The role of silicone ureteral stents in extracorporeal shock wave lithotripsy of large renal calculi. *J Urol* 1988; 139:15.

40

Extracorporeal Shock Wave Lithotripsy and Use of Stents

George W. Drach, M.D.

This 45-year-old man arrives from a town 60 miles away with a 1.8-cm stone impacted in the left ureteropelvic junction. Radiographs with contrast obtained 2 days ago also show an 8-mm stone in an unobstructed right renal pelvis. The ureters and bladder are normal. He wants to "get it all over with at one time," so you schedule him for bilateral extracorporeal shock wave lithotripsy (ESWL). The scheduling nurse asks whether you want to schedule him for stent placement before ESWL.

In the past I thought that the decision criteria for stents were simple and clear. I am no longer as certain. This patient insists on getting his left and right stones taken care of at one sitting. Elsewhere in this text I have mentioned that I do not like to do bilateral treatments simultaneously, because these patients seem to have more problems after therapy than the unilaterally treated patients. If, however, I have informed the patient of the possible increase in complications and he still insists on bilateral treatment at a single sitting, then I will certainly put a stent in one ureter. In this patient I would stent the left ureter, because the left kidney has a higher stone burden of 1.8 cm. I would expect the fragments of the 8-mm right renal stone to pass without difficulty.

What are the most recent thoughts on stents for shock wave lithotripsy? I agree with many authorities that one should have assured drainage, either by stenting or by percutaneous nephrostomy, when treating patients with solitary kidney. Even those patients with a stent in the ureter of their solitary kidney may become obstructed after shock wave lithotripsy, and the stent must then be changed or a percutaneous nephrostomy placed. One recent report[2] reveals a patient who had ureteral obstruction by stone fragments 7 weeks after lithotripsy and 4 weeks after stent removal.

How large a stone burden deserves stenting? One investigation[5] compared patients with stone burdens less than 3 cm. About 55 percent had stents. Outcomes in terms of freedom from stone did not differ between the two groups. Patients with stents had greater incidence of urinary frequency, urgency, and hematuria than patients without stents.[4] Incidence of steinstrasse was about equal in the two groups. On the other hand, these authors[5] agreed that stents may be useful in patients with large stone burdens (> 2.5–3 cm). Two earlier studies[1, 3] have shown that the incidence of complications in patients with stone burdens more than 2.5 cm decreased significantly when pretreatment stents were inserted.

Those who study shock wave lithotripsy and stents imply that they should be used when treating the kidney of patients with known urinary infection. Of course, all authorities recommend that any patient with infected urine, or those with histories of urinary infection, be treated with antibiotics before and during lithotripsy. Which one of these patients should have a stent inserted? I believe that patients with struvite calculi often deserve a ureteral stent, as do patients with recent pyelonephritis. It is certainly easier to insert the stent before the febrile episode than after it has occurred.

Another indication for use of stents arises when the stone or stones are poorly seen and a catheter or stent is passed to identify the ureter at the stone, or to inject contrast during the shock wave lithotripsy. This may be especially useful when one is treating radiolucent stones, such as uric acid. On other occasions, the stent may be used as an anatomic marker to position the patient properly on the lithotripter.

Some years ago, stents were passed to push ureteral stones into the kidney. If the stone would not push up, the stent was left alongside the stone to allow an "expansion chamber effect." This was supposed to improve the breakage of the stone. Many studies have since shown that ureteral calculi break well in situ without the need for any stents, so I no longer use them for this purpose.

SUMMARY

I would use a unilateral stent in this patient because of his bilateral treatment. Other accepted indications for stents include solitary kidney, stone burden greater than 2.5 cm, concomitant urinary infection, or need for stent or catheter to localize a stone.

REFERENCES

1. Bregg K, Riehle RA Jr: Morbidity associated with indwelling internal ureteral stents after shock wave lithotripsy. *J Urol* 1989; 141:510–512.
2. Cohen ES, Schmidt JD: Extracorporeal shock-wave lithotripsy for stones in solitary kidney. *Urology* 1990; 26:52–54.
3. Fine H, Gordon RL, Lebensart PD: Extracorporeal shock wave lithotripsy and stents: Fluoroscopic observations and a hypothesis on the mechanisms of stent function. *Urol Radiol* 1989; 11:37–41.
4. Pryor JL, Jenkins AD: Use of double-pigtail stents in extracorporeal shockwave lithotripsy. *J Urol* 1990; 143: 475–478.
5. Preminger GM, Kettelhut MC, Elkins SL, et al: Ureteral stenting during extracorporeal shock wave lithotripsy: Help or hindrance? *J Urol* 1989; 142:32–36.

41

Treatment of Staghorn Calculus With Extracorporeal Shock Wave Lithotripsy

Daniel M. Newman, M.D.

An internist in your office complex refers to you a 33-year-old woman with a long history of urinary tract infections associated with *Proteus mirabilis*. Each time he treats her with ampicillin for 2 to 3 weeks, the infection clears. Within several weeks, it returns. He obtained a voiding cystourethrogram (normal) and an intravenous pyelogram. This series shows an normal right upper system and bladder, but the left kidney is distorted by a partial staghorn calculus that fills the pelvis and has prongs extending into a middle and lower infundibulum. The patient has no other health problems. On your examination, there is mild deep tenderness to palpation of the left flank. Your urinalysis shows pH 7.0, glucose absent, albumin trace, 4 to 6 white blood cells/high-power field (HPF), and 10 to 15 red blood cells/HPF. Gram stain shows no bacteria (the patient finished a course of ampicillin 2 days ago).

This patient has a partial staghorn calculus associated with recurrent urea-splitting bacteriuria *(Proteus mirabilis)*. The stone most likely is a mixture of struvite and carbonate apatite. As every urologist knows, calculous material in the urinary tract provides a privileged sanctuary for bacteria from antimicrobials. As long as stone material exists in this patient's upper urinary tract, she will be at increased risk for reinfection with a urea-splitting organism and thus at increased risk for stone recurrence. Although many options exist for the management of patients such as this with staghorn calculi, we should not lose sight of our traditional goal in the management of such cases: to achieve a completely stone-free kidney if possible. A stone-free kidney will give the patient the very best chance in the long term of remaining free of recurrent infections and stones.[1, 2]

Options to be considered in this situation include:

1. Open surgery (extended pyelolithotomy or anatrophic nephrolithotomy.
2. Extracorporeal shock wave lithotripsy (ESWL) monotherapy, with or without a stent
3. A primary percutaneous approach, combined with ESWL if required

The choice of these various options depends on the degree of dilatation of the renal collecting system and the endourologic skills of the urologist.

Although most staghorn calculi are associated with significant anatomic changes in the affected kidney, an occasional partial staghorn calculus may be found in association with a relatively normal renal collecting system. Because this calculus is described as a partial staghorn, we will assume that the stone burden is not massive. Given the aforementioned findings, ESWL monotherapy, combined with ureteral stenting, is a reasonable option that is expected to yield a completely stone-free result in approximately 80% of cases. The ureteral stenting will minimize the morbidity associated with the large amount of gravel produced, and the presence of a relatively normal renal collecting system will greatly increase the likelihood that all stone particles produced during ESWL will be successfully expulsed from the kidney.

However, if the renal collecting system is dilated to any significant degree, the likelihood of residual fragments occurring after ESWL monotherapy increases dramatically. These fragments typically will accumulate in dependent calices and may contribute to persistent bacteriuria, as well as provide a nidus for future stone growth.[2, 3] On the other hand, our experience with an initial percutaneous approach to partial staghorn calculi demonstrates that greater than 90% of such kidneys can be rendered entirely stone free with such an approach. It is important, however, for urologists to be honest with themselves about the extent of their endourologic skills, because the results obtained with a percutaneous approach are directly dependent on the skill and persistence of the operating surgeon. A few aspects of technique are worthy of emphasis when staghorn calculi are treated:

1. During percutaneous debulking, an attempt should be made to remove as much stone material as is possible and to reduce any residual stones to less than 2 cm in diameter if possible. This then reduces the stone burden requiring fragmentation with ESWL.

2. At the time of initial percutaneous debulking, any calyx containing residual stone material that cannot be reached with the rigid nephroscope should be entered with the flexible nephroscope. Access to every involved calyx with the flexible nephroscope is important, because after ESWL, a secondary percutaneous procedure should be performed to visually inspect all calyces and to rinse out any residual fragments that remain. Secondary nephroscopy with a flexible instrument is easily performed under minimal or no anesthesia and is essential to achieving good results with this approach. If a calyx containing stone material cannot be accessed with the flexible nephroscope, additional access into this calyx should be created at the time of the initial debulking procedure. The point to be emphasized here is that when a percutaneous approach to a renal calculus is elected, a commitment should be made to achieve access sufficient for visual inspection of every part of the kidney known to contain stone material. If such an attitude is adopted, the likelihood of leaving stone fragments behind is greatly reduced.

3. Nephrostomy tubes should not be removed in the hope that residual stone material will pass after ESWL. Every effort is needed to make maximal use of the percutaneous access before the nephrostomy tube is removed. The results achieved with the percutaneous approach to staghorn calculi are directly related to the operator's skills in the use of flexible endoscopes. When I am performing a secondary percutaneous procedure with a flexible instrument, I always pressurize the irrigant because this greatly enhances the efficiency of rinsing out the stone fragments created by ESWL.

At our institution the complications associated with the percutaneous management of partial staghorn calculi, as described earlier, are minimal. Patients are genuinely appreciative of having their problem promptly resolved as opposed to the long and drawn-out course of events commonly associated with attempts to manage these problems with ESWL monotherapy. In addition, the morbidity associated with the presence of an indwelling ureteral stent for a lengthy period of time is avoided.

We should not forget that the results of open surgical procedures (extended pyelolithotomy or anatrophic nephrolithotomy) for this problem are excellent.[6, 7] It is unwise to substitute ESWL monotherapy for patients with partial staghorn calculi and a dilated renal collecting system. If the urologist's endourologic skills are insufficiently developed to achieve a high likelihood of a stone-free result with the percutaneous approach, open surgery would be a very appropriate option to offer to the patient.

Whatever approach is chosen, I usually administer culture-specific antibiotics for approximately 3 months after therapy. I recommend this because the risks of recurrent stone formation are increased greatly should recurrent urea-splitting bacteriuria occur during the first 3 months postoperatively.[2] In addition, these patients should be considered for metabolic evaluation because metabolic abnormalities commonly coexist in patients with staghorn calculi.[8]

SUMMARY

Urologists should not lose sight of the goals of therapy in the management of patients with infected partial staghorn calculi: to render the patient free of both stone and infection. Such results need to realize the limitations of ESWL monotherapy, which may be considered for patients with low-volume, partial staghorn calculi in nondilated renal collecting systems. For patients with large partial staghorn calculi or those with any degree of dilation of the upper urinary tract, superior results are obtained by an initial percutaneous approach combined with ESWL if needed. The endourologic approach should always be completed with flexible nephroscopy to actively remove all residual stone material before the nephrostomy tube is removed. Finally, in selected instances, open surgery remains a time-honored and excellent approach for the management of these difficult stone cases.

REFERENCES

1. Griffith DP: Infection-induced stones, in Coe FL: *Nephrolithiasis, Pathogenesis, and Treatment*. Chicago, Year Book Medical Publishers, 1978, p 203.
2. Patterson DE, Segura JW, Leroy AJ: Long-term follow-up of patients treated by percutaneous ultrasonic lithotripsy for struvite staghorn calculi. *J Endourol* 1987; 1:177.
3. Sonda LP, Wang S, Ellis J, et al: Resolution of bacteriuria in patients with infection stones: Comparison of results employing newer treatment modalities. *J Urol* 1988; 2:151.
4. Kahnoski RJ, Lingeman JE, Coury TA, et al: Combined percutaneous and extracorporeal shock wave lithotripsy for staghorn calculi: Alternative to anatrophic nephrolithotomy. *J Urol* 1986; 135:679.
5. Lingeman JE, Smith LH, Woods JR, et al: Staghorn calculi, in *Urinary Calculi: ESWL, Endourology, and Medical Therapy*. Philadelphia, Lea & Febiger, 1988.

6. Boyce WH: Nephrolithotomy, in Glenn JF (ed): *Urologic Surgery,* ed 3. Philadelphia; JB Lippincott Co, 1983.
7. Boyce WH: Surgery of urinary calculi and perspective. *Urol Clin North Am* 1983; 10:585.
8. Segura JW, Erickson SB, Wilson DM, et al: Infected renal lithiasis: Results of long-term surgical and medical management, in Smith LH, Robertson BW, Finlayson B (eds): *Urolithiasis.* New York; Plenum Press, 1981.

42

Stones in Children

William W. Bohnert, M.D.

You have just seen a 12-year-old girl with a 1.5-cm stone of the right kidney visible on plain abdominal radiograph. It is associated with intermittent flank pain and occasional nausea. There is no family history of stone disease, and prior evaluation by her pediatrician has not shown hypercalciuria or urinary tract infection. No other evaluation or treatment has been done.

EVALUATION

When one sees a patient with an abdominal calcification on a plain film compatible with a 1.5-cm renal stone, preliminary hematologic, bacteriologic, and biochemical data, including a complete blood cell count, urinalysis, urine culture, and a chemistry profile should be obtained. With a known normal blood urea nitrogen and creatinine determination, the entire anatomy of the urinary tract must be visualized. In the absence of an allergic history to intravenous (IV) contrast, the first step would be to get an excretory urogram to determine the location of the stone, the amount of obstruction created, the relative level of renal function, and whether there is any anatomic abnormalities and, thus, be able to recommend a treatment program. A renal ultrasound could be used as the primary imaging procedure in a child with renal insufficiency. With renal functional impairment, management of the stone problem would be best managed in a joint effort between the pediatric nephrologist and the urologist.[1]

In this case presentation, hypercalciuria and urinary tract infection have been ruled out by the patient's pediatrician. If the patient had a history of recurrent urinary tract infections previously, a voiding cystourethrogram (VCUG) should be done. If any radiologic signs or changes of prior infection are present on the IV pyelogram (IVP), one may want to order a VCUG as well to rule out vesicoureteral reflux.

Other metabolic causes of renal stones must be considered, including cystinuria and uric acid lithiasis. A nitroprusside test for cystinuria and a chemistry profile are appropriate. Uric acid lithiasis is unlikely because the stone was initially seen on the patient's plain film of the abdomen. A commercial kit called Urocystin is available from the Mission Pharmacal Company (San Antonio, Tex.) for office testing for cystinuira.

SURGICAL MANAGEMENT

With a 1.5-cm stone in a female adolescent, some form of surgical intervention will be needed. Today with the development of extracorporeal shock wave lithotripsy (ESWL),[2] less than 1% of patients with renal stones will require open surgery. This new technology has revolutionized the management of the majority of patients with urolithiasis. Initially developed for adults, many urologists have treated pediatric and adolescent patients safely and effectively with simple modifications of the equipment (Fig 42–1).[1, 3]

Extracorporeal shock wave lithotripsy, developed by Dornier Medical Systems, Limited, in West Germany, employs an underwater spark plug to generate high-energy shock waves that are focused by means of an ellipsoid reflector. After induction of anesthesia, the patient is positioned on a support system in a

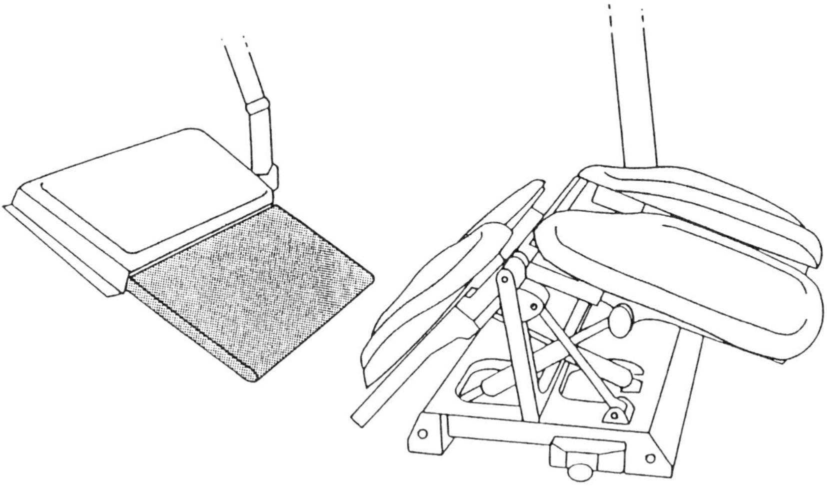

FIG 42–1.
Pediatric ESWL. Gantry modification. Padded lead shield *(shaded area)* is used to support the body and to protect lung fields from shock waves. (From Adams MC, Newman DM, Lingeman JE: *J Endourol* 1989; 3:245. Used by permission.)

water bath so that the calculus is located at the second focal point above the ellipsoid. At that focal point, F_2, the cumulative energy of the shock waves are sufficient to fragment the stones. The number of shocks delivered varies between 250 and 2,100, at discrete intervals synchronized with the R wave of the electrocardiogram. The kilovoltage (energy) delivered is user dependent (range 12–26 kV).

After completing the preliminary evaluation of this patient, she should be scheduled for ESWL, electively or urgently, depending on the amount and severity of her intermittent pain and nausea. At most lithotripsy centers in the United States today, she would be treated as an outpatient or an overnight stay.

General or epidural anesthesia would be required for treatment in this adolescent. No instrumentation, catheterization, or insertion of indwelling stents would be needed. Successful fragmentation can be expected in most patients, with spontaneous passage of all fragments within 1 to 3 months. Children and adolescents pass stone fragments quite easily with minimal morbidity and complications. In patients with large stone burdens (>2 cm), stents, secondary treatment with ESWL, or both and increased ancillary procedures are required[1, 3–6]

Complications include skin bruising at the entrance and exit sites, low-grade temperature elevations, distal ureteral obstruction caused by columns of stone fragments (steinstrassen) and, rarely, perirenal hematoma. Newman et al.[3] reported three steinstrasse events in 44 patients. Two developed after treat-

TABLE 42–1.
Experience With Pediatric ESWL*

Series	No. of Patients	No. of Stone Events	Average Shock Waves	Average kV	Stone Event Retreatment Rate (%)	Short-term Stone-free Rate (%)	Complications
Mininberg[7]	17	19	1,485	20	0	47	None
Kramolowsky et al.[8]	14	16	1,250	—	7	83	Pulmonary edema (1), ureterolithotomy (1)
Kroovand et al.[4]	18	22	1,800	21	27	82	Pulmonary contusion (2), percutaneous nephrostomy (2)
Sigman et al.[9]	38	44	1,295	18	11	70	Pulmonary contusion (1), sepsis (1)
Mosaad and El-Salamouni[10]	42	42	<900	18	21	86	None
Adams et al.[11]	44	55	1,186	19.6	11	79	Perirenal hematoma (1)
TOTAL	173	198	1,220†	19†	13.5	76	

From Adams MC, Newman DM, Lingeman JE: J Endourol *1989; 3:245. Used by permission.*
†Approximate.

ment of 1.5-cm renal pelvic stones in female patients. All steinstrassen resolved spontaneously within 48 hours of treatment without intervention (Table 42–1).[1]

After ESWL is completed and the patient leaves the recovery area for home or to the hospital floor, oral fluids in large quantities are encouraged and the urine is strained. It is extremely important to collect stone fragments for stone analysis.

After discharge, the patient returns 1 week after treatment for a follow-up urinalysis and repeat plain film of the abdomen. If significant steinstrassen are seen, an ultrasound can be done to see if significant hydronephrosis is present.

MEDICAL MANAGEMENT

Depending on the composition of the stone, determined by stone analysis, long-term recommendations can be made for stone prevention. Cystinuria is treated by alkalinization of the urine and adequate hydration. D-Penicillamine can be used for chemolysis of existing stones and in the occasional patient who does not respond to conservative measures. Uric acid lithiasis is managed with high fluid volumes and alkalinization. Dietary purine restriction and allopurinol can be used if needed. Infectious stone recurrence is prevented by maintaining a sterile urine and eliminating all existing stones and fragments. Congenital anomalies that promote urinary infection and stasis must be corrected. When hypercalcemia or hypercalciuria does occur, accurate diagnosis and appropriate therapy should be carried out. Controversy exists in the literature regarding extensive testing for metabolic abnormalities in children, because in certain series reported the recurrence rate was quite low.[12–14] In the absence of infection, congenital anomalies leading to stasis, and obvious metabolic abnormalities, high volume fluid intake and urine excretion, regardless of stone type, are the mainstay of therapy. Although no specific regimen is universally accepted, it seems reasonable to encourage an intake equal to calculated maintenance fluid requirements.[14] Stone activity should be monitored periodically with plain abdominal films for several years to detect recurrence or growth of small retained fragments.

There has been a great deal of concern and discussion about long-term safety regarding renal growth and somatic growth after shock wave lithotripsy. It has become apparent from the Newman et al.[3] series, as well as others, that ESWL is safe for children in the short term. With follow-up of as long as 3 years in a small number of pediatric patients, there has been no decrease in function or renal growth after ESWL, as measured by IVP or ultrasound. Long-term follow-up with these patients and their kidneys is mandatory, as is more basic research on the bioeffects of shock waves on the growing kidney.[1]

CONCLUSION

With the development of ESWL by Chaussey et al.[2] and the modifications in application to pediatric patients by Newman et al.,[3] the successful treatment of stones in children has improved dramatically. It is important to remember that ESWL is only part of the complete treatment of patients with stones. Although it has become easy simply to retreat a stone patient with ESWL, we must not forget that in many children urolithiasis is a complex problem that needs thorough anatomic, metabolic, and bacteriologic evaluation to try to prevent recurrent stone formation after successful treatment.[15]

REFERENCES

1. Adams MC, Newman DM, Lingeman JE: Pediatric ESWL: Long term results and effects on renal growth. *J Endourol* 1989; 3:245.
2. Chaussy CG, Schmiedt E, Jocham D, et al: Experience with extracorporeally induced destruction of kidney stones by shock waves. *J Urol* 1982; 127:417.
3. Newman DM, Coury T, Longeman JE, et al: Extracorporeal shock wave lithotripsy experience in children. *J Urol* 1986; 136:238.
4. Kroovand RL, Harrison LH, McCullough DL: Extracorporeal shock wave lithotripsy in children. *J Urol* 1987; 138:1106.
5. Mininberg DT: Extracorporeal shock wave lithotripsy in children: An overview. *J Endourol* 1989; 3:385.
6. Nijman RJ, Ackaert K, Scholtmeijer RJ, et al: Long term results of extracorporeal shock wave lithotripsy in children. *J Urol* 1989; 142:609.
7. Mininberg DT: ESWL in Children. Urologists' Correspondance Club, April 27, 1987.
8. Kramolowsky EV, Willoughby BL, Loening SA: Extracorporeal shock wave lithotripsy in children. *J Urol* 1987; 137:939.
9. Sigman M, Laudone VP, Jenkins AD, et al: Initial experience with extracorporeal shock wave lithotripsy in children. *J Urol* 1987; 138:389.
10. Mosaad A, El-Salamouni T: Results of extracorporeal shock wave lithotripsy in young children, in Lingeman JE, Newman DM (eds): *Shock Wave Lithotripsy II: Urinary and Biliary*. New York, Plenum Press, 1989.
11. Adams MC, Newman DM, Lingeman JE: Pediatric ESWL: Long term results and effects on renal growth. *J Endourol* 1989; 3:245.
12. Wolther PC, Lamm D, Kaplan GW: Pediatric urolithiasis: A ten-year review. *Pediatrics* 1980; 65:1068.
13. Stapleton FB, Noehn RS, Jerkins G: Hypercalciuria in children with urolithiasis. *Am J Dis Child* 1982; 136:675.
14. Polinsky MS, Kaiser BA, Balvarte HJ: Urolithiasis in childhood. *Pediatr Clin North Am* 1987; 34:683.
15. Diamond DA, Menon M, Lee PH, et al: Etiological factors in pediatric stone recurrence. *J Urol,* 1989; 142: 606.

43

Use of Blast Path Concept in Extracorporeal Shock Wave Lithotripsy

Robert C. Newman, M.D.

You have simulated a 312-lb male patient in your Dornier HM-3 bathtub lithotriptor (Dornier Medical Systems, Inc., Marietta, Ga.), but the 1.6-cm stone lies 2 cm outside the focal point when the patient is as close to the ellipsoid as possible. You know that the patient's previous stones have been analyzed as calcium oxalate dihydrate. He has been told that percutaneous stone removal should be done, but he is very fearful of any holes in his kidney.

PREPARATION

Given this scenario, this patient is technically not a candidate for extracorporeal shock wave lithotripsy (ESWL) because his weight is more than the manufacturer's maximum allowable weight of 297 lb. If the patient can loose 15 lb, he will become a candidate for treatment. In the interim, I would recommend placement of a double J stent. The stent should decrease the probability of his becoming obstructed from the stone. In addition, with stones greater than 1 cm, stent placement will decrease the potential need for fragment manipulation after ESWL from 10% to 15% to 1% to 2%. The patient should be advised that post-ESWL manipulation (e.g., percutaneous nephrostomy) may be necessary.

When ESWL is considered, there are two positive factors from the patient's standpoint. First, his previous stones have been composed of calcium oxalate dihydrate. When viewed on a radiograph of the kidneys, ureters, and bladder, these stones usually have a fluffy appearance and very indistinct margins. This contrasts with calcium oxalate monohydrate stones, which are more radiodense and tend to have sharply defined borders. If the patient's current stone is dihydrate, it will fragment more readily than one of primarily monohydrate composition. Presumably this is related to the higher water content of the calculus. Second, the stone is of modest size. The probability of adequately fragmenting a 1.6-cm stone is greater than with larger calculi.

Extracorporeal shock wave lithotripsy is not risk free. However, presuming that the patient is healthy, except for his obesity, there should be less risk associated with ESWL than with percutaneous nephrolithotomy (PNL). For example, the incidence of hemorrhage requiring transfusion is less than 1% with lithotripsy, whereas with PNL the risk may be as high as 10%.

SIMULATION

The concept of simulation before ESWL is important in the obese patient for two reasons. First, it allows the operator to find out if, in fact, the stone can be positioned at F_2. Conventional positioning at F_2 should be used for treatment whenever possible. In some circumstances, such as a stone overlying the sacroiliac joint, this may require placing the patient in a prone rather than a semi-sitting, supine position. When the stone is in the kidney, having the patient in the prone position usually does not facilitate positioning at F_2.

Second, it is important to know if the stone can be visualized. In the obese patient, radiographic resolution is likely to be suboptimal. It is not possible to treat stones that cannot be seen with the imaging equipment in the tub. If the stone is not well visualized but is known to be within the collecting system, placement of a ureteral catheter before ESWL will allow injection of dye and will most likely make it possible to localize the stone.

BLAST PATH THEORY

The blast path concept was conceived soon after lithotripsy treatments were begun in the United States.[1] The term is used to describe the alternative positions at which stones may be treated when the Dornier HM-3 lithotriptor is used. When the electrode fires at F_1, the major axis of the pressure wave passes through F_2. The path of the blast is inclined to the Z axis of the lithotriptor at an angle of about 14.3 degrees. The isobar map presented by Heine[2] demonstrates that the point of maximum impulse along this path is at F_2 (Fig 43–1). The astute observer will also note that the pressure is maintained distant to F_2 along the path of the blast.

The Dornier HM-3 monitors are depicted in Figure 43–2. The blast path may be drawn on the video monitors by sketching a line 25 degrees off the horizontal axis. Stones positioned along this axis will lie in the path of the blast.

Using the Blast Path

The practical importance of using the blast path relates to the fact that stones can be fractured during treatment when they are positioned distal to F_2 as long as they are on the blast path. As Figure 43–1 demonstrates, the amount of energy focused at varying points along this path diminishes as one moves away from F_2. Therefore, to achieve maximum benefit from the treatment, one must position the stone as close to F_2 as possible on both monitors.* The likelihood of stone fracture can be enhanced by either increasing the number of shocks administered or increasing the kilovoltage. When treating stones on the blast path, one might use 2,000 to 4,000 V more than one would if treating at F_2. For example, assume that you would usually treat the 1.6-cm stone at F_2 using 18 kV. Because of the patient's size, the closest you can get the stone is 2 cm from F_2 (in video space). To achieve optimal fragmentation, I would increase the kilovoltage to the 20- to 22-kV range. If the calculus were further out on the blast path, one might use 24 kV. Alternatively, the number of shocks delivered might be increased. If the stone lies 8 cm from F_2 on the blast path, the operator might increase the kilovoltage and the number of shocks delivered. (From the safety standpoint, there have been no reports of significant damage to the perinephric or muscular tissues when F_2 falls short of the kidney.)

One might reasonably ask, "Why can't I focus the stone at F_2 in the first

**The operator should be aware that the distance from F_2 to the point selected on the blast path as depicted on the video monitor is approximately twice the distance in real space. Stated another way, if the stone is 2 cm from F_2 as measured on the video monitor (video space), it is actually about 1 cm away from F_2 inside the patient (real space).*

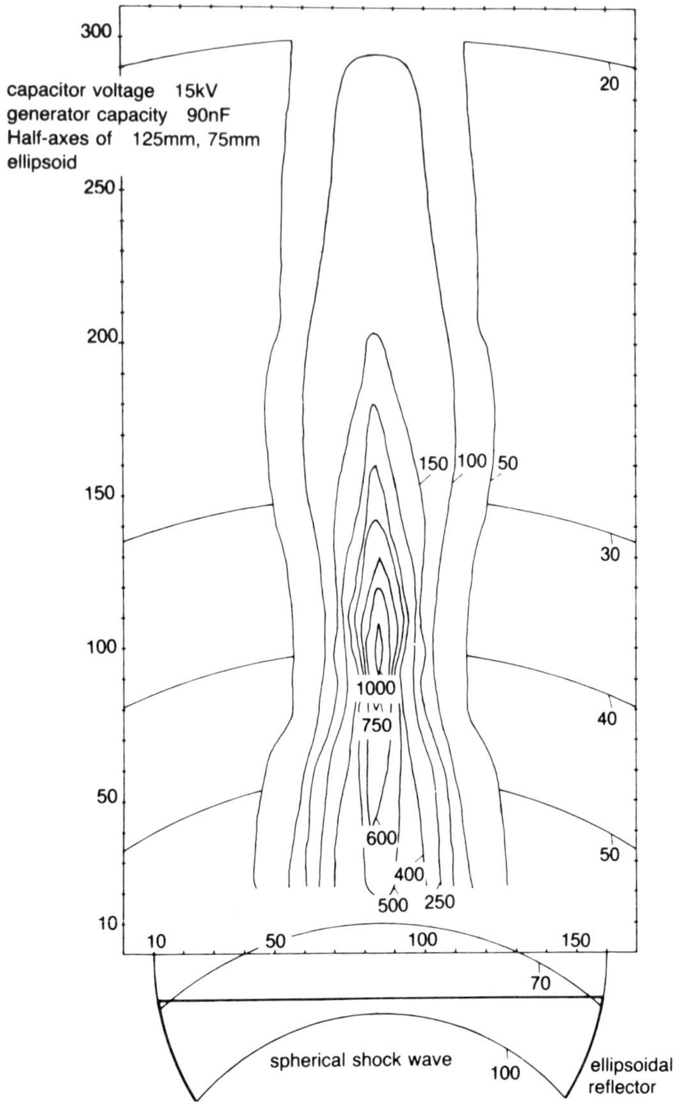

FIG 43–1.
Isobar map of pressure maxima showing elongation of isobars along major axis of hemiellipsoid. (From Heine G: Physical aspects of shock wave treatment, in Gravenstein JS, Peter K [eds]: *Extracorporeal Shock Wave Lithotripsy for Renal Stone Disease.* Stoneham, Mass, Butterworth, 1986, p 15. Used by permission.)

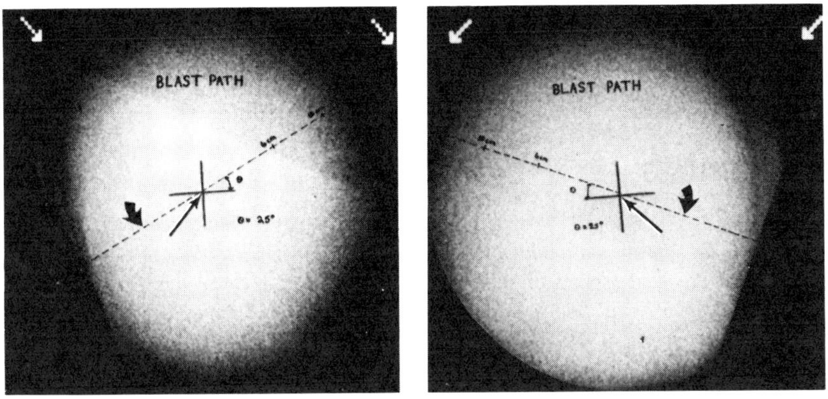

FIG 43–2.
Blast path *(large arrow)* depicted on Dornier HM-3 monitors I and II. The *small arrow* points to F_2. The path projects into the upper inner quadrant of each screen.

place?" The explanation is a matter of simple geometry. The distance from the top of the ellipsoid to F_2 is 13 cm; therefore, if the stone lies more than 13 cm from the patient's back, it will not be possible to position the stone at F_2. In most patients the pelvocalyceal system is closer to the patient's back than other parts of the collecting system (e.g., the ureter). Should the stone be lodged in the ureter when the patient is seen, it may be advantageous to manipulate the stone back up into the kidney.

There are a couple of other tricks that the operator can use when attempting to move the stone closer to F_2. One should be certain that the patient is maximally stretched out on the gantry. This can be accomplished by pushing the appropriate button on the gantry itself. This maneuver will sometimes elevate the patient enough so that positioning at F_2 will be possible.

When the stone is imaged, the balloons on the bottom of the tub should be inflated so that the medial-most portion of the balloon (as it relates to the center of the tub) does not project past the ellipsoid edge. If the balloons are inflated more than this, the patient's back may lie atop the balloons rather than on the ellipsoid. This is sometimes called "riding the balloons." Partially deflating the balloons may result in more optimal positioning of the stone.

Other Uses of the Blast Path

The blast path can be used in a variety of other circumstances in which positioning at F_2 is not possible. Fortunately, this is necessary less than 5% of all ESWL cases. These would include stones in pelvic, horseshoe, or transplant kidneys, calculi in the ureter, and calcifications in the biliary duct. The technique may be used in either semisitting (standard) or prone position. Using this adjunct, the urologist should be able to treat stones at virtually any location in the urinary tract.

REFERENCES

1. Whelan JP, Finlayson B, Welch J, et al: The blast path: Theoretical basis, experimental data and clinical application. *J Urol* 1988; 140:401–404.
2. Heine G: Physical aspects of shock wave treatment, in Gravenstein JS, Peter K (eds): *Extracorporeal Shock Wave Lithotripsy for Renal Stone Disease*. Stoneham, Mass, Butterworth, 1986, p 22.

44

Complications of Extracorporeal Shock Wave Lithotripsy

James E. Lingeman, M.D.

Three months ago, you treated this 54-year-old man for left renal urolithiasis in your bathless ("dry") lithotriptor. You apply 2,300 shock waves at 17 kV for 54 minutes to his 1.2-cm stone. Stone fragmentation is excellent, and the patient is free of stones at the 3-week examination. He does have some left abdominal and flank pain, but your physical examination is unremarkable. He believes it relates to his treatment. Magnetic resonance imaging (MRI) of the abdomen indicates no abnormality of the abdominal contents, including the kidneys.

Extracorporeal shock wave lithotripsy (ESWL) has appropriately revolutionized the management of the urolithiasis patient. Patients such as the one described in this case are ideal candidates for management with ESWL. However, although the benefits of ESWL were immediately apparent at the time of its introduction to both patient and physician alike, the fact that shock waves produce trauma to renal and surrounding tissue during virtually every lithotripsy treatment was much slower in being recognized. Early reports from Munich suggested that shock waves produced no pathologic effects in animals.[1] However, these animals received small numbers of shock waves and were not killed until 2 weeks after shock wave exposure. Subsequent animal studies from a number of different centers demonstrated that when therapeutic numbers of shock waves were applied to dog or pig kidneys, hemorrhage in and around the kidney could be routinely expected.[2, 3]

The rapid acceptance and adoption of ESWL have been facilitated partly by the false perception that this technology is entirely safe and that shock wave treatment does not induce severe, acute, or chronic side effects. Currently numerous clinical and experimental reports demonstrate that ESWL can cause marked acute and chronic effects in both animals and humans (Table 44–1).[1–11]

The most consistent observation associated with ESWL is gross hematuria, which is a direct reflection of renal parenchymal injury and not secondary to movement of stone particles during treatment.[3] In addition, significant increases in the levels of a number of serum and urinary enzymes have been documented 24 hours after ESWL: bilirubin, lactic dehydrogenase, serum glutamic oxaloacetic transaminase, creatine phosphokinase, *N*-acetyl-β-glucosaminidase, β-galactosidase, and γ-glutamyl transpeptidase.[4, 5] Several cases of clinically typical acute pancreatitis associated with a marked increase in serum amylase and lipase levels have been observed.[4] These data imply significant trauma to the kidney and adjacent tissues (liver and skeletal muscle) during ESWL. Most of these laboratory values begin to decrease within 3 to 7 days and are normal at 3 months.

The trauma to renal parenchyma associated with ESWL ranges from mild contusions localized in the parenchyma to large hematomas associated with sufficient bleeding to require blood transfusion.[6, 7] Several reports employing MRI have established that 63% to 85% of patients will exhibit one or more morphologic abnormalities in or around the kidney after ESWL.[7, 11] These data indicate that renal injury in ESWL-treated patients is considerably more common than originally appreciated.[13] The small veins in renal parenchyma appear to be particularly susceptible to shock wave injury.[14] A potential sequela of the intraparenchymal and perirenal hemorrhage associated with ESWL could be fibrosis with compression of the kidney, resulting in an alteration of renal hemodynamics. Such changes are known to occur in other forms of renal trauma and have

TABLE 44–1.
Clinical Side Effects of ESWL

Reference	Side Effect
	Acute changes
Chaussy[1] Knapp et al.[6], and Kaude et al.[7]	Hematomas (subcapsular or perirenal)
Knapp et al.[6] and Kaude et al.[7]	Low signal intensity perinephric fat changes (MRI)
	Loss of corticomedullary demarcation (MRI)
	Perirenal or capsular fluid (MRI)
Lingeman et al.[4]	Pancreatitis
	Increased bilirubin and lactic dehydrogenase levels
	Increased serum glutamic transaminase and creatine phosphokinase levels
Kaude et al.[7]	Partial to total ureteral obstruction
	Delayed to complete loss of renal function without ureteral obstruction
	Enlargement of kidney (excretory urography)
	Decrease in effective renal plasma flow in treated kidney
Delius et al.[3]	Hematuria
Chaussy[1]	Shock wave–dependent arrhythmias
Assimos et al.[5]	Increased *N*-acetyl-β-glucosaminidase levels
	Increase β-galactosidase levels
	Chronic changes
Lingeman et al.[12]	Increase in diastolic blood pressure
Williams et al.[10]	New onset of hypertension
Brito et al.[8] and Williams et al.[10]	Loss of renal function
Newman et al.[9]	Increased rate of new stone formation

similarities to the Page kidney.[15, 16] Studies performed in dogs have identified chronic changes consisting of fibrosis with loss of tubules and glomeruli and scar formation.[14] It is postulated that the traumatic effects of shock waves are caused by cavitation bubbles produced in the wake of the passing shock wave.[17]

In the case of the patient described in this example, it may be presumed that some degree of renal contusion occurred during his lithotripsy treatment and could well provide an explanation for the discomfort that he experienced after treatment. The previously described acute effects of shock wave lithotripsy typically resolve rapidly, and this patient should be assured that any discomfort related to his lithotripsy will resolve with time, particularly given the normal MRI. Magnetic resonance imaging seems to be the most sensitive test for detecting anatomic changes within the kidney after lithotripsy.[11]

Regarding the potential for chronic complications after ESWL, the picture is less clear. Certainly all nephrolithiasis patients need to be followed regularly because of their risk of recurrent stone formation. It would seem prudent to include periodic measurements of blood pressure and renal function as well. Extensive studies done at our institution to date do not demonstrate an increased incidence of new-onset hypertension, although we have been able to detect a slightly greater increase in diastolic blood pressure in ESWL patients when compared with stone disease patients not receiving ESWL.[12] Even if there would appear to be some slight risk of blood pressure changes after ESWL therapy, such findings do not detract from the overwhelmingly positive benefits of ESWL for a patient such as this. They merely indicate an additional responsibility for the treating urologist to be aware of the potential of such complications, to use the minimum dosage of shock wave energy necessary for stone fragmentation, and to follow patients appropriately looking for the possible development of such problems.

An important issue raised by the previously noted research is that the science of shock wave lithotripsy is currently still in its infancy and we truly do not yet know the safe limits for the application of this remarkable new technology. Caution regarding the maximum number of shock waves that may be administered in a single session of lithotripsy would therefore seem appropriate.

REFERENCES

1. Chaussy C: *Extracorporeal Shock Wave Lithotripsy: Technical Concept, Experimental Research and Clinical Application,* ed 2. Basel, S Karger, 1986.
2. Lingeman JE, McAteer JA, Kempson SA, et al: Bioeffects of extracorporeal shock wave lithotripsy. *J Endourol* 1987; 1:89.
3. Delius M, Enders G, Zuan Z, et al: Biological effects of shock waves: Kidney damage by shock waves in dogs—dose dependence. *Ultrasound Med Biol* 1988; 14:117.
4. Lingeman JE, Newman DM, Mertz JHO, et al: Extracorporeal shock wave lithotripsy: The Methodist Hospital of Indiana experience. *J Urol* 1986; 135:1134.
5. Assimos DG, Boyce WH, Furr EG, et al: Urinary enzyme levels after extracorporeal shock wave lithotripsy. Selective elevation of urinary enzyme levels after extracorporeal shock wave lithotripsy. *J Urol* 1989; 142:687.
6. Knapp PM, Kulb TB, Lingeman JE, et al: Extracorporeal shock wave lithotripsy–induced perirenal hematomas. *J Urol* 1988; 139:700.
7. Kaude JV, Williams CM, Millner MR, et al: Renal morphology and function immediately after extracorporeal shock wave lithotripsy. *Am JR* 1985; 145:305.
8. Brito CG, Lingeman JE, Newman DM, et al: Long-term follow-up of renal function in extracorporeal shock wave lithotripsy treated patients with solitary kidney [abstract]. *J Urol* 1990; 143:299A.
9. Newman DM, Scott JW, Lingeman JE: Two-year follow up of patients treated with extracorporeal shock wave lithotripsy. *J Endourol* 1988; 2:163.

10. Williams CM, Kaude JV, Newman RC, et al: Extracorporeal shock wave lithotripsy: Long-term complications. *Am JR* 1988; 150:311.
11. Knapp PM, Scott JW: Magnetic resonance imaging following extracorporeal shock wave lithotripsy [abstract]. *J Urol* 1987; 137:287A.
12. Lingeman JE, Woods JR, Toth PD: Blood pressure changes following extracorporeal shock wave lithotripsy and other forms of treatment for nephrolithiasis. *JAMA* 1990; 263:1789.
13. Chaussy C, Schmiedt E: Extracorporeal shock wave lithotripsy (ESWL) for kidney stone: An alternative to surgery? *Urol Radiol* 1984; 6:80.
14. Newman RC, Hackett R, Senior D, et al: Pathologic effects of ESWL on canine renal tissues. *Urology* 1987; 29:194.
15. Entel WJ, Page IH: Hypertension due to renal compression resulting from subcapsular hematoma. *J Urol* 1955; 73:735.
16. Sufrin G: The Page kidney: A correctable form of arterial hypertension. *J Urol* 1975; 113:450.
17. Fischer N, Muller HM, Gulhan A, et al: Cavitation effects: Possible cause of tissue injury during extracorporeal shock wave lithotripsy. *J Endourol* 1988; 2:215.

45

Cellular Effects of Extracorporeal Shock Wave Lithotripsy

Kenneth Bregg, M.D.
E. Darracott Vaughan, Jr., M.D.

A 25-year-old healthy man with no prior stone history has a 1.8-cm renal pelvic stone. Extracorporeal shock wave lithotripsy (ESWL) has been recommended as the treatment of choice, but he is concerned about the effects of ESWL on the kidney and other organs and seeks your opinion regarding its safety.

Extracorporeal shock wave lithotripsy was first introduced into clinical practice in Munich in 1980.[1–5] In 1984 Dornier introduced the HM-3 lithotriptor (Dornier Medical Systems, Inc., Marietta, Ga.) at six centers in the United States to cooperate in a Food and Drug Administration (FDA) cooperative trial.[1, 2] By December 1984, ESWL was approved by the FDA for general clinical practice.

It was initially hailed as an "authentic modern miracle," designed to treat renal calculi at a lower morbidity and cost without significant complications.[6] An underwater electrical discharge could be generated across a spark gap, with the formation of shock waves. These shock waves were then focused at the calculi by means of an ellipsoid reflector and a biplanar fluoroscopic system. Propagation of the shock waves through both water and human tissue occurs with little loss of energy because of similar acoustical impedances. On striking a substance of a different acoustical density, such as a stone, the shock waves undergo reflection and refraction. Compressive and tensile forces are generated capable of causing stone fracture.

Initial work by Chaussy et al.[4, 5] revealed few complications associated with ESWL.[1] Gross hematuria was observed in almost all cases. Chaussy et al.[5] were able to follow renal function iodine-hippuran clearance studies 2 years after ESWL and found an enhancement to 110% of the initial performance. Routine sonographic examinations revealed a 0.6% rate of renal or perirenal bleeding.

Animal experiments were performed in which 17 dog kidneys were implanted with human calculi. The animals were then killed 14 days after receiving 500 shocks, and no pathologic changes were evident in the kidney.[7] Despite these reports, more recent clinical, radiologic, and experimental data have raised concern significantly regarding the bioeffects of ESWL.[8–11]

ANIMAL STUDIES

Few studies have been done to evaluate pathologic changes in animal kidneys after ESWL. In contrast to the early studies by Chaussy and others, most investigators have determined varying amounts of damage to animal kidneys. Brendel[12] evaluated the effects of shock waves at three different "therapeutic doses" and found renal hemorrhage ranging from very small to 0.5 cm in diameter.

Newman et al.[13] performed a study to determine the margin of safety for lithotripsy in dog kidneys. Kidneys were shocked with a range between 48 and 72 hours and 28 to 32 days. The predominant histologic finding in kidneys examined shortly after lithotripsy was damage to thin-walled veins, with resultant cortical and medullary hemorrhage, as well as perirenal hemorrhage or hematoma. Bleeding was more prevalent in the kidneys that received 4,500, 6,000, and 8,000 shocks than in the kidney that received 1,776 shocks. Fibrosis was noted in both kidneys 1 month after ESWL and was much more extensive in the kidney that received 8,000 shocks (compared with 1,600 shocks).

Similarly, Delius et al.[14] found that the number and size of hematomas in ESWL-treated dogs directly correlated with the number of shock waves given; specifically, 1,500 to 3,000 shocks was much more damaging than 500 shocks. Abrahams et al.[15] used the Medstone lithotriptor to shock canine kidneys with a range between 1,000 and 2,000 shocks. A variety of pathologic changes were noted, including numerous hemorrhages, organizing hematomas, linear fibroblastic scars, and chronic interstitial nephritis.[15] This study is limited by the lack of control animals and by the concern that pathologic changes were present in canine kidneys that were operated on even without ESWL.

Morphologic and radiographic changes have also been appreciated in the rat kidney.[16, 17] Recker et al.[17] noted morphologic changes, including glomerular bleeding, tubular dilation, atrophy, and partial necrosis. Most of these changes resolved in the rats killed 35 days after ESWL, but a few localized glomeruli and tubules showed dose-dependent sclerosis. Neuerburg et al.[16] killed rats 14 to 35 days after ESWL and found fibrotic shrinkage of the parenchyma in 10 of 26 kidneys. This fibrosis was much more common in kidneys receiving 2,000 or 5,000 shocks compared with kidneys receiving 500 or 1,000 shocks.

Injury to other organ systems after ESWL has been controversial in animal models. Abrahams et al.[15] examined multiple organs and found only one hematoma in the wall of the large intestine. Chaussy,[7] however, reported thoracic bleeding in rats, and a recent report[18] in rabbits demonstrated changes in bone consisting of aseptic marrow necrosis 1 to 2 months later.

These animal studies allow several conclusions to be drawn. Renal injury occurs acutely after shock wave administration, is quite common, and is directly related to the number of shock waves. Although often hemorrhage and edema will resolve with time, chronic fibrosis has been demonstrated in a significant number of animals. The exact threshold at which irreversible damage occurs has unfortunately not yet been determined, although minimal damage occurs when 500 or 1,000 shocks are applied, with progressive damage occurring as the number of shock waves are increased above this level. The range of voltage applied varied in these experiments but was comparable with the 18 to 24-kV range used to treat human kidneys.

DIRECT CELLULAR EFFECTS

Several mechanisms have been proposed to explain shock wave injury.[19–21] Thermal injury is unlikely, because shock wave energy is comparable to diagnostic ultrasound. Shock waves may also have a direct effect, because the compressive and tensile forces of the shock wave may overcome the cohesive properties of the cell. Delius[19] has proposed that cavitation, the expansion and motion of bubbles in the shock wave field, may cause cell injury. Tissue damage increases as the rate of shock rate administration increases, and this supports cavitation as the means of injury. An interaction between waves by a direct shock wave action would be difficult to account for, with the interval between waves being 1,000 times the wave duration.[19]

Russo et al.[22] demonstrated that exposure to high-energy shock waves resulted in decreased cell viability and significant inhibition of cell growth in vivo and in vitro. Exposure to ESWL has been shown to potentiate the efficacy of cytotoxic agents.[23]

CLINICAL EFFECTS

Multiple studies employing laboratory, radiologic, and clinical modalities have assessed the bioeffects of ESWL. The studies demonstrate a variety of enzymatic and radiologic derangements that tend to revert toward normal with time. What remains unclear is how much renal function can permanently be lost by ESWL and whether or not ESWL can cause new-onset hypertension.

Several studies have consistently demonstrated laboratory abnormalities after ESWL. The initial cooperative FDA trial reported elevated levels of lactic dehydrogenase, serum glutamic oxaloacetic transaminase, creatine phosphokinase, and bilirubin.[2] More recently, Assimos et al.[24] monitored the levels of three urinary enzymes, *N*-acetyl-β-glucosamidase, β-galactosidase, and γ-glutamyltransferase before and after treatment. Both *N*-acetyl-β-glucosamidase and β-galactosidase levels were increased significantly after ESWL and were highest on days 1 and 3 after lithotripsy and returned to baseline by day 28. Haput et al.[25] monitored increased serum levels of serum glutamic pyruvic transaminase, lactic dehydrogenase, and total bilirubin. Elevations in these enzymes were clearly related to greater kilovoltage and number of shocks (>2,000 shocks at 20 kV) or to treatments on the right side, indicating liver damage as well.

Initial reports using routine post-ESWL ultrasonography revealed less than 1% incidence of significant bleeding.[2, 3, 5] The advent of both computed tomography (CT) scanners and MRI have shown the true incidence to be much higher. Rubin et al.[26] performed CT scans in 50 patients before and after ESWL treated with a mean of 2,100 shocks. Scanning after ESWL revealed subcapsular hematomas in 15% of patients and intrarenal hematomas in 4% of patients. Perinephric "soft tissue stranding and facial thickening" of varying degrees seen in 70% of patients was believed to be secondary to perirenal edema.

Kaude et al.[27] found that magnetic resonance imaging (MRI) revealed abnormalities in 63% of 38 treated kidneys, including hemorrhage in 29% of kidneys. The authors state that follow-up radiographs revealed resorption of perirenal fluid and eventually of subcapsular fluid. Besides more sensitive imaging modalities, these studies reveal significantly more bleeding than earlier studies because more shock waves were applied (2,100, 1,800 vs. 978, 1,270).

Knapp et al.[28] reported that patients most likely to hemorrhage after ESWL were those with hypertension, especially if not well controlled. Of patients with poorly controlled hypertension, 3.8% developed significant perirenal bleeding. Grantham et al.[29] observed 3 out of 100 patients after ESWL whose kidneys had no or minimal function, and all 3 had significant hemorrhage or edema documented by MRI.

In contrast to earlier studies, more recent studies have shown a decrement in renal function after ESWL. Gilbert et al.[30] demonstrated a reversible acute decrement in renal function in cases where obstruction was not a factor. Kaude et al.[27] showed that although total effective renal plasma flow (ERPF) was not affected by ESWL, 30% of the treated kidneys had a decrease in their ERPF by greater than 5%. Renogram curves displayed partial parenchymal obstruction in 25% of patients and total parenchymal obstruction in 22%. Because the scans were done shortly after ESWL and the radioactivity remained in the parenchyma, this pattern was interpreted to result from a direct effect on the renal parenchyma as opposed to obstruction.

Similarly, Williams et al.[8] found that the ERPF to the treated kidney decreased by more than 5% in 24% of patients, and a statistically significant decrease in the percentage of ERPF to the treated kidney was present 17 to 21 months after ESWL. Thomas et al.[31] found a significant decrease in renal function shortly after ESWL only when the number of shocks exceeded 1,500 or when the power index (kV $\times$ shocks) is greater than 25,000. Although patients who underwent follow-up scans generally had no significant loss over the long-term period, the authors believe long-term function will be adversely affected at a 45,000-power index. In summary, the studies of both Williams et al.[8] and Thomas et al.[31] imply that short-term changes in renal function may not be totally reversible and may be dose related.

Other complications have been sporadically reported. These include pancreatitis, chest x-ray changes possibly related to a lung contusion, ESWL-induced gastric or duodenal erosions, and formation of perinephric abscesses.[2, 3, 32, 33]

Recently significant concern and controversy have arisen as to whether ESWL may cause new-onset hypertension. Both MRI and CT scanning have demonstrated a relatively high incidence of subcapsular and perirenal bleeding after ESWL, analogous to what may occur after acute renal trauma. This raises the possibility that a "Page kidney" may result. The Page kidney refers to renovascular hypertension that results from an ischemic kidney compressed by fluid, blood, or fibrosis. Since first described in 1939, several reports have described the development of a Page kidney after renal trauma and subsequent cure by nephrectomy or decortication.[34–36] No study to date has looked at renal vein renins in patients who have developed hypertension after ESWL.

Lingeman and Kulb[37] followed 295 patients at least 1 year after ESWL. New-onset hypertension that required drug therapy was present in 8.2% of patients. Although not requiring pharmacologic therapy, an additional 15.2% of patients had an increase in their diastolic blood pressure averaging 16.7 mm Hg. No significant difference between the groups was present in terms of renal function or power index delivered. Peterson and Finlayson[38] reviewed the charts of 79 patients who underwent ESWL and discovered new-onset hypertension in three patients (4%). Two of these patients had significant perirenal bleeding. Williams et al.[8] reported on seven patients (8%) who had developed severe hypertension and required treatment within 21 months.

Review of the medical literature reveals the annualized incidence of hypertension to be between 3% and 6% in men between 30 and 60 years of age, suggesting that ESWL may be increasing new-onset hypertension.[39] These studies are of limited value, however, because to demonstrate ESWL causes new-onset hypertension, one must compare these patients to stone disease patients who did not undergo ESWL, especially because stone patients have higher incidence rates of hypertension.[40]

A subsequent study undertaken at Methodist Hospital of Indiana[41] revealed an annualized incidence of new-onset hypertension of 2.4% in patients after ESWL compared with 4.0% in the group of non-ESWL stone formers. The annualized increase in diastolic pressure of 0.78 mm Hg in ESWL patients was, however, statistically significant when compared with controls.

In summary, the data are retrospective and conflicting regarding the association between ESWL and new-onset hypertension. Further prospective studies with adequate control patients need to be carried out. The concept of the Page kidney after ESWL should be further investigated by careful renin studies in both patients and animal models.

SUMMARY

Certainly ESWL remains the treatment of choice for most upper urinary tract calculi, with more than 1 million treatments having been performed worldwide. Evidence is increasing, however, that ESWL is associated with multiple acute complications that may lead to the development of reduced renal function and hypertension in a small number of patients.[42] The exact threshold at which point

ESWL becomes detrimental has yet to be determined, but certainly measurable damage can occur at less than the FDA recommendation of a maximum of 2,000 shocks during treatment. Shock waves should be administered judiciously and limited wherever possible.

Lithotripsy in the future will in general be performed on machines that will impart less power and energy to the kidney; however, more treatments and greater numbers of shock waves will be required. Whether or not these new lithotriptors will be as damaging to the kidney remains to be seen, and careful clinical trials must be conducted in the future.

REFERENCES

1. Jocham D: Historical development of ESWL, in Riehle RA Jr (ed): *Principles of Extracorporeal Shock Wave Lithotripsy*. New York, Churchill Livingstone, 1987.
2. Drach GW, Dretler SP, Fair WR, et al: Report of the United States cooperative study of extracorporeal shock wave lithotripsy. *J Urol* 1986; 135:1127.
3. Riehle RA Jr, Fair W, Vaughan ED Jr: Extracorporeal shock wave lithotripsy for upper urinary tract calculi: One year experience at a single center. *JAMA* 1986; 255:2043–2048.
4. Chaussy C, Schmiedt E, Jocham D, et al: First clinical experience with extracorporeally induced destruction of kidney stones by shock waves. *J Urol* 1982; 127:417.
5. Chaussy C, Schmiedt E, Jocham D, et al: Extracorporeal shock wave lithotripsy (ESWL) for treatment of urolithiasis. *Urology* 1984; 23:59.
6. Mulley AG Jr: Shock-wave lithotripsy. *N Engl J Med* 1986; 314:845.
7. Chaussy C (ed): *Extracorporeal Shock Wave Lithotripsy. New Aspects in the Treatment of Kidney Stone Disease*. Basel, S Karger, 1982.
8. Williams CM, Kaude JV, Newman RC, et al: Extracorporeal shock wave lithotripsy: Long-term complications. *AJR* 1988; 150:311–315.
9. Ackaert KSJW, Schroder FH: Effects of extracorporeal shock wave lithotripsy (ESWL) on renal tissue. *Urol Res* 1989; 17:3.
10. Lingeman JE, McAteer JA, Kempson SA, et al: Bioeffects of extracorporeal shock wave lithotripsy. *J Endourol* 1987; 1:89.
11. Lingeman JE, McAteer JA, Kempson SA, et al: Bioeffects of extracorporeal shock wave lithotripsy. *Urol Clin North Am* 1988; 15:507.
12. Brendel W: Effect of shock-waves on canine kidneys, in Gravenstein JS, Peter K (eds): *Extracorporeal Shock Wave Lithotripsy: Technical and Clinical Aspects*. Stoneham, Mass, Butterworth, 1986, p 141.
13. Newman R, Hackett R, Senior D, et al: Pathologic effects of ESWL on canine renal tissue. *Urology* 1987; 29:194.
14. Delius M, Enders G, Yvan Z, et al: Biological effects of shock waves: Kidney damage by shock waves in dogs—dose dependence. *Ultrasound Med Biol* 1988; 14:117–122.
15. Abrahams C, Lipson S, Ross L: Pathologic changes in the kidneys and other or-

gans of dogs undergoing extracorporeal shock wave lithotripsy with a tubless lithotriptor. *J Urol* 1988; 140:391.
16. Neuerburg J, Dals HJ, Reckow, et al: Effects of lithotripsy on rat kidney: Evaluation with MR imaging, histology, and electron microscopy. *J Comput Assist Tomog* 1989; 13:82.
17. Recker F, Rubben H, Bex H, et al: Morphological changes following ESWL in the rat kidney. *Urol Res* 1989; 17:229.
18. Graff J, Pastor J, Richter KD: Effect of high energy shock waves on body tissue [abstract]. Proceedings of the Fifth World Congress on Endourology and ESWL, Cairo, Egypt, 1987, p 260.
19. Delius M: Effect of extracorporeal shock waves on kidney. *J Urol* 1988; 140:390.
20. Holmes RP, Yeaman LD, Taylor, et al: Enhanced adriamycin uptake by neutrophils exposed to shock waves [abstract]. *J Urol* 1987; 138:3044.
21. Russo P, Mies C, Huryk R, et al: Histopathologic and ultrastructural correlates of tumor growth suppression by high energy shock waves. *J Urol* 1987; 137:338.
22. Russo P, Stephenson RA, Mies C, et al: High energy shock waves suppress tumor growth in vitro and in vivo. *J Urol* 1986; 135:626.
23. Oosterhof GON, Smits GHHJ, Ruyter JE, et al: The in vitro effect of electromagnetically generated shock waves (lithoster) on the Denning R 3327 PAT-Z rat prostatic cancer cell line. *Urol Res* 1989; 17:13.
24. Assimos DG, Boyce WH, Farr EG, et al: Selective elevation of urinary enzyme levels after extracorporeal shock wave lithotripsy. *J Urol* 1989; 142:687.
25. Haupt G, Haupt A, Donovan JM: Short-term changes of laboratory values after extracorporeal shock wave lithotripsy: Comparative study. *J Urol* 1989; 142:259.
26. Rubin JI, Arger PH, Pollack HM, et al: Kidney changes after extracorporeal shock wave lithotripsy: CT evaluation. *Radiology* 1987; 162:21.
27. Yaick JV, Williams CM, Millnor MR, et al: Renal morphology and function immediately after extracorporeal shock wave lithotripsy. *AJR* 1985; 145:305.
28. Knapp PM, Kelb TB, Lingeman JE, et al: Extracorporeal shock wave lithotripsy-induced perirenal hematomas. *J Urol* 1988; 139:700.
29. Grantham JR, Millner MR, Kauck JV, et al: Renal stone disease treated with extracorporeal shock wave lithotripsy: Short-term observations in 100 patients. *Radiology* 1986; 158:203.
30. Gilbert BR, Riehle RA Jr, Vaughan ED Jr: Extracorporeal shock wave lithotripsy and its effect on renal function. *J Urol* 1988; 139:482.
31. Thomas R, Roberts J, Sloane B, et al: Effect of extracorporeal shock wave lithotripsy on renal function. *J Endourol* 1988; 2:141.
32. Karow MHA, Mohamed ARE, Ketab EE, et al: Extracorporeal shock wave lithotripsy (ESWL) induced erosions in upper gastrointestinal tract. *Urology* 1987; 30:224.
33. Karamalegos AZ, Dioleno HC, Moylan DF: Formation of perinephric abscess following extracorporeal shock wave lithotripsy. *Urology* 1989; 34:277.
34. Grant P, Gifford W, Piduan WR, et al: Renal trauma and hypertension. *Am J Cardiol* 1971; 27:173.
35. Sufrin G: The Page kidney: A correctable form of arterial hypertension. *J Urol* 1975; 113:450.

36. Engel WJ, Page IH: Hypertension due to renal compression resulting from subcapsular hematoma. *J Urol* 1955; 73:735.
37. Lingeman JE, Kulb TB: Hypertension following extracorporeal shock wave lithotripsy [abstract]. *J Urol* 1987; 137:45A.
38. Peterson JC, Finlayson B: Effects of ESWL on blood pressure, in Gravenstein J, Peter K (eds): *Extracorporeal Shock Wave Lithotripsy for Renal Stone Disease,* Stoneham, Mass, Butterworth, 1986, p 145.
39. Dannenberg AL, Garrison RJ, Kannel WB: Incidence of hypertension in the Framingham study. *Am J Public Health* 1988; 78:676.
40. Robertson WG, Peacock M, Baker M, et al: Studies on the prevalence and epidemiology of urinary stone disease in men in Leeds. *Br J Urol* 1983; 55:595.
41. Lingeman JE, Woods JR, Toth PD: Blood pressure changes following extracorporeal shock wave lithotripsy and other forms of treatment for nephrolithiasis. *JAMA* 1990; 263:1789.
42. Evan AP, Willis LR, Connors BA, McAteer JA, et al: Renal injury by shock wave lithotripsy, *J Endourol* 1991; 5:25.

46

Renal Changes Related to Extracorporeal Shock Wave Lithotripsy

John M. Donovan, M.D.

This 47-year-old female has just undergone bilateral ESWL treatment for a 7-mm left renal stone, and a 1-cm right renal stone. A stent was placed in the right ureter without difficulty. Although you had planned to send her home after the treatment, she has severe bilateral colic. You observe her in the hospital overnight. The next morning, the pain persists, and her hematocrit has fallen from 41% to 30%. She also is mildly hypertensive (144/98) compared to her preoperative blood pressure of 130/80. CAT scan of the abdomen indicates a 5-cm hematoma at the lower pole of the left kidney, and significant subcapsular hemorrhage around the right kidney. You question her carefully, but she denies taking any drugs which might affect coagulation and clot formation. Over the next 2 days, her pain decreases, and the hematocrit remains at 30%. Her blood pressure returns to normal.

Questions for the consultant: How do you analyze this complication of ESWL therapy? What are your recommendations for continued evaluation, therapy, and follow-up?

The shock waves of extracorporeal shock wave lithotripsy (ESWL) travel at the speed of sound in water, and the pressure at the target is 5,000 to 8,500 psi. This much force could potentially injure the soft tissue of kidneys. Indeed, the prevalence of acute gross injury to kidneys from ESWL in clinical practice ranges from 63% to 74% as monitored with magnetic resonance imaging or computed tomography (CT) scan. However, the renal injury is usually clinically insignificant. More recently, studies have suggested a dose-dependent threshold for renal injury. Namely, energy levels used during ESWL over a theoretical threshold for safe ESWL treatments of 2,000 shock waves at 20 kV result in kidney injury, adjacent tissue injury, or both.

INITIAL EVALUATION AND TREATMENT

The current incidence of postlithotripsy renal hematomas and subcapsular hemorrhage requiring transfusion ranges from 0.25% to 0.66%. The primary risk factors for the development of postlithotripsy hemorrhage or hematomas are hypertension, urinary tract infection, and simultaneous bilateral treatments. Coagulation disorders and ingestion of medications that affect coagulation or platelet function are other factors as well. Patients with hypertension have a fivefold increased risk for bleeding.

Because this particular patient had no significant hypertension at the time of lithotripsy or recent use of drugs that might affect her platelet function, such as aspirin or nonsteroidal anti-inflammatories, attention needs to be given to the possibility of an unsuspected coagulopathy or an excessive number of shock waves delivered at high kilovoltage, exceeding the theoretical threshold for safe lithotripsy.

Consultation with a hematologist is appropriate, as well as measurements of liver function tests, prothrombin time, partial thromboplastin time, bleeding time, fibrinogen level, and fibrin split products. If no correctable coagulopathy can be found to explain this patient's complication, further evaluation of this patient's lithotripsy procedure should be undertaken. It may be necessary to have the lithotriptor unit evaluated by the lithotriptor's engineering staff to assure proper function of this particular unit.

Her areas of hemorrhage and subcapsular hematoma have arisen from renal contusions or bruises that have resulted from blunt renal trauma of lithotripsy (Fig 46–1). Consequently, the management should be conservative, as for any patient suffering blunt renal trauma with renal contusions. A urine culture should be obtained to rule out infection. Renal function should be evaluated with appropriate laboratory studies and renal scans when indicated. Bilateral renal contusions can result in short-term acute renal failure. Short-term hemodialysis has occasionally been required after lithotripsy. Serial blood cell counts

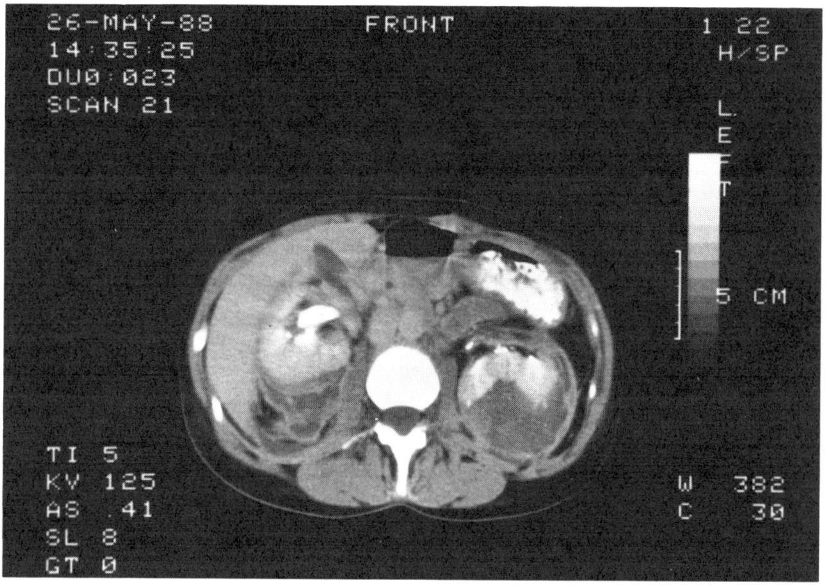

FIG 46–1.
Computer tomographic scan at midlevel of kidneys shows bilateral intrarenal and perirenal hematomas.

should be obtained to ascertain or confirm that the bleeding has stopped and that the patient's condition has stabilized. Blood transfusions may be required to stabilize the patient until tamponade effect controls the bleeding. Rarely, arterial embolization has been required to stop renal bleeding. On one occasion a patient required a nephrectomy to control bleeding after unsuccessful embolization. The patient should be kept at bed rest until her gross hematuria has cleared. It is unreasonable to expect that this patient's microhematuria will clear until all stone fragments have cleared. Serial radiographs and ultrasound images will be necessary to monitor both the passage of stone fragments and the size of hematomas. Patients can be discharged once their pain is controllable and hematocrit stabilizes. They should be hemodynamically stable for 48 hours before discharge.

Hypertension after ESWL is uncommon but is a recognized complication of renal contusions, especially those associated with subcapsular hematomas or cortical scarring. Early complications after blunt renal trauma can occur within the first 4 weeks of injury and include delayed bleeding, abscess, sepsis, and hypertension. Consequently, the patient should be followed in the office or clinic every 1 to 2 weeks for the first 6 weeks for monitoring of blood pressure, for a physical examination, and for urinalysis and urine cultures when indicated, as well as renal ultrasound, to follow the hematoma and stone burden.

After this time the patient should be followed monthly for the first year with blood pressure measurements. An intravenous pyelogram (IVP) is generally recommended 3 months after the injury. The IVP should be evaluated for cortical scarring or obstruction of the upper ureter or the ureteral pelvic junction by either fibrosis or stone fragments.

LONG-TERM CARE AND FOLLOW-UP

Recent animal studies have demonstrated an association between high-energy lithotripsy and subsequent focal interstitial fibrosis and capsular fibrosis, which suggests that some of the tissue damage that occurred after lithotripsy is irreversible and analogous to blunt renal trauma seen clinically. This could conceivably result in a Page kidney phenomenon, with partial renal ischemia resulting in a renin-mediated type of hypertension. Some would suggest that all patients should be evaluated for any evidence of blunt renal contusions with ultrasound and should have hematocrit tested after lithotripsy. Those patients with moderate to severe pain after ESWL or a significant decrease in hemoglobin levels definitely require a renal ultrasound the day after ESWL. If a hematoma is found, a CT scan should be obtained to evaluate the degree of parenchymal injury and site of hematoma.

Because delayed hypertension can occur up to 15 years after renal trauma, should patients be followed for the development of hypertension for an extended period of time after lithotripsy? Certainly those patients found to have evidence of renal contusions, hemorrhage, or subcapsular hematomas should be followed more closely. Long-standing hypertension after renal trauma is usually a result of partial renal ischemia, resulting in a renin-mediated type of hypertension. Most of these patients can be managed medically, but surgical intervention may be necessary in unresponsive patients.

CONCLUSION

It is up to the individual lithotriptor operator to identify those patients who are at increased risk for the development of subcapsular hematomas and to correct those risk factors before lithotripsy. Patients with hypertension must have their blood pressure under adequate medical control at the time of treatment. Patients who have a coagulopathy should have their coagulopathy corrected, and those who are taking medications affecting clotting function should stop taking such medications for 2 weeks before treatment. All patients should be free of infection. Those patients who have large stone burdens should probably receive staged treatments, especially if they have a history of hypertension. It is the responsibility of the lithotriptor operator to manage the patient prudently, to recognize that a safe threshold for lithotripsy does exist, and to stay within this threshold. For those patients who do develop bleeding complications after lithotripsy, they, like patients with blunt renal trauma, require immediate support with hydration and transfusions as needed, regular evaluation of blood pressure and renal function, and correction of any abnormal coagulation factors that may contribute to the underlying stone disease. Finally, long-term evaluation of blood pressure, renal function, and metabolic factors contributing to underlying stone disease should be done on a regular basis.

BIBLIOGRAPHY

Baumgartner BR, Dickey KW, Ambrose SS, et al: Kidney changes after extracorporeal shock wave lithotripsy: Appearance on MR imaging. *Radiology* 1987; 163:531–534.

Donahue LA, Linke CA, Rowe JM: Renal loss following extracorporeal shock wave lithotripsy. *J Urol* 1989; 142:809–811.

Drach GW, Dretler S, Fair W, et al: Report of the United States cooperative study of extracorporeal shock wave lithotripsy. *J Urol* 1986; 135:1127–1133.

Gunasekaran S, Donovan JM, Chvapil M, et al: Effects of extracorporeal shock wave lithotripsy on the structure and function of rabbit kidney. *J Urol* 1989; 141:1250–1254.

Haupt G, Haupt A, Donovan JM, et al: Short-term changes of laboratory values after ESWL: Comparative study. *J Urol* 1989; 142:259–262.

Hunter PT, Finlayson B, Hirko RJ, et al: Measurement of shock wave pressures used for lithotripsy. *J Urol* 1986; 136:733–738.

Kaude JV, Williams CM, Millner MR, et al: Renal morphology and function immediately after extracorporeal shock wave lithotripsy. *AJR* 1985; 145:305–313.

Knapp PM, Kulb T, Lingeman JE, et al: Extracorporeal shock wave lithotripsy-induced perirenal hematomas. *J Urol* 1988; 139:700–703.

Lingeman JE, Kulb TB: Hypertension following extracorporeal shock wave lithotripsy. *J Urol* 1987; 137:142A.

Page IH: The production of persistent arterial hypertension by cellophane perinephritis. *JAMA* 1939; 113:2046–2048.

Rubin JI, Arger PH, Pollack HM, et al: Kidney changes after extracorporeal shock wave lithotripsy: CT evaluation. *Radiology* 1987; 162:21–24.

Spark RF, Berg S: Renal trauma and hypertension. The role of renin. *Arch Intern Med* 1976; 136:1097–1100.

VonKnorring J, Fyhrquist F, Ahonen J: Varying course of hypertension following renal trauma. *J Urol* 1981; 126:798–801.

Williams CM, Kaude JV, Newman RC, et al: Extracorporeal shock wave lithotripsy: Long term complications. *AJR* 1988; 150:311–315.

47

Extracorporeal Shock Wave Lithotripsy of Ureteral Stones

Alan D. Jenkins, M.D.

You consult in the care of a 36-year-old man with a 5-mm stone impacted in the ureter 3 cm above the right ureterovesical junction. He has been transferred to your care after two unsuccessful attempts at stone retrieval in a remote hospital. His most recent intravenous pyelogram (IVP) (2 days ago) shows delayed function to 3 hours, with ureteral dilation to the level of the stone. Aside from this stone, his general health is excellent.

The management of this patient before the development of ureteroscopy and extracorporeal shock wave lithotripsy (ESWL) would have been straightforward. If the stone did not pass spontaneously and blind manipulation was unsuccessful, a ureterolithotomy would have been performed. The approach is not so simple in the 1990s. The optimum management of this patient is controversial, especially in North America.

The best treatment is that which minimizes the patient's pain, relieves the obstruction, and minimizes any residual damage to the kidney and ureter. The options for treating this patient are observation with the hope that the stone will pass spontaneously, ESWL, endoscopic manipulation, or ureterolithotomy.

The likelihood that a stone will pass spontaneously is related to its size, location within the ureter, and its shape. More than 80% of stones less than 4 mm in diameter will pass spontaneously, especially if they are in the lower half of the ureter. Spontaneous passage of stones with a diameter equal to or greater than 6 mm is unlikely, especially if they are in the upper ureter. Approximately 50% of lower ureteral stones with a diameter between 4 and 6 mm will pass.

Because this patient's stone is 5 mm in diameter, the likelihood of spontaneous passage is 50%. The two unsuccessful attempts at stone manipulation, however, will alter this statistic. A stone may pass after an unsuccessful attempt at basket extraction, but the resultant edema of the ureteral mucosa makes this unlikely for at least several days. The delayed function on IVP and the ureter dilated to the stone implies that the stone is tightly impacted in the ureter and probably will not pass.

Waiting for this stone to pass is a viable option only if the patient has little or no discomfort and the ureter was not injured during the unsuccessful manipulation. Ureteral integrity can be ascertained with a retrograde ureterogram, but this requires an invasive cystoscopy and a formal anesthetic in a young man. Another IVP, if the 2-day-old IVP had been obtained before the manipulation, would help evaluate the ureter, but the least invasive study would be a plain abdominal radiograph and a sonogram. The stone may be in a different location if it has been pushed through the ureteral wall, but this happens more commonly with ureteroscopy than with simple basketing. An ultrasound examination that uses a full bladder for a sonographic window can localize lower ureteral stones, identify ureteral dilation above a stone, and detect a perivesical collection of blood or extravasated urine.

If this patient has no evidence of a ureteral injury, the decision must be made whether to intervene immediately or wait for the stone to pass. High-grade ureteral obstruction does not have to be relieved emergently to preserve renal function. Irreversible renal injury does not occur after up to 2 weeks of complete ureteral obstruction. If the patient's pain can be controlled comfortably with oral analgesics, it would not be unreasonable to follow him and hope for spontaneous passage.*

Further observation is unlikely to happen in the real world, because the patient has had enough trouble that he wants something done, and he was referred to you for a definitive solution. Such patients should be told that the procedure with the greatest chance of success removing the stone is a ureterolithotomy. Although less invasive than open surgery, ureteroscopy and ESWL are associated with more uncertainty. Most patients, however, want to avoid surgery.

The choice between ureteroscopy and ESWL is very controversial. Most urologists in North America would treat this stone ureteroscopically. An attempt would be made to negotiate a floppy-tipped guidewire around the stone. Even if this were not possible, the ureter distal to the stone would be dilated with a balloon and the ureteroscope advanced to the stone. If there were adequate space between the stone and the ureteral wall, the stone would be engaged in a basket and extracted whole. An impacted stone would be fragmented with ultrasonic, pulsed dye laser, or electrohydraulic lithotripsy under direct vision. A double pigtail catheter would be left to drain the kidney for several days.

Although ureteroscopy is the procedure of choice in North America, ESWL would be used in Western Europe and at a few stone treatment centers in the United States. A major reason for this disparity is that the most readily available type of lithotriptor is the Dornier HM-3 (Dornier Medical Systems, Inc., Marietta, Ga.), which usually requires a formal regional or general anesthetic. If the patient already is anesthetized, most American urologists believe that ureteroscopic extraction of a distal ureteral stone is more expeditious than ESWL. This situation will change as more anesthesia-free lithotriptors become available. My prediction is that in situ ESWL will become the optimal treatment of all ureteral calculi, even in North America.

Ureteral stones treated in situ appear to be more resistant to the effects of shock waves than freely floating renal pelvic stones. This concept has become well-accepted lithotriptor folklore, even though little, if any, data exist to formally support it. Therefore, most urologists attempt to manipulate ureteral stones back to the kidney before ESWL. In situ ESWL is performed only if this manipulation is unsuccessful.

The mechanism of stone fragmentation by lithotripsy is thought to be spalling, whereby successive layers of superficial stone material are torn off by

---

**Another option would be to place a percutaneous nephrostomy to drain the kidney. Relief of the ureteral dilation might permit more efficient peristalsis and subsequent passage of the stone. It is unlikely that any patient would accept this approach unless he were septic, in which case drainage of the upper urinary tract would be the procedure of choice.*

each shock wave. If a stone is impacted in the ureter, the initial sand cannot disperse, and the multiple fragment-fluid interfaces may prevent subsequent shock waves from reaching the core of the stone. This theoretical problem possibly can be overcome by placing a ureteral catheter adjacent to the stone to create an expansion space. An artificial expansion space also can be created by instilling saline through a ureteral catheter that has been placed just distal to the stone.

In spite of the widespread acceptance of these concepts, they have little experimental support. An alternative explanation is that ureteral stones that can be manipulated back to the kidney would respond readily to in situ ESWL. Tightly impacted stones that might respond poorly to in situ ESWL probably cannot be pushed back to the kidney. The effect of ureteral catheterization would not be therapeutic but simply selection. A disadvantage of pre-ESWL manipulation of ureteral stones is that renal parenchyma probably is more sensitive to shock wave–induced injury than is the ureter. Why expose the kidney to potential injury if a ureteral stone will fragment readily with in situ ESWL?

Early experience with in situ ESWL of distal ureteral calculi was not encouraging. Eight of the first 36 patients with solitary juxtavesicular calculi treated with in situ ESWL at the University of Virginia needed additional post-ESWL procedures: repeat ESWL, ureteroscopic extraction of fragments, or temporary percutaneous nephrostomy drainage. One factor may have been responsible, in part, for these disappointing initial results. Virtually all of these patients had pre-ESWL manipulation with a ureteral catheter or a ureteroscope. In situ ESWL was a last resort before ureterolithotomy. The vigorous manipulation may have caused even more edema of the ureteral mucosa, thereby resulting in a more intensely impacted stone.

The Dornier HM-3 lithotriptor was designed to treat stones in the kidney and upper ureter, but lower ureteral stones can be treated if the patient is placed in the proper position. Patients with stones in the juxtavesicular ureter (between the ureterovesical junction and the lower border of the sacroiliac joint) are placed in an almost jackknife position. The shock waves are directed through the left or right buttock. Juxtavesicular stones have been treated at the University of Virginia with a mean of 2,200 shock waves at a mean of 24 kV.

Patients with stones in the presacral ureter (between the lower and upper margins of the sacroiliac joint) are placed in a prone position. This may require mechanical modification of the patient chair on older models of the Dornier HM-3. Prone treatment of presacral stones is easier and more effective than standard supine treatment, because the shock waves do not have to traverse the thick sacral and iliac bones.

Most patients treated with Dornier HM-3 lithotriptors have an epidural or general endotracheal anesthesia. If a patient with a distal ureteral stone is anesthetized already, ureteroscopic manipulation is an unavoidable temptation. Why

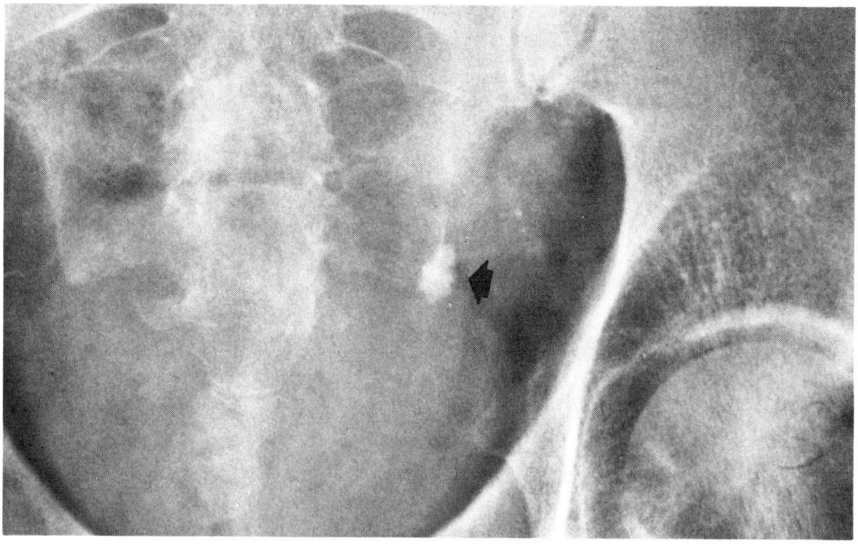

FIG 47–1.
A 7-mm diameter stone is impacted in the lower left ureter *(solid arrow).*

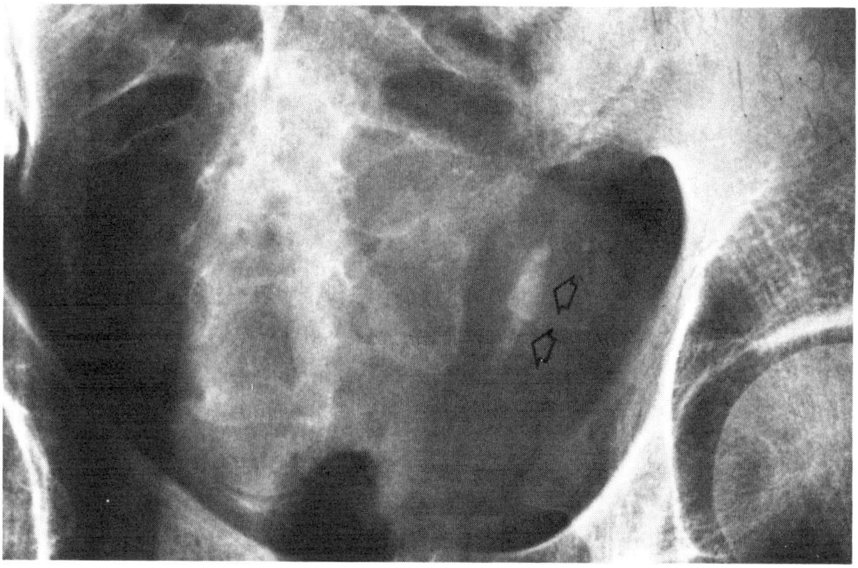

FIG 47–2.
Immediately after treatment with 5,000 shock waves (16–19 kV) on a Siemens Lithostar. Sandlike material is visible in the ureter *(open arrows).*

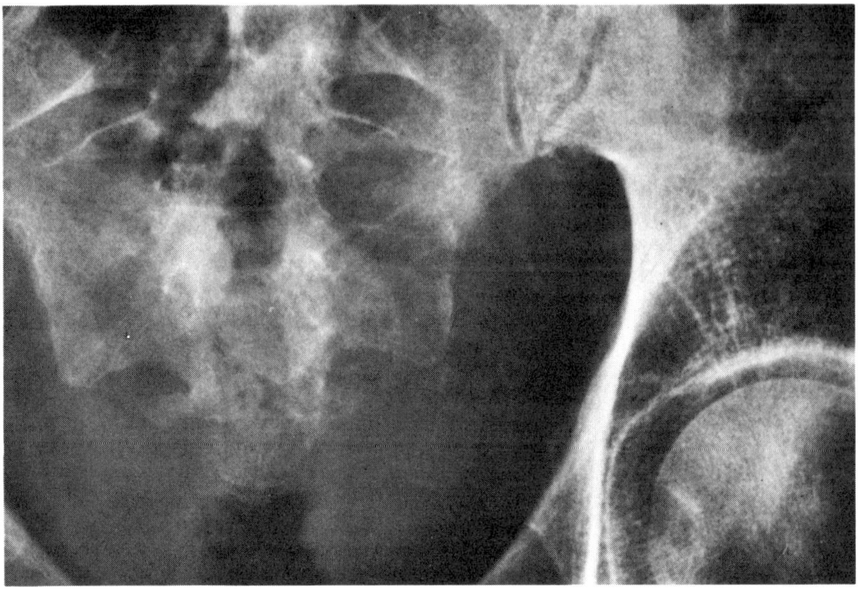

FIG 47–3.
No retained stone material is visible 24 hours after in situ lithotripsy.

bother with the uncertainties of in situ ESWL when the stone can be removed ureteroscopically?

The advent of newer lithotriptors that require little, if any, anesthesia diminishes the appeal of an ureteroscopic approach. In situ ESWL of distal ureteral calculi, without pretreatment manipulation, becomes more appealing than ureteroscopy. Urologists and patients can dispense with anesthesia, ureteroscopy, and aggravating double pigtail catheters.

Treatment of lower ureteral calculi is surprisingly easy with the Siemens Lithostar. The angled shock head can be placed on a patient's buttock and the shock waves directed through the sacroiliac window. Stones can be localized with the biplanar fluoroscopic system without a ureteral catheter. Although the treatment can be accomplished without any anesthesia, a typical apprehensive patient is more comfortable with IV sedation.

Eight patients with juxtavesicular ureteral stones have been treated with a Siemens Lithostar at the University of Virginia. Anesthesia was provided with a transcutaneous electrical nerve stimulation unit whose four electrodes were placed on the patient's buttock surrounding the shock head and IV sedation with fentanyl and midazolam was administered. Only one patient required ureteroscopic extraction of a fragment 3 weeks after ESWL. The remaining patients were rendered stone free with ESWL alone.

An exemplary patient is shown in Figures 47–1 to 47–3. This man had a 7-mm stone wedged in the lower left ureter (see Fig 47–1). The stone was treated with 1,500 shock waves at 16 to 19 kV. There was some concern that the stone appeared incompletely pulverized on an immediate spot radiograph (see Fig 47–2), so an additional 3,500 shock waves were given. The appearance of the fragmented stone on another spot radiography was no different, and the treatment was stopped. Little, if any retained sand was visible on a radiograph obtained 24 hours after in situ lithotripsy (see Fig 47–3).

Even if the 24-hour posttreatment plain radiograph shows no definite pulverization, it is best to follow the patient for a couple of weeks before retreatment is considered as long as the patient is afebrile and relatively asymptomatic. Edematous ureteral mucosa may prevent immediate dispersion of the sand. The fragments will pass when this edema resolves.

BIBLIOGRAPHY

El-Faqih SR, Husain I, Ekman PE, et al: Primary choice of intervention for distal ureteric stones: ureteroscopy or ESWL? *Br J Urol* 1988; 62:13–18.

Jenkins AD: Dornier extracorporeal shock-wave lithotripsy for ureteral stones. *Urol Clin North Am* 1988; 15:377–384.

Miller K, Bubeck JR, Hautmann R: Extracorporeal shock wave lithotripsy of distal ureteral calculi. *Eur Urol* 1987; 12: 305–307.

48

Electrohydraulic Lithotripsy of Ureteral Calculi

Bernard Lytton, M.B., F.R.C.S.

A 23-year-old man is hospitalized on your service because of a 7-mm stone impacted in the right ureter at the level of the pelvic brim. He has had severe colic, nausea, and vomiting. This continues for 3 days, and repeat films indicate that the stone has not moved at all.

Ureteral calculi account for about two thirds of upper urinary tract stones; two thirds of these are held up in the lower ureter. About 70% of ureteral stones less than 10 mm will pass spontaneously if the patient is treated with analgesics and high fluid intake. Infection, intractable pain, and progressive or severe persistent obstruction are indications for immediate treatment and removal of the stone.

Several options are available in the management of this man. I would favor an endoscopic approach as my first choice. The patient should be given a low spinal or epidural anesthetic and prepared for cystoscopy on a table with radiologic capability, preferably including fluoroscopy.

An attempt should be made to negotiate a floppy-tip guidewire or glidewire past the stone, and if successful, a double J stent is placed over the guidewire into the renal pelvis to bypass the stone. This should relieve the patient of his acute symptoms and obstruction and allow the edema of the ureter to subside. Occasionally this results in spontaneous passage of the stone, but usually it will require operative removal. The presence of a draining ureteral stent allows this to be carried out as an elective procedure. Should it not be possible to manipulate the guidewire past the stone, ureteroscopy should be performed. When this is being done to treat a stone, it is advisable to dilate the intramural ureter first. A no. 7 French Gruntzig balloon catheter with a 4-cm balloon that can be inflated to a no. 12 or 15 French size should be passed over the guidewire and positioned so that the distal ureter and its orifice can be dilated. The balloon is inflated for 60 seconds. Huffman and Bagley[1] recommend the use of a pressure gauge to monitor balloon dilation to minimize the potential for ureteral injury that can occur if the balloon bursts as a result of excessive pressure. A pressure of 8 atm is believed to be sufficient to ensure adequate dilatation of the intramural ureter. The balloon catheter is then removed, leaving the guidewire in place. A no. 6.9 French mini-ureteroscope is introduced into the ureter either alongside or over the guidewire to see if the stone can be visualized. If the ureter is edematous and the stone cannot be adequately visualized, a percutaneous nephrostomy should be established, which will promptly relieve the patient's symptoms and allow the acute reaction to subside. Again, this may allow the stone to pass spontaneously, but more often it will need to be removed endoscopically or treated by extracorporeal shock wave lithotripsy (ESWL). The latter is preferred by some urologists, especially if a stent can be passed alongside the stone into the bladder from above. Imaging of the calculus will be obscured by the sacrum in this patient's case, and there is probably only a 50:50 chance of disintegrating the stone. The preferred method of management therefore is endoscopic removal with the aid of lithotripsy if necessary. If the stone is not obscured by edema of the ureteral wall, a further attempt may be made to maneuver the guidewire past the stone stone under direct vision. This should be done with caution; it is easy to perforate the ureter under these circumstances, because the wall at the site of an impacted stone is usually very friable. Fluoroscopic monitoring is helpful in preventing or recognizing this complication. Successful passage of a guidewire should allow passage of a double J stent. Sometimes however, it proves impossible to pass a stent over the guidewire because the ureteral wall is too rigid to accommodate it.

If the stone is well visualized and a stent cannot be passed, an attempt may be made to either extract it with a three-pronged wire grasping forceps (a basket should not be used under these circumstances) or disintegrate it by electrohydraulic lithotripsy (EHL). This must be done with caution under direct vision all of the time. If the stone does not break easily, it is best to establish a percutaneous nephrostomy and remove the stone at a later date.

ELECTROHYDRAULIC URETERAL LITHOTRIPSY

When the stone is thought to be too large to be extracted intact, if it is firmly impacted, or if it is very spiculated, the stone should be disintegrated. One of the most effective and readily available methods is EHL.[2] Ultrasound probes can be used only under direct vision through large special ureteroscopes and are not very efficient.[3] The pulse dye laser is another method for disintegrating stones but is vastly more expensive and less available.[4] It is no more effective than EHL but is much smaller and has less potential for ureteral injury. However, with the development of the no. 3 and 1.9 French EHL probes, the potential for injury is minimal so that the laser no longer has any significant advantage.

The no. 3 French electrode can be passed through the no. 3.4 French operating port in the mini-ureteroscope, which is already in place. A no. 1.9 French electrode fits easily through the other operating port, which is 2.3 French in size. Electrohydraulic lithotripsy is safe only if done under direct vision so that the operator can be certain that the electrode does not come into contact with the wall of the ureter at any time and that a constant flow of irrigating fluid is maintained. The lithotriptor unit is set at 60 to 70 V on short bursts of 0.1 second's duration for each activation of the foot pedal. The continuous mode should not be used. The irrigant should be 0.15% saline solution, which allows for generation of an adequate spark at the tip of the electrode. One must remember that the usual gravity flow of irrigant through the ureteroscope is diminished by about 60% to 70% when the operating port is occupied by an electrode or instrument. To improve the flow rate, one may apply a pressure bag to the plastic bag so that the irrigating fluid can be delivered under increased pressure, or preferably one can connect the inflow into the ureteroscope to a three-way stopcock and use a 30-mL syringe to augment the flow by frequently flushing the ureteroscope channel to clear debris and bubbles generated by the lithotripsy. It is important to keep a continuous flow of fluid through the instrument so as to prevent thermal injury to the ureteral wall by heat generated from the electrode. Care should be taken to keep the electrode tip a few millimeters away from the end of the ureteroscope to avoid damage to the fiber optic lens. The spark at the end of the electrode produces a cavitation bubble, the expansion and collapse of which creates a shock wave sufficient to break the stone. A smaller electrode produces a more localized but equally effective cavitation bubble but generates less heat. This helps to focus the energy on the stone rather than on the ureteral wall. As the electrode erodes with use, the pulse repetition frequency increases, necessitating some increase in the voltage setting. It is probably better to replace the electrode when this occurs. If the stone is tightly impacted, it may be more difficult to disintegrate because much of the energy of the hydraulic shock wave is attenuated. There is also some increase in the risk of injury to the ureteral wall, so that if the stone does not start to break up easily, the procedure should be discontinued and a percutaneous nephrostomy established to allow the edema to subside. Stones composed of calcium oxalate monohydrate are harder to disintegrate with EHL, as they are with ESWL.[5] We have failed to break a stone by EHL on two occasions, and in both cases they were composed of calcium oxalate monohydrate. Sometimes the first fragments to be broken off will have to be removed using a three-prong wire grasping forceps before the rest of the stone can be engaged. It is our practice to remove the larger fragments and leave the smaller ones to be passed spontaneously. After lithotripsy, a guidewire is reinserted under direct vision and a double J ureteral stent placed over it. The patient is then sent home the next day, and the internalized stent is left indwelling for 1 week. We havc disintcgratcd morc than 50 urctcral stones by EIIL. It has proved to be both safe and effective for all types of urinary calculi, including cystine and uric acid stones. Careful long-term follow-up using excretory urography or renal ultrasonography on 24 patients showed no evidence of any ureteral injury or other long-term complications attributable to the lithotripsy.

REFERENCES

1. Huffman JF, Bagley DH: Balloon dilation of the ureter for ureteroscopy. *J Urol* 1988; 140:954–956.
2. Green DF, Lytton B: Early experience with direct vision electrohydraulic lithotripsy of ureteral calculi. *J Urol* 1985; 133:767–770.
3. Huffman JL, Bagley DH, Schoenberg HW, et al: Transurethral removal of large ureteral and renal calculi using ureteroscopic ultrasound lithotripsy. *J Urol* 1983; 130:31–34.
4. Dretler SP, Watson G, Parrish J, et al: Pulsed dye laser fragmentation of ureteral calculi: Initial experience. *J Urol* 1987; 137:386–389.
5. Dretler SP: Stone fragility: A new therapeutic distinction. *J Urol* 1988; 139:1124–1127.

49

Electrohydraulic Lithotripsy of Bladder Stones

Hubert G.W. Frohmüller, M.D., M.S., F.A.C.S.

This 72-year-old man had a transurethral resection of the prostate 4 years ago. He passed a small urinary stone after an episode of left renal colic 20 years ago. Recently, he has noticed decreased urinary stream and, on two occasions, blood in the urine. You confirm microscopic hematuria on an otherwise normal urinalysis. Urine culture indicates no growth. Intravenous urogram reveals normal upper urinary tracts, three radiodense bladder calculi (largest 2 cm, smallest 1.4 cm), and an apparent bladder neck contracture. You confirm these findings cystoscopically.

The incidence of calculi of the urinary tract in the population of the Northern Hemisphere is about the same as that of diabetes mellitus, with considerable geographic differences. With rare exceptions stones in the upper and lower urinary tract originate as renal calculi. The recurrence rate of urinary calculi during a patient's life time is, within a wide range, around 50%.

Bladder neck contractures subsequent to transurethral resection of the prostate occur in about 1% to 2% of the cases.[3] Located either at the vesical neck or in the prostatic urethra, they range from large-caliber strictures to tiny openings hardly permitting the passage of a no. 3 French ureteral catheter. The likely causes of these contractures are extensive resection of the smooth muscle and the fibrous structures at the vesical neck, as well as excessive fulguration of bleeding points in this circumference. In some patients a bladder neck contracture may develop within a few months after transurethral resection, whereas in others it can take years until the characteristic symptoms of decreased urinary stream occur.

This patient belongs to the unfortunate minority in whom a vesical neck contracture developed after transurethral resection of the prostate. The fact that he had passed a urinary stone many years ago makes him highly susceptible to form recurrent calculi. When gravel originating in the kidneys passed through the ureters into his bladder, the vesical neck contracture formed a barrier, preventing the spontaneous passage of these tiny particles into the urethra. Behind, in other words, proximal to the obstacle formed by the contracture, the gravel gradually clots together into stones of the sizes described. Though rare as a cause of bladder stone development, prostatic fragments retained after transurethral resection can function as nuclei for such calculi. Calcium-containing stones are radiodense which are usually easier to fragment than the harder radiolucent calculi, which consist of uric acid. Still, when broken apart, such stones may be composed of layers of different material, such as uric acid and calcium oxalate or calcium phosphate. Cystitis can be excluded in this case because of the negative urine culture.

Because the presence of vesical calculi, as well as the diagnosis of bladder neck contracture, was confirmed cystoscopically, the stricture at the vesical neck appears to be of moderate degree, permitting at least the passage of the instrument into the bladder.

Cystoscopic examination is of great importance in determining the best approach for treatment of this patient. Whereas the majority of vesical calculi can be disintegrated and removed by transurethral means, exceptions to this approach are extremely large stones and calculi within bladder diverticula. In these cases a suprapubic cystolithotomy is indicated.

Because the sizes of the lithotrite and resectoscope used for removal of the bladder neck contracture are usually larger than those of the cystoscope used for inspecting the bladder, difficulties may arise when such instruments are introduced through the contracted bladder neck. In this case one can dilate the vesical neck with van Bueren sounds or incise it with an internal urethrotome.

Generally, transurethral bladder neck surgery and fragmentation of the bladder stones can be performed at the same time with the patient under general anesthesia. Most urologists prefer using spinal or peridural anesthesia for doing transurethral procedures.

Lithotripsy should be carried out before the resection of the bladder neck, because bleeding caused by the resection can interfere with the lithotripsy procedure.

In 1950, Yutkin, a Russian engineer, discovered the destructive effect of electrohydraulic shock waves, and in 1959 Goldberg performed the first successful transurethral electrohydraulic lithotripsy.[1] The armamentarium used is shown in Figures 49–1 and 49–2.

The impulses for the electrohydraulic shock waves are formed in a generator that produces a maximum discharge of 8 kV. The impulses can be regulated in three power levels, the frequency can be modified in a range of 1 to 70 per second, and the duration of the impulses can be adjusted between 1 and 5 seconds. A foot switch is used to trigger the impulses. The energy is transmitted through a polytetrafluoroethylene-isolated electrode mounted in a guide element that prevents the operating telescope from being damaged. At our institution a no. 24 French continuous irrigation resectoscope sheath is used, which also can be fitted with a punch lithotrite, a direct vision aspiration attachment, and a resection element. Thus, the sheath of the instrument can remain in place throughout the entire operation.[1]

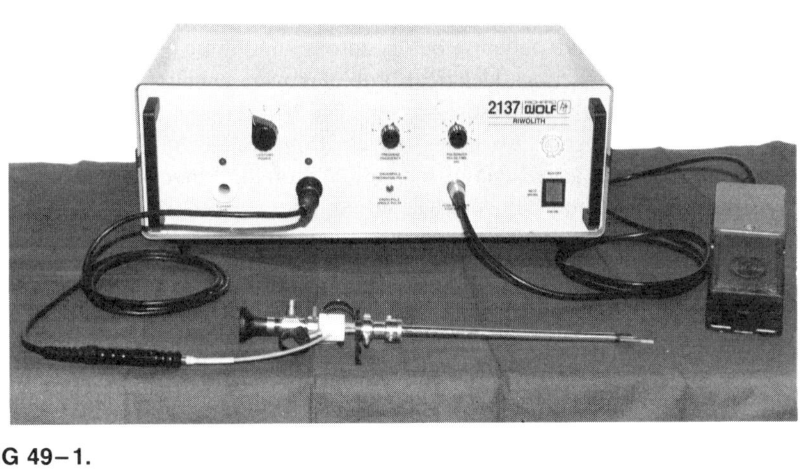

FIG 49–1.
Impulse generator for electrohydraulic lithotripsy with foot switch, high-voltage cable, and electrode connected to a no. 24 French operating cystoscope.

The lithotrite probe is advanced toward the calculus with a handle. When contact with the stone is achieved, electrohydraulic shock waves are emitted by activating the foot switch. The discharge is repeated as often as necessary. Once the stone fragments have been broken down sufficiently to be removed through the instrument sheath, the guide element carrying the lithotrite probe and the observation telescope are removed and replaced by a direct vision aspiration attachment that allows observation of the aspiration procedure.[2] By dispensing with an observation telescope, one can use the entire lumen of the instrument sheath for removal of the stone fragments. Aspiration itself is done with the aid of a vacuum pump in a closed system. If this special equipment is not available, the stone fragments can be removed blindly by means of an Ellik evacuator.

To avoid damage to the bladder wall, one must take care to touch only the stone when discharging the electrode and not the bladder wall itself. When a large stone is broken down by electrohydraulic lithotripsy into fragments that are still too large to be evacuated through the lumen of the instrument, it may hasten the further destruction of the calculus by switching from the electrohydraulic procedure to punch lithotripsy (Figs 49–2 and 49–3). Using this element which can be introduced through the same sheath, one can easily crush the fragments into small particles that can be aspirated as described earlier.

A report from our institution on 345 consecutive cases of bladder stones treated by electrohydraulic lithotripsy alone or combined with punch lithotripsy demonstrated that the method is safe and simple and can be accomplished rapidly.[1] The average age for male patients was 68.5 years, the oldest being 102 years, and for female patients was 63.9 years. None of the patients died postoperatively. The weight of the transurethrally removed stones ranged from 1 to 135 g. The operation was completed in an average of 26 minutes. Bladder perforations occurred in five patients, but cystotomy and drainage were necessary in only one. In 12 operations technical problems were encountered, with damage of the electrode in 9 of these 12 cases. The hemorrhage in the majority of cases was negligible. In a few cases the electrohydraulic lithotripsy could be performed using local anesthesia of the patient's urethral mucosa.

As mentioned earlier, bladder neck surgery can be accomplished after electrohydraulic lithotripsy. While the sheath of the instrument remains in place, the guide with the electrode is removed and the electroresection element is introduced for subsequent resection of the bladder neck contracture.

As pointed out by Greene and Leary,[3] cold punch resection is preferable to electroresection in vesical neck contracture because it eliminates thermic injury to the tissue. Also, the gritty consistency of the cicatricial tissue can be appreciated with the tip of the cold punch resectoscope, and the limits of resection can be judged when the grittiness is gone and the tissue appears soft and pli-

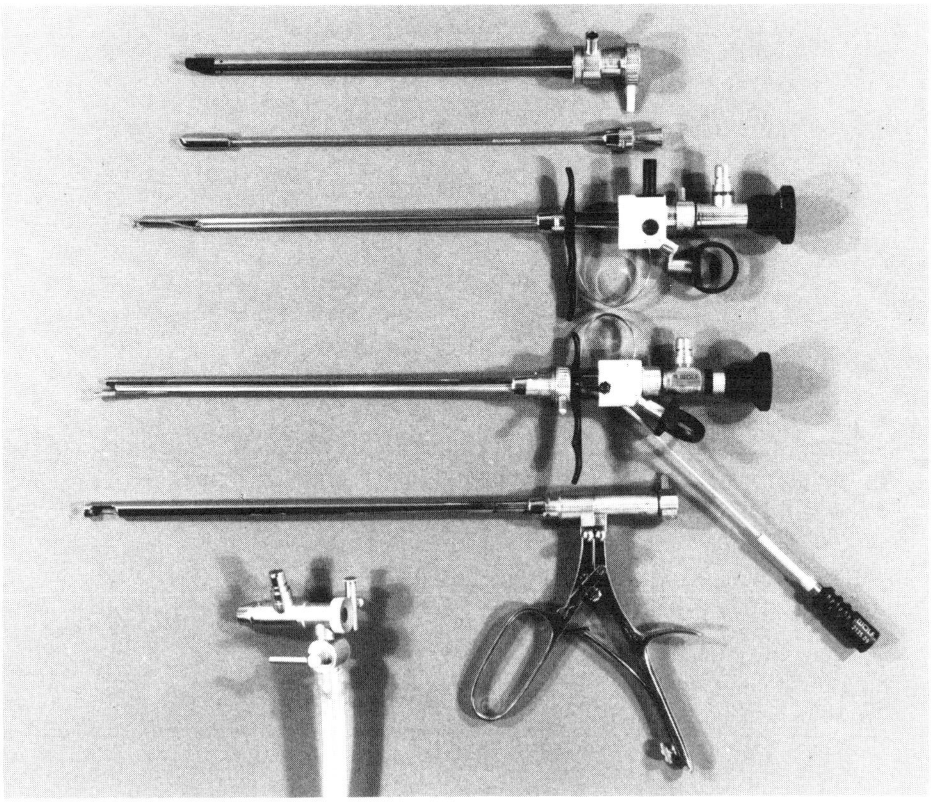

FIG 49–2.
A no. 24 French cystoscope sheath that fits *(from top)* obturator, electroresection element, electroprobe element for electrohydraulic lithotripsy, punch lithotrite, and aspiration attachment with direct vision observation window.

able. Fulguration should be as minimal as possible. When bleeding is slight or nonexistent, often no electrocautery is necessary.

Even though the efficacy of anti-inflammatory corticosteroid injection has not been proved, some urologists recommend the injection of a water-insoluble corticosteroid agent into the areas of resection after removal of the contracted tissue at the vesical neck.[4] Whatever method of treatment was used, the peril of recurrence of a vesical neck contracture is considerable.

After completion of the electrohydraulic lithotripsy and the resection of the bladder neck contracture, a no. 24 French balloon catheter is inserted. Because of its excellent tissue compatibility, a catheter made of pure silicone is preferred. It may stay in place for up to 10 days. Antibiotic therapy should be

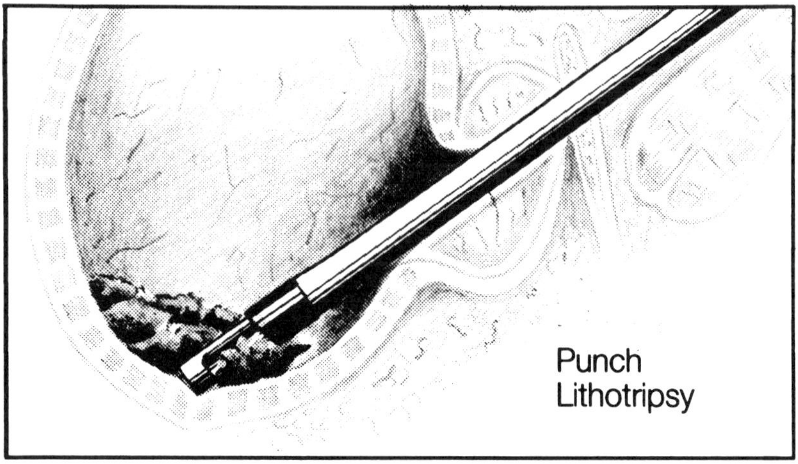

FIG 49–3.
Punch lithotripsy.

given until a few days after the catheter is removed. Urine culture is performed thereafter to ensure the urine is sterile. Because of the danger of recurrence of bladder neck contracture, the patient should be followed routinely. As soon as the patient complains of difficulties urinating, a retrograde urethrogram and a cystoscopic examination should be performed.

REFERENCES

1. Bülow H, Frohmüller HGW: Electrohydraulic lithotripsy with aspiration of the fragments under vision—304 consecutive cases. *J Urol* 1981; 126:454.
2. Frohmüller H: Elektrohydraulische Lithotripsie mit Direktsicht-Aspiration der Konkrementtrümmer. *Urologe* 1971; 10:64.
3. Greene LF, Leary FJ: Contracture of the vesical neck following transurethral prostatic resection. *Surg Gynecol Obstet* 1967; 124:1277.
4. Malek RS, Greene LF: Corticosteroid therapy of postoperative contractures of the vesical neck. *J Urol* 1973; 110:297.

50

Management of a Ureteral Stone by Laser Lithotripsy

Stephen P. Dretler, M.D.

One of your medical colleagues comes to your office because he has developed severe right renal colic. He states that he passed a stone on the left about 3 years ago and "knows this is the same thing." He takes no medications and has no allergies. Physical examination reveals a slim man writhing in pain. He has marked palpation and percussion tenderness of the right flank. Urinalysis is unremarkable except for more than 30 red blood cells/high-power field. Intravenous (IV) pyelogram shows a radiodense 3 by 6 mm stone impacted in the ureter at the inferior edge of the iliac bone. Moderate hydroureteronephrosis exists above the stone. You prescribe tablets for pain relief, and the patient improves over the next week. Your repeat abdominal film indicates that the stone has not moved, and renal ultrasound continues to show moderate hydronephrosis. The patient is concerned because he believes he is losing renal function because of obstruction.

The issues raised by this case presentation include the likelihood of spontaneous passage of a calculus, the time one may allow hydronephrosis to continue before renal damage may occur, the factors that may influence the choice of a method of intervention, the technique of laser fragmentation, and posttreatment management.

SPONTANEOUS STONE PASSAGE

Three factors affect the likelihood of spontaneous stone passage: the width of the stone, the length of the stone, and the level of ureter in which it is first discovered. Figure 50–1 demonstrates that a 3-mm wide calculus has approximately the same rate of passage (85%) within 1 year as does a 6-mm long calculus. A 5-mm wide calculus has approximately the same rate of spontaneous passage (55%) as an 8-mm long calculus, and a 6-mm wide calculus has a 35% rate of passage equivalent to that of a 10-mm long calculus.[1] A stone that becomes symptomatic and is discovered in the lower ureter has an 86% chance of passage, but if it comes to clinical attention in the upper ureter, the likelihood of spontaneous passage falls to 43%. However, in this particular clinical situation, we do not have the luxury of waiting 1 year for passage, and what becomes the rate-limiting step in the intervention decision process is the degree of hydronephrosis.

TIME OF INTERVENTION

The completely obstructed kidney has a permanent decrease in both tubular and glomerular function within a 2-week period. Pressures above ureteral stones have been measured in the 40 to 50 mm Hg range and as high as 70 mm Hg during colic. Intrapelvic pressures are elevated to an average of 20 to 30 mm Hg for the first 12 to 16 weeks of partial ureteral obstruction.[2] The increase in pelvic pressure for a long period results in significant impairment of renal function, which does not return to normal even after the release of obstruction. There is no information that pinpoints the specific amount of time a kidney may be partially obstructed and return to normal function. An animal model was never able to be developed that allowed a reproducible partial obstruction to be created. However, it is known that after 2 weeks of complete ureteral obstruction, release allows the concentrating ability to return to normal. After 4 weeks of complete ureteral obstruction, release results in some permanent impairment of concentrating ability. Thus, it appears that after 4 weeks of partial obstruction, a permanent deficiency in renal function could occur. Because no definitive information is available, it seems prudent to intervene for a ureteral stone,

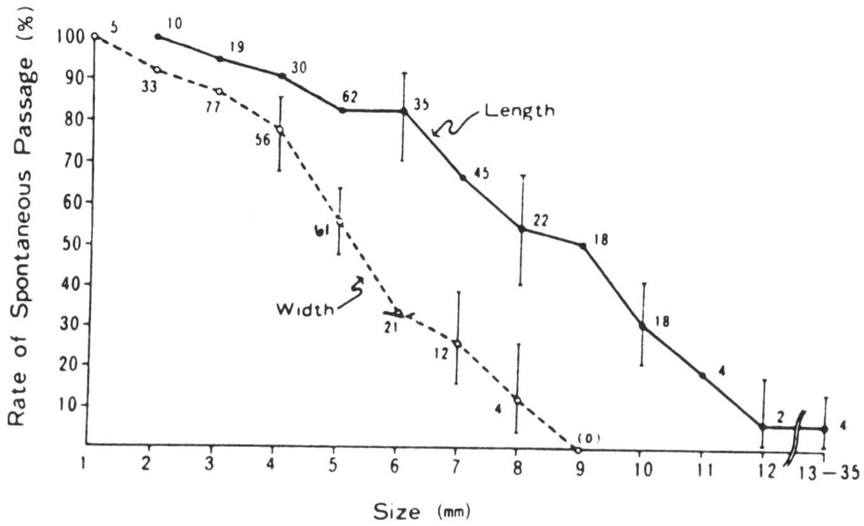

FIG 50–1.
Rates of spontaneous passage of ureteral calculi within 1 year in successive 1-mm intervals of length and width. Vertical bars indicate 90% confidence intervals. Numbers in parentheses indicate those of calculi passed spontaneously.

regardless of size, after partial obstruction (moderate hydronephrosis) has been present for 4 weeks. One might stretch that out another week or 2, but that is entirely dependent on the degree of hydronephrosis.

CHOICE OF INTERVENTION

The choice of method of intervention will depend on the patient's symptoms, the level, size, and composition of the calculus, the equipment available, and the skill of the individual physician. If the patient is febrile, a drainage procedure must be done (retrograde stent or percutaneous tube). In an afebrile, nonseptic patient, a calculus in the upper ureter will probably be best treated by stent and extracorporeal shock wave lithotripsy (ESWL); calculi larger than 1 cm and composed of the denser calcium oxalate monohydrate or calcium phosphate dihydrate are best treated by stent and ESWL in the upper ureter and ultrasonic lithotripsy when over the sacrum or in the lower ureter. If a Siemens Lithostar (Siemens Lithostar Medical Engineering Group, Erlangen, Germany), or a multiple-function Dornier 5000 (Dornier Medical Systems, Inc., Marietta, Ga.) machine (experimental) is available, preliminary anesthesia-free ESWL may become appropriate as primary therapy for all sizes of lower ureteral stones, because this treatment will likely be associated with an 80% overall success rate.[3] However, it is both an expensive alternative and one not universally available. A calculus over the sacrum or at the lower level of the iliac bone may be difficult to visualize on Dornier HM-3 or HM-4 lithotriptors (Dornier Medical Systems, Inc.) without the use of a ureteral catheter to assist in localization.[4] Therefore, if instrumentation is necessary and stents have to be placed to visualize these lower ureteral calculi, and the success rate of ESWL treatment is only 80%, it seems prudent to use a no. 7.2 French ureteroscope and a laser to fragment the calculus, with the likelihood of 99% success[5] at one half the cost of ESWL.[6]

TECHNIQUE OF LASER LITHOTRIPSY

Except for cystine calculi, which do not fragment with laser lithotripsy, essentially all lower ureteral stones of this size may be successfully treated using the no. 7.2 French semirigid ureteroscope and the pulsed dye laser. This laser operates at a wavelength of 504 nm and a pulse duration of 1.2 μsec and is well absorbed by stone and not by tissue; therefore, its use is rarely, if ever, associated with tissue injury. This wavelength is, however, well absorbed by hemoglobin, and if it is discharged on a ureteral vein, the vein will rupture and cause minor bleeding at that point. The laser is used at an energy of 80 mJ/pulse via a 200-μm core fiber for fragile stones (calcium oxalate dihydrate, mixed calcium oxalate monohydrate and calcium oxalate dihydrate, struvite, and some uric acid stones) or 140 mJ/pulse via a 320-μm core fiber for less fragile brushite or black calcium oxalate monohydrate stones. The higher energy used through the larger fiber has a greater fragmenting ability without any significant increase in the likelihood of tissue injury, and I now use this for all calculi, hard or soft. The use of higher energy via the larger fiber results in the formation of a longer-lived cavitation bubble with a higher pressure (~1,000 bar) than that produced with 60 mJ via a 200-μm core fiber (600 bar).[7] Calcium oxalate monohydrate stones are able to be fragmented by the higher pressure generated by the 140-mJ energy. I have treated over 100 patients with the higher energy without evidence of tissue injury.

With the patient under general or regional anesthesia, a cone-tip retrograde is done, under C-arm or continuous fluoroscopy, to assess the patency of the distal ureter and the degree of impaction. A 0.038-in. guidewire (use one accompanying a stent set for easier postoperative stent placement) is passed by the stone to the renal pelvis as both a safety wire and to pass a stent at the termination of the procedure. If a wire cannot be passed by the stone, it is placed at the level of the stone and then advanced as fragmentation proceeds. Using the no. 7.2 French semirigid ureteroscope, the operator enters the bladder, being careful not to allow the narrow tip of the no. 7.2 French uretero-scope to create a false passage in the prostatic urethra. An introducer sheath may be used but is not necessary. The ureteral orifice is entered beside the 0.038-in. guidewire without the need for ureteral dilatation except in the rare instance of meatal stenosis. The no. 7.2 French semirigid ureteroscope has two channels, both 0.028 in. in diameter, and each will accept a 0.025-in. guidewire. Hand irrigation with saline is used through one channel, and the laser fiber is passed through the second channel. If it is difficult to advance the instrument and forceful irrigation will not dilate the ureter in front of the ureteroscope, two methods are useful. The first I call "riding the wire." The ureteroscope is placed directly on the 0.038-in. guidewire and very slowly advanced, even if the only things seen are the coils of the wire. The second method is to advance a 0.025-in. guidewire through the working channel. The use of the second guidewire will usually open the ureter enough to advance the ureteroscope. In the rare circumstance when the no. 7.2 French instrument cannot be advanced, it is removed. Balloon dilatation of the ureter is carried out, and then the no. 7.2 French semirigid instrument is again inserted. If the ureteral curvature is still too great to allow use of the no. 7.2 French instrument, a flexible, steerable ureterorenoscope is used (rarely necessary in the lower ureters, male or female).

Care should be taken to minimize the hand irrigation pressure during ureteroscope insertion to prevent dislodgement of the calculus. Placement of Fogarty catheters or stone baskets above the stone to prevent migration are not easily performed and add significantly to the overall French size of instruments in the ureter. Rarely does gentle irrigation through the no. 7.2 French instrument cause cephalad migration of the calculus from the lower ureter to the kidney; however, migration of fragments may occur after initiation of fragmentation.

When the stone is in view, a 200- or 320-μm core fiber is chosen, depending on the appearance of the stone. Yellow, fragile calculi may be fragmented with either fiber; however, black, dense monohydrate calculi are fragmented only with 120 to 140 mJ passed via the larger 320-μm fiber. The fiber is placed directly on and perpendicular to the surface of the stone. Unless the stone is particularly fragile, the laser will not work when placed at an oblique angle. If the stone is nodular, the laser is aimed at the junction of the nodules, because this is the weakest point; in the case of monohydrate, it is where the dihydrate "glue" is located. In homogeneous yellowish brown calculi (which are admixtures of calcium oxalate monohydrate and calcium oxalate dihydrate), the operator places the laser at one point and continues to discharge energy at that point until fragmentation begins. The outside of these calculi are harder than the inside, and once the outer surface is breached, fragmentation is easier. Now that higher energies are available, most calculi can be fragmented to 2- to 3-mm pieces so that basket removal of fragments is rarely required. Laser energy does not cause the "kick" that electrohydraulic lithotripsy (EHL) causes, and, therefore, it is rare that fragments migrate cephalad.

If the laser will not completely fragment the calculus or the fragments are not broken to a size that can pass spontaneously, a no. 9.5-French instrument is passed to allow removal by a no. 5 French basket. A no. 2 French basket is able to be placed in the no. 7.2 French ureteroscope, but initial designs have not been very sturdy, and only small fragments may be removed. Recently, a no. 6.9 French semirigid meteroscope with a no. 3.4 French has become available. This allows use of larger baskets for fragment removal.

Electrohydraulic lithotriptor probes are now available in no. 1.6 French and 1.9 French sizes. These fit through these smaller calibre ureteroscopes and are competitive with the laser in stone fragmenting efficiency. However, tests comparing the laser and various EHL units show that 10 to 20 times the energy is needed by the electrohydraulic lithotriptor to deliver fragmentation equivalent to the pulsed dye laser (Table 50–1).[8] The requirement for high energy levels is the reason that the electrohydraulic lithotriptor causes significantly more tissue damage during stone fragmentation than does the pulsed dye laser.

If a rigid ureteroscope cannot reach the stone because of a narrow, scarred, or tortuous ureter, a retrograde or an antegrade approach with a flexible ureterorenoscope may be necessary. Rarely, if ever, is it impossible to reach a stone by one of these methods. I use prone ESWL (in the Dornier HM-3) for the rare patient who fails ureteroscopy and has an adequate ureter below the stone.

Many alternatives are available for the treatment of each lower ureteral calculus. The laser is particularly helpful if the stone is impacted, because it can be discharged directly on the calculus without creating adjacent mucosal injury. Contrarily, the electrohydraulic lithotriptor, because of its propensity for tissue injury, is a poor choice when the stone is impacted. The ultrasound is also dif-

TABLE 50–1.
Comparison of Pressure Generated by Various Lithotriptor Devices

	mJ	Fiber	Maximum Pressure (bar)
Candela laser	60	200 μm	600[7]
	120	320 μm	~1,000
ACMI	200	no. 1.9 French	~500[7]
Wolf	830–1,230	no. 3.3 French	620–1,270[8]
Northgate	120	no. 3.0 French	255–370[8]
Storz	620	no. 3.0 French	480–1,020[8]
Dornier HM-3			
Old	18–24 kV	—	900–1,100
New	18–24 kV	—	600–850

ficult to use for impacted calculi, because unless the stone is held within a basket, the pressure can push the stone through the ureteral wall. The advantages of the laser are the small-caliber fiber that allows small-caliber instrumentation and the use of small amounts of energy (60–140 mJ) to create a large amount of fragmentation pressure (600–1,000 bar) with minimal tissue injury.

AFTER FRAGMENTATION

Most patients who have ureteroscopy and laser lithotripsy are treated as outpatients and have a self-retaining stent (with an external pull-out string) placed after the procedure. If the ureter has been perforated or split by balloon dilatation and it is essential that the ureteral stent remain in place, the string is cut just inside the urethral meatus so it is easily reached but difficult to inadvertently remove. The average time the stent is left in an uncomplicated, asymptomatic patient is 3 to 5 days.

All patients are given an IV dose of a broad-spectrum antibiotic before insertion of the ureteroscope, and oral antibiotics are prescribed while the stent is in place. If the patient has an infection, antibiotics are given for 24 hours before instrumentation.

FUTURE OF LASER LITHOTRIPSY

Work is currently in progress to allow laser lithotripsy to be performed without anesthesia and without the need for a ureteroscope. A flexible cystoscope will allow the 320-μm fiber to be placed within a steerable no. 5 French guidewire and be placed in the ureter without anesthesia. The laser will be placed at the level of the stone by fluoroscopic control, and the laser energy will be discharged. If "fluoresence" or a "plasma" (colliding calcium ions) is being created by absorbtion of the laser light by the stone, it will be recorded on an oscilloscope and the internal computer will allow the laser to fire.[9] If fluoresence or a plasma is not being recorded, the laser will automatically shut off after delivering only a harmless 10 to 15 mJ of energy. Because the laser light itself is an essentially painless form of energy, anesthesia-free, fail-safe laser lithotripsy may be performed. It is expected that after appropriate animal studies this will be in clinical use.

SUMMARY

A patient with a moderate hydronephrosis from a ureteral stone should have intervention within 4 weeks. Calculi below the level of the pelvic bone may be treated by ESWL if adequately visualized, with the expectation that in the second-generation lithotriptors, an 80% success rate will be achieved. An alternative that offers a higher success rate for less cost is the use of a small-caliber ureteroscope and the pulsed dye laser. The choice of treatment will depend on the availability of equipment.

REFERENCES

1. Ueno A, Kawamura T, Ogawa A, et al: Relation of spontaneous passage of ureteral calculi to size. *Urology* Vol. X, 1977; 10:544–546.
2. Gillenwater JY: The pathophysiology of urinary obstruction, in *Campbell's Urology,* ed 5. Philadelphia, WB Saunders, 1986, vol 1, pp 542–571.
3. Holden D, Rao PN: Ureteral stones: The results of primary in situ extracorporeal shock wave lithotripsy. *J Urol* 1989; 142:37–39.
4. Chaussy CG, Fuchs GJ: Extracorporeal shock wave lithotripsy of distal ureteral calculi: Is it worthwhile? *J Endourol* 1987; 1:1.
5. Dretler SP: An evaluation of ureteral laser lithotripsy: 225 consecutive cases. *J Urol* 1990; 143:267–272.
6. Nesbitt JA, Drago JR: Cost comparison of extracorporeal shock wave lithotripsy vs ureteroscopic laser destruction of distal ureteral stones. *J Urol* 1988; 139:292A.
7. Bhatta KM, Rosen DI, Dretler SP: Unpublished data, 1990.
8. Rosen DI, Willscher M: Unpublished data, 1989.
9. Bhatta KM, Rosen DI, Watson GM, et al: Acoustic and plasma guided lasertripsy (APGL) of urinary calculi. *J Urol* 1989; 142:433–437.

Index

C

D

E

M

N

O

P

Q

R

S

T

U

W